Theory, Practice, and Trends in Human Services

An Overview of an Emerging Profession

Ed Neukrug
Old Dominion University

Brooks/Cole Publishing Company
Pacific Grove, California

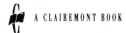

ITP™ The trademark ITP is used under license.

A CLAIREMONT BOOK

Brooks/Cole Publishing Company
A Division of Wadsworth, Inc.

© 1994 by Wadsworth, Inc., Belmont, California 94002. All rights reserved.
No part of this book may be reproduced, stored in a retrieval system, or tran-
scribed, in any form, or by any means—electronic, mechanical, photocopying,
recording, or otherwise—without the prior written permission of the publisher,
Brooks/Cole Publishing Company, Pacific Grove, California 93950, a division of
Wadsworth, Inc.

Printed in the United States of America
10 9 8 7 6 5 4 3 2 1

Library of Congress Cataloguing-in-Publication Data
Neukrug, Ed.
    Theory, practice, and trends in human services : an overview of an
emerging profession / Ed Neukrug.
        p.   cm.
    Includes bibliographical references (p.   ) and index.
    ISBN 0-534-22278-1
    1. Human services personnel.   2. Human services.   I. Title.
HV40.35.N485   1993
361.3'2'02373—dc20   93-20941
                                                                CIP

Sponsoring Editor: *Claire Verduin*
Marketing Representative: *Bob Podstepny*
Editorial Associate: *Gay C. Bond*
Production Editor: *Nancy Shammas*
Manuscript Editor: *Betty Duncan*
Permissions Editor: *Carline Haga*
Photo Editor: *Diana Mara Henry*
Interior Design: *Anne Draus, Scratchgravel Publishing Services*
Cover Design: *Sharon L. Kinghan*
Cover Illustration: *Diana Ong/SuperStock*
Production Service and Typesetting: *Scratchgravel Publishing Services*
Cover Printing: *Color Dot Graphics, Inc.*
Printing and Binding: *Arcata Graphics/Fairfield*

Photo credits:
14, UPI/Bettmann; **37,** Courtesy Carl Rogers Memorial Library; **41,**
Courtesy, Dr. Harold McPheeters; **90,** © Bettye Lane; **119,** Joel Becker;
123, Courtesy, Harvard Graduate School of Education; **132,** © Michael
Siluk; **152,** Courtesy, Avanta Network, Issaquah, WA; **159,** Joel Becker;
187, Courtesy, Cheryl Evans; **189,** Joel Becker; **204,** Mike Spinelli/
Courtesy of NEA Today; **219,** The Bettmann Archive; **245,** Ed Kamper
Photography, Courtesy Charles M. Super; **250,** © Diana Mara Henry,
Carmel, CA; **267L,** The Bettmann Archive; **267R,** UPI/Bettmann; **269,**
© Michael Siluk; **271,** Anna Beetham Goldenberg; **275,** Courtesy, Lisa
Lyons.
Lyrics credit: **61,** Song lyrics from "The Boxer" copyright © 1968
Paul Simon. Used by permission of the Publisher.

THIS BOOK IS PRINTED ON ACID-FREE RECYCLED PAPER

In Memory of My Father

Preface

I mentioned to my friend that my publisher asked me to write a preface. I went on to say, "Nobody ever reads a preface." At that point he responded, "I do!" A preface, he said, gives him a better sense of how the chapters are interconnected and a better idea of the whole. He then noted, "It's kind of like looking at a person's face. What if you looked only at a person's earlobes, eyes, mouth, and so on, and you saw all those things before seeing the face? You really would have a different perspective. The preface gives you a sense of the whole book, and then the parts become more meaningful." I said, "Well, I guess I never looked at it from that viewpoint. Maybe I'll try reading a preface or two and see if it will give me a different perspective on the book." So, for those of you who will read this, let me give you an overview of this text.

Theory, Practice, and Trends in Human Services is unique in a number of ways when compared to other survey texts in the human service field. The writing style is down-to-earth, concise, and to the point. You will find that relatively difficult concepts are presented in readable—some might say simplistic—ways. This uncomplicated style of presentation is designed to engage students. I have also tried to highlight concepts by adding a "human touch," weaving in personal experiences and presenting vignettes of others' experiences throughout the text. I hope you find these scenarios interesting and informative.

This text approaches the field of human services as a unique profession with a defined body of knowledge, a profession that has its roots in the fields of social work, counseling, and psychology. Similarly, this text approaches the work of the human service worker as that of a professional, not a paraprofessional as some in the field have advocated. I believe it is time that we acknowledge the uniqueness of our profession and the importance of the professional training that human service workers receive.

Continuing with the theme of professionalism, I have included in Chapter 2 ways of contacting a number of professional organizations in the mental-health field. As you begin your long and hopefully fulfilling professional journey, I encourage you to join the professional associations such as the National Organization of Human Service Education (NOHSE). In Appendix B I have included a summary sheet on the Council for Standards in Human Service Education (CSHSE) as this organization has been a driving force in setting standards in the field.

Similarly, for instructors and interested students, I have included in Appendix D a copy of CSHSE's National Standards for Human Service Worker Education and Training Programs. If your program is not currently approved, you might find this information particularly useful, and students can use these standards as an outline for understanding the profession.

Whereas other texts interweave many themes common to the human services throughout the various chapters, each chapter in this text presents an overview of one unique area of the human services profession. I believe this helps you, the reader, more easily organize your thoughts about the profession. Although some themes run throughout the text, you will find that each chapter can stand on its own. Some of the chapters discuss material that is generic to human services and has been widely discussed in the classic textbooks of the field. These chapters may have a familiar tone, though perhaps presented in a novel way: Chapter 1, The Development of the Human Service Worker; Chapter 2, The Human Service Profession: History and Current Issues; Chapter 4, The Counseling Interview; Chapter 6, Systems: What Are They, and How Do We Work with Them; and Chapter 10, A Look to the Future. Other chapters in the book are either new to a text of this kind or present a unique approach to the material: Chapter 3, Theoretical Approaches to Human Service Work; Chapter 5, The Development of the Person; Chapter 7, The Human Service Worker in a Pluralistic Society; Chapter 8, Research, Program Evaluation, and Testing; and Chapter 9, The Human Service Worker and the World of Work. I believe these chapters contain essential knowledge for the potential human service worker.

A quick note on Chapter 7, The Human Service Worker in a Pluralistic Society. Our society is changing, becoming increasingly more diverse. Yet I am continually amazed at how little many of us know about the varying subcultures with whom we share our daily lives. Despite this fact, few texts have broached this subject. In teaching about diversity, I continue to find this to be a very sensitive topic. I believe covering and *discussing* issues of diversity are crucial to the effective functioning of the human service worker as well as to the survival of our society. The first part of Chapter 7 offers some background information on the multitude of subcultures in our society. You may find it dry, yet it is crucial to understand the roots of many of these subcultures. Generally, when I teach Chapter 7, I encourage students to read the first section of the chapter, but I do not test them on it. I want students to get a "sense" of the differing cultures, and I am less concerned that they memorize facts and figures. The second part of this chapter speaks more directly on how to work with clients from diverse backgrounds. The material in this section is important for students to know in their work with diverse clients.

If you are an instructor of this course, you may find that one or two chapters are not as relevant to your view of human services as you may wish. This may be particularly true of Chapter 8, Research, Program Evaluation, and Testing, and Chapter 9, The Human Service Worker and the World of Work. These chapters can easily be skipped; there is plenty of material in the rest of the book for a semester course and little continuity would be lost. However, I personally feel that skipping these chapters would be a mistake; they contain vital information for any professional in human services. Any human service professional today will come in contact with test results, should be reading about new research, and will be asked to evaluate a program or client outcomes. Similarly, any human service worker should be aware of the importance of work and career for the self-esteem of his or her clients and should be aware of how to generate career options for clients.

A unique aspect of this text is that near the end of each chapter you will have an opportunity to reflect on your own level of developmental maturity. You will be able to compare yourself to what might be considered the "ideal" human service worker, who embodies the best characteristics of the professional in the field. Life is a continual growth process, and instructors can encourage students to view these sections as offering a model that we can all strive to emulate while discouraging students from feeling inadequate if they do not currently embody some of these traits. If you are an instructor, prior to having your students read Chapter 1, you might encourage them to complete the questionnaire entitled Assessing Your Adult Developmental Level, which can be found at the end of the chapter. I have found this to be a good exercise during the first class.

Near the end of each chapter is a section on ethical and professional issues. The human service profession has too long paid far too little attention to this extremely important aspect of our work. These sections discuss ethical and professional concerns that are relevant to the chapter topics. Usually, the experiential exercises at the end of each chapter offer ethical and professional dilemmas, vignettes, and/or questions so that students can continue to reflect upon these important issues. Finally, the proposed NOHSE/CSHSE Code of Ethics is presented in Appendix A; all students are encouraged to read it and discuss these guidelines in class.

Each chapter ends with experiential exercises that can further the understanding of the material presented. If you are an instructor, you may want your students to complete some of these exercises before they read the chapter. There is usually not enough time to do all of the exercises, so you may want to assign those activities that best augment your teaching style. I encourage students to read each exercise and complete as many as they can.

Acknowledgments

I owe much to many people in the writing of this text. First, I'd like to acknowledge a number of individuals who reviewed the chapters in the text. A special thanks to Susan Soule-Smith who reviewed most of the text and assisted me in some of the "nitty-gritty" work that needed to be done. Second, to Mark Blagen, Judith Justice, Anna Goldenberg, Pat Lunger, Dr. Robert Daniel, and my mother, thank you for your careful review of various chapters. Appreciation also goes to Elise Cosby, who assisted me in some of the final technical aspects of the book.

Many others reviewed the manuscript and/or provided materials, and they, too, are greatly appreciated: Dr. Michelle Kelly, Old Dominion University; Dr. Chris Lovell, Old Dominion University; Dr. Radha Parker, Old Dominion University (Chapter 5); Cheryl Evans, Old Dominion University; Dr. John Lanci, Stonehill College; Dr. Lee Manning, Old Dominion University; Dr. Marty Muguira, Old Dominion University (Chapter 7); Dr. Garrett McAuliffe, Old Dominion University (Chapter 9); David Cross, Houston Community College; Margaret J. French, Pitt Community College; Jeffery S. Haber, Metropolitan State College; John R. Heapes, Harrisburg Area Community College; Mary Kay Kreider, St. Louis Community College; Richard Reiner, Rogue Community College; and Cynthia Tower, Fitchburg State College.

A number of students also helped me with various aspects of the text and were instrumental in the writing and development of the proposed ethical guidelines of NOHSE/CSHSE. They include Vicki Clyman, Craig Dupuis, Sarah Hite, Kim Lombart, Randy Sowala, and Cheryl Strode. Also, in preparing the text I had the opportunity of using a rough draft of it in some of my classes. Thanks to all of my students who gave me feedback, found typos, and made valuable suggestions.

I would also like to give my sincere thanks to the staff at Scratchgravel and Brooks/Cole for their hard work and pleasant attitudes. I always felt that I could go to them for advice and suggestions. Particular thanks go to Anne Draus at Scratchgravel, to Betty Duncan, and to Adrienne Carter, Diana Henry, Carline Haga, Gay Bond, and Nancy Shammas at Brooks/Cole. A special thanks to Claire Verduin, publisher, without whom this book would never have been written.

Most of all, this text could not have been written without my family and friends: my mother and father who gave me sensitivity and resilience and planted the seeds for me to run my life the way I want to; my sister, Carole, and my brother, Howard, who have always been there for me; Joseph, my very special nephew who let me put him in the book; my sister-in-law, Amy, and my brother-in-law, Ray, who provided ongoing support; and my many friends who have helped me through life—a special thanks to Allan, Lenny, David, John, Jonathan, Dianne, Garrett, Mike, Bob, and Bill.

Finally, thank you to Cindy Frazer, my friend, personal editor, and a person I love very much. Cindy taught me how to write and helped me to love. And thanks to Cindy's children, Matthew and Courtney, who enliven both our lives.

Contents

9 The Human Service Worker and the World of Work   238

10 A Look to the Future: Trends in the Function and Roles of the Human Service Worker   264

Appendix A
Proposed Ethical Standards of Human Service Workers (NOSHE)

Appendix B
Council for Standards in Human Service Education: Summary Information Sheet

Appendix C
Proposed Cross-Cultural Competencies and Objectives (AMCD)

Appendix D
Council for Standards in Human Service Education: National Standards for Human Service Worker Education and Training Programs

Glossary

References

Index

1

The Development of the Human Service Worker

Defining the Human Service Worker
What Is the Human Service Field? / Who Is the Human Service Worker? / Who Is *Not* a Human Service Worker?

Characteristics of the Effective Human Service Worker
The Empathic Person / The Nondogmatic Person / The Person Who Is Internally Oriented / The Person Who Is Accepting of Others / The Introspective Person / The Person Who Is Genuine / The Person Who Is an Experiencer of Life and Lives Life as a Process / The Person Who Is an Acquirer of Knowledge

Personality Development of the Effective Helper
An Adult Development Approach / Perry's Scheme of Adult Cognitive Development / Kegan's Constructivist View of Adult Cognitive Development

Acquiring the Characteristics of the Effective Helper: A Values Clarification Approach

Ethical and Professional Issues
The Development of Ethical Guidelines—Who Decides What's Ethical?

The Developmentally Mature Human Service Worker: Willing to Meet the Challenge

Summary

Experiential Exercises

High school was a rough time in my life. Although I did well in school, my personal life was less than satisfactory. I was overweight, afraid of dating, particularly concerned with how I appeared to my friends, and had low self-esteem. I spent little time thinking about what major I would choose when I went to college. Although my mom would periodically threaten to take me to a psychologist (a threat that today I wish she had carried out), I mostly kept my fears to myself. My school counselor, although nice, did not seem tuned in to my problems and instead appeared more concerned with my schedule. In fact, one time when facing a problem, I found I had no one to whom I could turn. I considered going to my physical education teacher because he seemed like a nice guy, but instead I went to my father. Thankfully, he came through for me. I hoped things would change in college.

Having done well in the sciences in high school, I decided to start college as a biology major. With little personal reflection and a lack of adequate career services at my college, I decided dentistry was the way to go. At least I would make some money. It was 1969, the end of the '60s. Turmoil abounded around college campuses; drugs for "consciousness raising" were everywhere. Hare Krishnas and Zen Buddhists enticed you to follow them to "the answer." (If you did let them lead you down the path, you soon found out that the answer was that there was no answer). "The times, they were a changin'." It was a time to confront the traditional values of society, and soon I found myself confronting my own choices in life—my own traditional values. Did I really want to be a dentist or was there another path for me? Suddenly, studying psychology seemed to be my natural path. Why, of course, didn't I want to help people, help mankind (later to be called humankind), help the evolution of the planet? I quickly changed my major. Was I disappointed—I wasn't learning how to help others; I was memorizing the anatomy of the brain and the eye, learning how rats find their way through mazes, and exploring theories on why people do the things they do. Although I was promised that this knowledge was the basis of the helping professions, I wasn't convinced. Indeed, even today I'm not convinced.

During those times, I was never taught how to respond to someone in a "counseling" way. I felt displaced and disappointed. Unfortunately, during the 1960s, there were few human service programs. What led me on my search for a field that hardly even existed at that time? What intuitive sense did I have that there was another career path for me, in which I would be teaching 20 years later? What characteristics did I possess at the time that made me an effective human service worker, and what skills would I need to develop? In this chapter, we will explore many of these questions as we discuss the skills, characteristics, and values of the human service worker, as well as the broad field of human service work.

Defining the Human Service Worker

What Is the Human Service Field?

Having its origins in the mid-1960s, the human service field is relatively new. The profession grew out of an increased sense of social responsibility toward the poor, minorities and women, and the mentally ill. This sense of social awareness was one factor that led to President Johnson's Great Society initiatives and resulted in the establishment of federal grants for a variety of social welfare programs (Fullerton, 1990). With the social welfare system greatly expanding, it soon became apparent that the established graduate programs in counseling, psychology, and social work would not be able to handle the increasing need for trained human service professionals. Thus, we saw the beginnings of the human service degree. Although both associate's and bachelor's programs arose at this time, their orientations were somewhat different. The associate's degree was geared toward training the mental-health aide, or paraprofessional, whereas the bachelor's degree was seen as more broadly based and considered a professional degree (Fullerton, 1990). As the field has expanded over the years, those in it have worked to give it an identity of its own—an identity that borrows from other mental-health fields, yet with its own unique perspective. Today, there are close to 1200 human service programs offered at the associate's, bachelor's, and doctoral levels and at non-degree sites such as mental hospitals (McGrath, 1991–1992).

Who Is the Human Service Worker?

Generally, the **human service worker*** is a person who has an associate's or bachelor's degree in human services or a closely related field. Although specific course work varies from program to program, most human service degree programs offer an introductory course in human services as well as course work in interviewing, family counseling, group counseling, crisis intervention, and counseling skills. Other major areas that are sometimes covered include career development, testing, counseling theories, ethics, and multicultural issues (McGrath, 1991–1992).

Today, there are dozens of places where one might find human service workers, although some of the more prominent fields include mental health, mental retardation, substance abuse, aging/gerontology, domestic violence, youth service, child care, correction/criminal

*Boldface terms are defined in the glossary at the end of the book.

justice, education/schools, health care, recreation/fitness, and vocational rehabilitation (McGrath, 1991–1992).

With tens of thousands of human service workers employed in a
variety of social services agencies, professional associations such as
the **National Organization for Human Service Education** (NOHSE)
were established to address some of their common concerns. Some of
the more important functions of these associations will be addressed
in more detail in Chapter 2.

Who Is *Not* a Human Service Worker?

Although many professionals in the social service fields have training
that overlaps, some major differences exist among the fields. For instance, the human service worker is *not* any of the following:

Psychiatrist. Psychiatrists are physicians who generally have completed a residency in psychiatry. This means that they have completed extensive training in some kind of mental-health setting.
Being physicians, psychiatrists have expertise in prescribing medication for emotional problems. Their affiliated professional association is the **American Psychiatric Association** (APA).

Psychologist. Psychologists generally have doctoral degrees in
psychology, have completed internships at a mental-health facility,
and have passed specific state requirements to obtain licensure as
psychologists. Their professional association is the **American Psychological Association** (APA).

Social worker. Although the term *social worker* can apply to a person holding either an undergraduate or graduate degree in social
work or a related field (for example, human services), more generally social workers have master's degrees in social work (M.S.W.).
With additional training and supervision, social workers can become members of the Academy of Certified Social Workers (ACSW).
In addition, most states have specific requirements for becoming a
licensed clinical social worker (LCSW). Their professional association is the **National Association of Social Workers** (NASW).

Counselor. Although many individuals may call themselves counselors, generally a counselor is an individual who has a master's
degree in counseling. Many subspecialties exist in the counseling
field. A few of the more common ones are school counseling (for-
merly called guidance counseling), mental-health counseling, college counseling, and rehabilitation counseling. Many states today
have licensure for counselors, which usually requires additional
training and supervision to practice as a licensed professional
counselor (LPC). Their professional association is the **American
Counseling Association** (ACA).

Psychotherapist. Because most states do not have laws that regulate the term *psychotherapist*, individuals with no training, experience, or even a degree can call themselves psychotherapists. On a practical level, psychotherapists usually have advanced degrees in psychology, social work, or counseling and work in mental-health settings or in private practice, providing individual, group, or marital counseling.

Characteristics of the Effective Human Service Worker

Whether you are thinking about entering or have already decided to enter the human service field—as I did 20 years ago—you probably have some intuition that this field somehow fits your sense of who you are. You may have some image of the human service worker. Perhaps you think that he or she is a person who wants to help others; cares about people and the state of the world; is introspective, intuitive, and social; or has other similar qualities. On the other hand, you probably also think that the human service worker is *not* a cold person, does *not* hold rigidly sterile views, and is *not* concerned only with himself or herself. These qualities—the qualities of the human service worker—have been researched over the years.

Research shows that the effective human service worker embodies many of the characteristics discussed in the following pages. For instance, he or she is likely to be empathic, nondogmatic, internally oriented, accepting of others, introspective, genuine, an experiencer of life who lives life as a process, and an acquirer of knowledge.

The Empathic Person

Empathic individuals have a deep understanding of another person's point of view. These people can "get into the shoes" of another. For those of you who watch *Star Trek: The Next Generation*, the "counselor" character is the epitome of the empathic person, with her ability to understand another's perspective on the world. Carl Rogers (1957) liked to say that the empathic person could sense the private world of clients as if it were his or her own, without losing the "as if" feeling. Empathic individuals can accept people in their differences and can communicate this sense of acceptance.

The Nondogmatic Person

Nondogmatic people allow others to express their points of view. Although these individuals may have strong opinions of their own, they do not feel as if they need to change others to their viewpoints. Also, nondogmatic people are open to criticism, open to change, and open to hearing the views of others in a way that will allow them to adapt their own values and beliefs.

Certainly, one readily thinks of people like Hitler or Stalin as examples of dogmatic individuals, but these people are the extreme. Most of us have a kind of tempered dogmatism—there are areas in which we have extremely strong convictions, yet we aren't constantly trying to convince people to change to our point of view. It is important to look at our dogmatic areas and ask ourselves "Why do I have so much energy in this area?" Extreme dogmatism prevents one from listening effectively to another. If I am trying to convince you of something, how can I hear your point of view? Some research shows an inverse relationship between dogmatism and empathy; that is, dogmatic people tend not to be empathic (Neukrug & McAuliffe, 1993).

The Person Who Is Internally Oriented

Individuals who have more of an **internal locus of control,** as compared with an **external locus of control,** tend to rely on their own inner sense in making decisions. Shostrum (1974) notes that the healthy individual has a 3:1 ratio of "inner directedness to other directedness." This means that usually more importance is placed on internal thoughts and beliefs, although other people's opinions may sometimes be taken into account in decision making.

Individuals who have a high degree of **internality** are less likely to be affected by the views of significant people in their lives or by societal values. They are free thinkers. These individuals, however, do not just "go with their feelings." On the contrary, these individuals often have a high regard for how their actions affect others. Research shows that people who have a high degree of internal locus of control do not have a need to convince others of how to be (Neukrug & McAuliffe, 1993).

The Person Who Is Accepting of Others

People who have high regard for others can accept people in their differences regardless of dissimilar cultural heritage, values, or belief systems. When in a helping relationship, individuals with a high regard for others are able to accept the helpee (the person needing help) unconditionally, without having "strings attached" to the relationship. Rogers (1957) calls this **unconditional positive regard**. Leo Buscaglia calls this responsible love: "Responsible love is accepting and understanding. . . . [L]ove helps us to accept the fact that the other individual is behaving only as he [or she] is able to behave at the moment" (1972, p. 119).

Having high regard for others does not mean that one necessarily likes everything a person has done. For instance, one would most certainly not like the actions of the convicted murderer or rapist; however, the person with high regard can come to understand how the felon came to do the actions he or she committed. This deep understanding comes from being empathic and is like having a window that leads deep inside the soul of the other individual—a window that allows the helper to see the hurts and pains of the other. This window into the other's being assists the helper to accept the helpee unconditionally and with high regard.

The Introspective Person

Effective helpers are willing to look deeply within themselves. This means that they have the courage to receive feedback from others and are willing to be self-critical. Introspective individuals are open to their deeper feelings and are willing to examine their own hurts and pains. In researching the ability of helpers to be self-examining, investigators have examined helpers' rates of attendance in therapy. Generally, the results have been positive. For instance, one study found that 83% of psychologists had been in therapy (Prochaska & Norcross, 1983); another survey found that 71% of psychologists, psychiatrists, and clinical social workers had been in therapy (Norcross, Strausser, & Faltus, 1988). Similarly, Deutsch (1984) found that 34% of a cross section of psychotherapists had not sought out therapy for various problems. Finally, in another study of counselors, Neukrug and Williams (1993) found that 80% of them had been in individual, group, marital, or family therapy.

Being willing to look at oneself is extremely important in preventing what is called countertransference. **Countertransference** is the process in which the helper's own issues interfere with effectively helping his or her clients. If a helper has "unfinished business" of his or her own, then countertransference will likely occur. If that person has attended therapy, though, countertransference issues will less likely arise. Studies by Neukrug and Williams (1993) and Guy and Liaboe (1986) show that a fairly large percentage of helping professionals had been in therapy prior to entering training programs. This indicates that many helpers may have wounds from childhood that they have been willing to examine. This is important, for it is essential that these wounds do not interfere with the helpers' day-to-day dealings with clients.

The Person Who Is Genuine

At times I am caught in the dilemma of saying and acting in the way that I feel versus saying and acting in the way that I think another person wants me to be. Do I express my true feelings, or do I hide them in order to protect another person—or perhaps, more accurately, to protect myself? Do I tell my boss that I am angry at her and take the chance that I might get fired? Do I tell my client that what he shares with me makes me feel sad and take the chance that such a revelation might make him feel uneasy? Do I risk a friendship by telling my friend that I feel manipulated by him? Rogers (1961, 1980) felt that being in sync with your feelings and behaviors, being **genuine** or **congruent**, was crucial to healthy relationships. Individuals who embody such characteristics are **transparent**; that is, they readily show their feelings to others. Although it may be prudent at times not to share certain feelings with your boss, friend, or client, a relationship that emphasizes nongenuineness can have little substance and, in the case of the helping relationship, will be less likely to promote growth in clients.

As opposed to the individual who is congruent and real, nongenuine people do not have their feelings, thoughts, and actions in sync. How they feel is not represented by what they say or how they act. These individuals are fake—living life with subtle deceptions, oftentimes deceiving themselves. Afternoon soap operas for example, represent the exaggeration of nongenuineness. Here we see individuals "acting" at life—being terribly dishonest in their relationships—not for fear of hurting the other but for fear that their lives would be ruined if they were truthful. These "lies" are often not conscious. They have become part of the individual's way of living in the world.

Unless people are horribly caught up in a nongenuine way of living, they usually have a sense that they are living incongruently. There is a slight (sometimes more than slight) internal tug saying "something's not right inside" or "I know I'm trying to put something over on this person." Clients often come for help to have the human service professional assist them in becoming more in sync. Therefore, if the helper is nongenuine, assisting the client along his or her path would be difficult.

In the book *People of the Lie*, Peck (1985) felt that what can begin as "small white lies" could snowball over time, become a nongenuine lifestyle, and eventually represent evil. He felt that, at times, this nongenuine lifestyle could take over one's life and lead to possession by Satan. He sees therapy as "mini-confessionals" where people can cleanse themselves of their incongruities. Although, you may not believe that lying can lead to possession by the devil, most people would agree that living a nongenuine lifestyle is not healthy. "Abandon the show of saintliness and relinquish excessive prudence, then people will benefit a hundredfold. Abandon ostentatious benevolence and conspicuous righteousness, then people will return to the primal virtues of filial piety and parental affection. Abandon cleverness and relinquish gains, then thieves and robbers will disappear." (Lao-tzu, 1919, pp. 19–20).

The Person Who Is an Experiencer of Life and Lives Life as a Process

I remember when I was in college I was so anxious to finish and move onto graduate school that I never let myself enjoy the experience. I didn't enjoy learning, I didn't enjoy dating, I didn't enjoy me! Well, I later learned that dating could be fun, and unfortunately, not until years later did I come to realize that learning could be fun.

Working with clients can be tedious, and often change occurs very slowly. It is important to be able to be in the moment with one's client without pushing him or her too fast. If you are pushing yourself so fast that you're not taking time to experience life, chances are you will do the same with your clients. Not allowing clients to experience themselves and their plights prevents them from acquiring the insight necessary to produce change. This does not mean that mild confrontation may not be appropriate at times. However, confrontation is a tricky tool to be used only when the client can hear you, which usually is after he or she has gained a measure of insight.

Many of the existential psychologists like Carl Rogers (1980) and Rollo May (May, Angel, & Ellenberger, 1958), as well as the eastern philosophers, have highlighted the importance of experiencing life in the moment and allowing individuals to recognize their own inner qualities as their lives unfold with time.

I remembered one morning when I discovered a cocoon in the bark of a tree, just as a butterfly was making a hole in its case and preparing to come out. I waited a while, but it was too long appearing and I was impatient. I bent over it and breathed on it to warm it. I warmed it as quickly as I could and the miracle began to happen before my eyes, faster than life. The case opened, the butterfly started slowly crawling out and I shall never forget my horror when I saw how its wings were folded back and crumpled; the wretched butterfly tried with its whole trembling body to unfold them. Bending over it, I tried to help it with my breath. In vain. It needed to be hatched out patiently and the unfolding of the wings should be a gradual process in the sun. Now it was too late. My breath had forced the butterfly to appear, all crumpled, before its time. It struggled desperately and, a few seconds later, died in the palm of my hand.

That little body is, I do believe, the greatest weight I have on my conscience. For I realize today that it is a mortal sin to violate the great laws of nature. We should not hurry, we should not be impatient, but we should confidently obey the eternal rhythm. (Kazantzakis, 1952, pp. 120–121)

The Person Who Is an Acquirer of Knowledge

Although embodying many of the above-mentioned personality characteristics is crucial to being an effective human service worker, knowledge about effective helping skills is equally important. Learning how to listen and reflect accurately, how to use questions appropriately, when to interpret a client's behavior, and how to determine whether a client should be confronted are just some of the skills that may be crucial for the effective helper. Therefore, many individuals have devised methods of teaching such skills (Ivey, 1980; Miller, Morrill, & Uhlemann, 1970; Neukrug, 1980). Also, knowledge of specific techniques is crucial when working with certain types of clients (Frank, 1979). Therefore, having the desire to learn skills as well as the specific techniques needed to work with certain problems is essential for the effective human service worker. During my years of teaching counseling and helping skills, I have found that some students seem reluctant to learn these necessary skills. They seem to think that their personality characteristics are enough to "get them by." The truly effective human service workers have a thirst for knowledge. They exhibit this through their studies, their desire to join professional associations and read professional journals, and their ability to broaden and deepen their own approach to clients.

These eight characteristics of being empathic, nondogmatic, internally oriented, accepting of others, introspective, genuine, an experiencer of life who lives life as a process, and an acquirer of knowledge are qualities to which human service workers should strive. Few, if any, of us are "already there." More likely, each of these qualities should be viewed as road signs as we travel our own unique paths through life. Eventually, as we gain a little more knowledge than before, we may even feel comfortable just traveling the road. But how do we begin to acquire some of these qualities? The next section discusses this issue.

Personality Development of the Effective Helper

Are some of us born with the previously described characteristics that lead us toward the human service field, or can they be learned, or even still, are these qualities the combination of genetic and acquired traits? When I became a psychology major and still felt something was amiss, was I searching for this elusive human service field because I already possessed some of these characteristics and it was a natural place for me to be? Or, perhaps because of my own emotional wounds, I unconsciously sought out a field that dealt with emotional pain. In the latter case, it might mean that I didn't already possess these characteristics and needed to cultivate them.

Many theorists and philosophers have struggled with trying to understand this nature of the person. Carl Rogers and Abraham Maslow (1954), two of the founders of the field of **humanistic counseling and education**, thought we were born with a natural **actualizing tendency**, and if we were reared in a nurturing environment, many of the described characteristics would naturally develop. They also thought that even if the nurturing environment was not present in early childhood, the qualities could still develop if such an environment was available later in life. On the other hand, Sigmund Freud, the founder of **psychoanalysis,** thought that people constantly struggled with instinctual aggressive and sexual drives and that these drives, in combination with early childhood experiences, determined our temperament. Therefore, he would have believed that a human service worker's personality is formed in early childhood. Others, such as B. F. Skinner (1953), the famous behaviorist, and Albert Ellis (1988), the well-known cognitive therapist, believed that, although we may not be born with these qualities, they could be developed through certain learned experiences. These differing views of human nature and how they relate to the helping professions will be discussed in more detail later. However, whatever you believe, these qualities are clearly important for the effective helper.

An Adult Development Approach

Recently, adult developmental theorists—such as William Perry (King, 1978), Robert Kegan (1982), and Gail Sheehy (1976)—have proposed that the way individuals view the world can change throughout the life span if the individual is afforded opportunities for personal growth. They would state that many of the human service characteristics listed earlier are an outgrowth of a natural developmental process—that is, if given an environment that supports and yet challenges the individual's way of constructing reality, he or she would naturally develop many of these characteristics. Borrowing from some of the other developmental theorists such as Jean Piaget (1954), who examined child development, and Lawrence Kohlberg (1969), who examined moral development, these adult developmental theorists state that adult cognitive abilities are sequential and hierarchical—that is, current learning is based on what we have learned in the past, and as we are exposed to new learning, we can broaden and expand our way of viewing the world.

Adult cognitive theorists such as William Perry and Robert Kegan hypothesize that the way we think moves in stages—from a concrete, rigid type of thinking toward an abstract, more flexible, "relativistic" type of thinking. Recent research on adult cognitive development seems to support some of Perry's and Kegan's hypotheses because it shows that individuals who are at higher stages of adult cognitive development tend to embrace many of the characteristics of the effective helper (Benack, 1988; Bowman & Allen, l988; Bowman & Reeves, 1987; Neukrug & McAuliffe, 1993; Reeves, Bowman & Cooley, 1989). Therefore, it would seem to be imperative for human service programs to afford students opportunities to move forward on these cognitive schemes.

Perry's Scheme of Adult Cognitive Development

Perry's theory of intellectual and ethical development (King, 1978) has particularly emphasized the learning process of college students. His theory has three stages encompassing nine positions. In **dualism**, the first stage, students view the world as black or white, or right or wrong, and have little tolerance for ambiguity. Students in this stage might believe the professor has "the answer" and would expect learning to come mostly from the professor teaching to the student.

The second stage is **relativism**. Here students move away from viewing the world in an absolutist, right or wrong fashion. The relativist thinks abstractly, allows for differing opinions, and understands that there may be many ways of viewing the world. Students in this stage expect learning to be more of a sharing process and would explore the opinions of others to formulate their own outlook on life.

The final stage is **commitment to relativism**. Individuals in this stage maintain their relativistic outlook *and* can commit to specific values and behaviors in which they live their lives. In other words, they may take specific religious stances, job orientations or personality characteristics while maintaining an accepting attitude toward others' lifestyles (Widick, 1975). Students in this stage have their own strong opinions, yet they are still open to learning from others.

Research on the Perry scheme seems to indicate that the higher the stage one is in, the more likely it is that he or she embodies many of the characteristics important in the human service worker (Benack, 1988; Neukrug & McAuliffe, 1993). Also, it has become clear that as students go through college and graduate school, they advance on the Perry scheme (Magolda & Porterfield, 1988).

Kegan's Constructivist View of Adult Cognitive Development

Similar to Perry but using a more interpersonal model, Kegan (1982) suggests there are six stages of cognitive development (stages 0 through 5), with stages 3, 4, and 5 representing ways in which most adults view the world. Kegan's incorporative, impulsive, and imperial stages (stages 0, 1, and 2) deal mostly with child development and focus on how the individual moves from total self-involvement toward the beginning awareness of a shared world with other people (although some adults can still be seen acting out these earlier states). These stages will be dealt with in more detail in Chapter 5. Kegan's third stage is the **interpersonal stage** which represents the individual who is embedded in his or her relationships. Individuals in this stage cannot truly separate their sense of who they are from their families, friends, and/or community groups. Kegan's fourth stage, the **institutional stage**, represents the person who has separated his or her values and sense of self from parents, peers, and/or community groups. These individuals have a strong sense of personal autonomy and self-reliance. Kegan's final stage is the **interindividual stage**. Here individuals are able to maintain a separate sense of self and have the capability of incorporating feedback from others, feedback that allows for growth and change. They are not embedded in their autonomous self-reliant way of living as are stage 4 institutional persons.

The Woody Allen movie *Zelig* clearly shows an individual in transition from stage 3 to stage 4. Zelig is the epitome of stage 3, the interpersonal person. He takes on the persona of whomever he is around. He is afraid to be himself. If he's around an African-American, he becomes African-American; if he's around a Chinese person, he speaks fluent Chinese. He becomes obese when around someone who is obese, and he becomes a psychiatrist attempting to treat the psychiatrist he is with. What seems to be a lighthearted movie soon becomes serious when we see the reasons why Zelig becomes whomever he is around. Under hypnosis Zelig reveals the reasons he becomes the person he is with—he is afraid to be himself. A lifelong history of ridicule every time he expressed his own opinion made him too scared to be himself. After intensive therapy, Zelig becomes "cured." Finally, the big day arrives when Zelig is to meet a number of renowned psychiatrists who will examine him to see if he is actually cured. At first, things seem successful because Zelig does not take on the persona of the psychiatrists. But as the meeting continues, one of the psychiatrists remarks what a beautiful day it is. Zelig, who has become his "own person" and is now very assertive, states "It is not a nice day." Indeed, Zelig has become too much of his own person because he soon starts a fight with the psychiatrist in order to prove his point. Although Zelig has changed and grown, he is now embedded in another developmental level—Kegan's stage 4, the institutional stage.

If this film were to show Zelig moving into Kegan's final stage, the interindividual stage, we would see him being able to hear other points of view and incorporate them into his view of the world, if he so chooses. In Maslow's terms, he would then be the **self-actualized person**—a person who is in touch with himself, can hear feedback from others, is nondogmatic, has an internal locus of control, is empathic and introspective—in other words, an individual who embodies many of the characteristics of the effective human service worker.

Although Zelig represents a comedic example of movement through the Kegan stages, finding a real-life illustration is not difficult. Consider, for example, the life of Malcolm X (Haley, 1992). As a

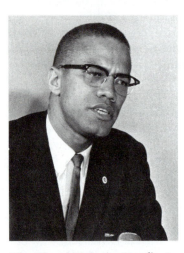

young adult, Malcolm X found himself involved in a life of crime and drug addiction. While serving a 10-year prison sentence for robbery, he was introduced to the Nation of Islam, the Black Muslim religion headed by Elija Muhammad. Malcolm readily gave up his former lifestyle and became embedded in the values of the Nation of Islam. He lived, slept, and breathed *their* values, and his identity became the values held by the Nation of Islam (Kegan's interpersonal stage). However, as he developed as a person, he realized that he did not agree with some of their ideas and he moved from embeddedness in their values to a strong sense of his own religious, cultural, and moral values. Still somewhat closed to other points of view, Malcolm X had matured to the point in which he was now embracing his own set of values (institutional stage).

The life of Malcolm X reflects movement through Kegan's stages of development.

Following a pilgrimage to Mecca, he changed his name to Al Hajj Malik al-Shabazz and again modified his views "to encompass the possibility that all white people were not evil and that progress in the black struggle could be made with the help of world organizations, other black groups, and even progressive white groups" (*Encyclopedia of Black America*, 1981, p. 544). Clearly, Al Hajj Malik al-Shabazz had evolved to Kegan's interindividual stage (and Perry's commitment in relativism stage). He now could hear other points of view, be open to feedback, and yet have a clear sense of his own uniqueness in the world.

Acquiring the Characteristics of the Effective Helper: A Values Clarification Approach

Helping students develop the characteristics of the effective human service worker is crucial if they are going to graduate as skilled professionals who have social consciousness. Embodying the characteristics of empathy, genuineness, introspection, internality, nondogmatism and learning to become an acquirer of knowledge, an experiencer of life, and one who has positive regard for others is no easy task. To develop these characteristics, you usually have to gain some form of feedback concerning how others view you. These characteristics need to be slowly nurtured and developed within a supportive yet somewhat challenging environment. For instance, Zelig needed to discover the therapeutic setting to feel the support and challenge that allowed him to transcend his previous way of living.

Although therapy is certainly one avenue people can use to facilitate personal growth, change can also occur through other experiences. For instance, college can offer the environment conducive for growth, with the classroom potentially being the needed supportive environment that is also challenging to the student. **Values clarification**, one approach easily used in the classroom, challenges students to understand and embrace their unique perspectives while offering potential new lenses from which to view the world. This supportive yet challenging classroom environment can assist students in their development as successful human service workers who embody the eight characteristics listed earlier. At the same time, this environment can assist the development of the emerging adult personality as represented by Perry and Kegan. The values clarification process is seen as a three-step process whereby individuals are challenged to (1) *choose their values*, (2) *prize their choices*, and (3) *act on the choices* they make (Raths, Harmin, & Simon, 1966).

Understanding the valuing process was brought home to me when I participated in a 5-day workshop sponsored by Sid Simon, one of the founding figures of the values clarification movement. During that time we were asked *not* to reveal some essential components of what made us who we were. Therefore, it was suggested that we not reveal to other workshop participants basic facts such as our level of education, the type of work we did, and other major identifying features. Because I was a doctoral student at the time, I soon realized how much of my ego was wrapped up in being in a doctoral program. I began to ask myself some basic questions: "Would people still like me if they didn't know I was highly educated?" More important, "Would I like myself without the persona of the doctoral degree?" As the workshop continued, certain exercises were designed to bring us increased awareness. For instance, we all participated in a 2-hour blind walk in which we had an assistant who aided us. During those 2 hours, we ate lunch (my aide fed me) and walked around the grounds with the help of our assistants. This exercise showed me how I take my able body for granted, how I don't use my senses to the fullest, and how I limit my capabilities in general.

Workshops like these help us understand what we value and how we define ourselves. They help us focus on those things in our lives that our important to us. For instance, through this workshop, I began to ask myself the following questions: "How important is my doctoral degree in defining me as a person?" "How important is a healthy and able body?" "If it is important, do I tend to treat my body in healthy ways?" Values clarification exercises like these help us identify those parts of ourselves that we pride and can challenge us to prize, cherish, and treat sacredly those parts of ourselves that we have identified as important. In addition, these exercises teach us to examine why we may not be prizing certain identified values and help us make decisions either to change our values or to find ways in which we can act to embrace those identified values.

Activity 1-1   Values Clarification

First, find a partner—someone you don't know well. Tell him or her a little about your life. You might want to talk about such things as how you perceive your future career path, what is important to you in life, how you find meaning in your life, people who have influenced you the most, and events that have had a great impact on you. Try to listen carefully to each other, and when you are finished, do the activity listed below.

1. Of the eight human service worker characteristics, rate how important you think each characteristic is toward the effective functioning of the human service worker. (Although *I* believe these qualities are all essential, *you* may have a varying opinion.)

2. Rate yourself next on how well you think you embody these characteristics.

3. Now, here comes the hard part. Have your partner rate you on how well he or she thinks you embodied the characteristics during the role play. (Remember, a person who is stage 3 on the Kegan scale will want to be liked and will be reticent to rate low, even if he or she really feels that the student should be rated low.)

4. Next, rate yourself based on whether you think you exhibited those qualities as you went through your life today.

5. When you have completed your ratings, examine the scores. Are there areas that you state you value but do not exhibit through your behavior? In other words, have you prized and cherished the things you state you value, or are there areas you can improve?

6. Because we all can improve parts of our lives, what ideas do you have to work on those areas? Write them in the space provided. In other words, what action can you take to enhance the values that you state you prize?

Activity 1-1 is an example of a values clarification exercise that pulls together many of the major themes of this chapter. To determine how you value the eight characteristics of the human service worker, whether you embrace the characteristics you value, and what action you can take to enhance the values you identify as important, take a moment to complete this activity.

When rating, use the scale below. A high rating indicates that you embody the characteristic, believe it is important, or exhibited the particular characteristic today.

1. An extremely high rating
2. A very high rating
3. A moderately high rating
4. A somewhat high rating
5. Neither high nor low

6. A somewhat low rating
7. A moderately low rating
8. A very low rating
9. An extremely low rating

Self-Inventory

	Importance	Self-Rating	Other Rating	Exhibit Today?	What You Can Do to Improve Scores
Empathic					
Genuine					
Nondogmatic					
Positive regard					
Introspection					
Internality					
Life as process					
Knowledge acquirer					

Because these exercises are important to help you stretch developmentally and, concurrently, cultivate the human service worker's characteristics, there will be experiential exercises at the end of each chapter to facilitate your own personal growth while you learn some of the basic facts and principles of the human service field.

Ethical and Professional Issues

The Development of Ethical Guidelines— Who Decides What's Ethical?

The fields of social work, counseling, and psychology have a long history of fighting social injustices while supporting what some might consider to be "moral correctness." Deciding what is morally correct, however, is not always easy. Consider the varying laws on obscenity around the country. The U.S. Supreme Court stated that local municipalities have the right to set their own standards concerning what is considered obscene (*Miller* v. *California*, 1973). Apparently, the Court recognized that the various municipalities around the country might view obscenity differently. Look at how the many religions of the world vary on their stands on such issues as abortion, homosexuality, premarital sex, the right of suicide for the terminally ill, and alcohol consumption. What may on the surface appear to be a matter of "black and white" or "right or wrong" is filled with complexities and a lot of gray.

In the development of ethical guidelines, those charged with the formation of such standards have likely wrestled with which societal and professional values the guidelines should reflect. Despite this fact, it is interesting to note that the three major helping professions—psychology, counseling, and social work—have all developed ethical guidelines that share similar values while serving a number of other general purposes:

1. They protect consumers and further the professional stance of the organizations (Corey, Corey, & Callanan, 1993).

2. They serve "as a vehicle for professional identity and [as] a mark of the maturity of the profession" (Mabe & Rollin, 1986, p. 294). As such, they denote the fact that a particular profession has a body of knowledge and skills that it can proclaim and that a set of standards can be established that reflect this knowledge (Ansell, 1984).

3. They profess a belief that the professional should exhibit certain types of behaviors that reflect the underlying values considered de-

sirable in the professional (Corey, Corey, & Callanan, 1993; Loewenberg & Dolgoff, 1988; VanZandt, 1990).

4. They offer the professional a framework in the sometimes difficult ethical and professional decision-making process (Corey, Corey, & Callanan, 1993).

5. They represent, in case of litigation, some measure of defense for professionals who conscientiously practice in accordance with accepted professional codes (Corey, Corey, & Callanan, 1993).

Although ethical guidelines can be of great assistance in the practitioner's ethical and professional decision-making process, as Mabe and Rollin (1986) note, there are limitations to the use of a code of ethics:

1. Some issues cannot be handled in the context of a code.

2. There are some difficulties with enforcing the code, or at least the public may believe that enforcement committees are not tough enough on their peers.

3. There is often no way to bring the interests of the client, patient, or research participant systematically into the code-construction process.

4. There are parallel forums in which the issues in the code may be addressed, with the results sometimes at odds with the findings of the code (for example, in the courts).

5. There are possible conflicts associated with codes: between two codes, between the practitioner's values and code requirements, between the code and ordinary morality, between the code and institutional practice, and between requirements within a single code.   .

6. There is a limited range of topics covered in the code. Because a code approach is usually reactive to issues already developed elsewhere, the consensus requirement prevents the code from addressing new issues and problems on the cutting edge.

The establishment of ethical guidelines are relatively new to the mental-health professions. For instance, the American Psychological Association (APA) first published its *Ethical Standards of Psychologists* in 1953, the American Counseling Association (ACA) developed its ethical guidelines in 1961, and the National Association of Social Workers (NASW) established its guidelines in 1960. However, because ethical standards are to some degree a mirror of the values inherent in the culture, they should not be considered static guidelines. Therefore, over the years, the associations' guidelines have undergone a number of major revisions that reflect these ever-changing values (see ACA, 1988; APA, 1989; NASW, 1990).

NOHSE, in collaboration with the **Council for Standards in Human Service Education** (CSHSE), has always supported the concept of a code of ethics (Linzer, 1990), and has recently supported the development of its own set of ethical guidelines, which may be adopted in 1994 (see Appendix A for a draft of these guidelines) (Neukrug & Bonner, manuscript submitted). Although these guidelines will no doubt have much in common with other codes of ethics (see ACA, 1988; APA, 1989; NASW, 1990), they will also reflect the unique perspective and job requirements of the human service worker.

Throughout this text we will raise various professional and ethical issues that relate to these codes of ethics. Ethical guidelines are moral, not legal, documents, and our professional associations expect us to be bound by them. Sometimes, when a person violates the codes of ethics, he or she will be dismissed from the professional association. In some instances, states have made part or all of a code of ethics into a legal document. In these cases, stiffer penalties such as fines or even imprisonment could result from an ethical violation. Of course, this depends on the seriousness of the violation.

The Developmentally Mature Human Service Worker: Willing to Meet the Challenge

The developmentally mature (Kegan's, stage 5) human service worker looks at his or her own behavior, risks obtaining feedback from others, and is open to change. This person views life as affording opportunities for growth and transformation. Although this individual's goal may be to embody the characteristics of the effective human service worker, he or she realizes that the "healthy" individual is always "in-process"—that is, realizes that life is a continual, never-ending growth process.

As Perry notes, the developmentally mature individual has commitment in relativism. As this applies to ethical codes, we would expect the developmentally mature human service worker to adhere almost always to ethical guidelines while realizing that ethical guidelines are ever-changing documents that do not hold "the answer." The developmentally mature human service worker is willing to explore ethical issues with a sense of openness and can imagine these guidelines changing over time.

Finally, developmentally mature human service workers are committed to excellence in themselves and in the profession. Therefore, they look for avenues of personal and professional growth and are willing to give of themselves in order to promote the profession.

Summary

We examined some of the origins of the human service field as well as those characteristics shown to be important for the effective functioning of the human service worker. The human service profession is relatively young, having its origins in the mid-1960s. Partly as a result of changing societal attitudes as well as increased funding for social welfare programs, a great need arose for more social service workers. Thus, we saw the beginnings of the associate's and bachelor's degrees in the human services. This training was contrasted with the training of other social service professionals.

We examined the importance of the human service worker embodying the eight characteristics of empathy, nondogmatism, being accepting of others, internality, introspection, genuineness, being an experiencer of life, and becoming an acquirer of knowledge. We discussed how those qualities were related to the cognitive development theories of Perry and Kegan. We also discussed ways of enhancing our personality characteristics while increasing our developmental level. Avenues such as therapy and values clarification exercises were seen as potential vehicles for change because they support and challenge our perceptions of the world. It was suggested that values exercises be interwoven throughout this course to assist the student in increasing self-knowledge.

We discussed the development of ethical codes and sources of ethical guidelines. The concept was raised that adhering to ethical guidelines is a "commitment in relativism." This means that we *choose* to embrace the guidelines and view them as ever-changing documents that do not necessarily hold "the answer."

Finally, we examined what it means to be a developmentally mature human service worker, noting that he or she is open to change and views life as a continual transformational process. Mature human service workers are personally and professionally committed to excellence and willing to expend the energy needed to improve both themselves and the profession.

Experiential Exercises

1. Who Is the Human Service Worker? What Is the Human Service Field?

1. We often have varying perceptions of the training, education, and salary of the different social service fields. To see whether your perceptions are correct, fill in the items requested for the following social service professionals.

	Education	Type of Courses	Additional Training?	Licensed? (Yes/No)	Salary
Psychologist					
Psychiatrist					
Mental-health counselor					
School counselor					
Mental-health aide					
Social worker					
Psycho-therapist					
Human service worker					

2. Obtain a Sunday newspaper and circle all the want ads that are social service oriented. In class, make a list of the types of jobs being advertised; the education, training, and experience needed for the job; and the salary being offered.

2.   The Characteristics of the Effective Human Service Worker

The following sets of activities have to do with the characteristics you think make an effective human service worker, as well as which qualities you possess that will make you an effective human service worker. To each question, write responses that you can bring to class. In class, you will be given the opportunity to discuss your responses in small groups.

1. Make a list of the personality characteristics you believe the effective human service worker should embody.

2. Make a list of the skills and techniques you think the effective human service worker should have.

3. What personality characteristics do you currently possess that will make you a successful human service worker?

4. What skills do you currently possess that will make you a successful human service worker?

5. Choosing one of the quotes from the chapter, (a) analyze its meaning and (b) discuss, in class, its meaning relative to the eight characteristics of the effective human service worker.

3. Acquiring the Characteristics of the Effective Human Service Worker

The following sets of questions concern the acquisition of the qualities of the effective human service worker. Write responses for each question that you can bring to class. In class, you will be given the opportunity to discuss your responses in small groups.

1. How have the influences listed below affected your desire to enter the human service field? (If you are not entering the field, base your response on the field you think you will eventually enter.)

   a. Parents' education

   b. Parents' occupations

   c. Placement in family (for example, middle child, youngest child)

   d. Educational experiences

   e. Work experiences

   f. Volunteer experiences

   g. Your values and beliefs

   h. Your gender and/or ethnic background

2. Often, individuals enter the helping professions because they have gone through their own painful experiences and want to assist others with theirs. What personal experiences have made you sensitive to other individuals' difficult life situations?

3. Many of the eight characteristics of the effective human service worker are developed through modeling the behavior of people who have significantly affected our lives. In the space provided in the charts, write the names of four people in your life that have most affected you in a positive way. These individuals can be friends, parents, religious leaders, politicians, movie figures, literary figures, and so on. Then, fill in the chart, noting how the individuals modeled one or more of the characteristics. Finally, in class, share with another student how much of the behavior of the other person you have taken on for yourself.

Significant Person

Characteristic	1.	2.	3.	4.
Empathy				
Genuinenesss				
Nondogmatic				
Positive regard				
Introspection				
Internality				
Life as process				
Knowledge acquirer				

4.   Assessing Your Adult Developmental Level

This self-inventory is designed to give you a general sense of your adult cognitive developmental level. (See pp. 11–14 for a more complete explanation of adult cognitive development as defined by Perry and Kegan.) The inventory is designed to examine your degree of dogmatism, empathy, internality, commitment in relativism, and openness to feedback. *This is not a scientifically proven instrument;* therefore, view your results very tentatively. However, your responses should give you a *rough* sense of your adult developmental level. Use the following scale when responding to each item:

1. Strongly agree   4. Slightly agree

2. Slightly agree   5. Strongly agree

3. Neither agree nor disagree

_____   1. I believe that my opinions are almost always right.

_____   2. It is not unusual for people to seek me out to talk about their problems.

_____   3. When I receive feedback from a professor, I usually learn something from it.

_____   4. The professor almost always has the answer.

_____ 5. In making major life decisions, I usually trust my own "inner sense."

_____ 6. In life, others usually are better at decision making than I am.

_____ 7. Usually, when I try to listen to someone, I make it a point to ask a lot of questions.

_____ 8. The best type of learning takes place when the professor gives us the facts.

_____ 9. If my church or synagogue espouses certain views, I am positive that I will agree with them.

_____ 10. When I am listening to someone, I usually know from the opening statement what that person is going to say.

_____ 11. Based on an individual's appearance, I can almost always determine the value of his or her beliefs.

_____ 12. Usually, my friends' opinions are more important than my own.

_____ 13. In determining my views on life, I have spent much time gathering information from others, reflecting, and being introspective.

_____ 14. Usually, when I am listening to someone who is struggling with an issue, I try to tell him or her what would be the best solution to the problem.

_____ 15. My views are solid, and no one can change them!

_____ 16. Things that happen in my life are out of my control.

_____ 17. I have chosen my values following deep reflection; however, I am still open to examining them further.

_____ 18. Life is what I make it to be.

_____ 19. When listening to someone, I usually disregard the person's feelings and listen more to "the facts" of the situation.

_____ 20. Generally, I think students can offer much to the knowledge base of a class.

Scoring the inventory. For items 2, 3, 5, 13, 17, 18, and 20, give yourself 1 point if your response was a 5, 2 points if your response was a 4, 3 points if your response was a 3, 4 points if your response was a 2, and 5 points if your response was a 1. For all other items, give yourself the number of points that you rated the item.

The highest score on this inventory is an 100. The closer you are to this score, the more you are empathic, internally oriented, non-dogmatic, open to feedback, and committed in relativism. This also is an indication of higher levels on the Perry and Kegan scales.

In class, (anonymous) hand your score to the instructor and then compare your score with the rest of the class. This will give you a sense of your adult cognitive development level as it compares with your peers.

5.   Assessing Our Values

In class, divide into triads. In your triad, you will be given the number 1, 2, or 3. Those who have been given the number 1 will be "pro," and those who have been given the number 2 will be "con." Number 3s are to help out numbers 1 and 2 if they have trouble doing the task.

Your task is to take one of the situations listed below (or come up with one of your own) and *role-play* your feelings about the situation. If you are pro, role-play the situation as if you are for it, even if you actually are against it. If you are con, role-play the situation as if you are against it, even if you are for it. It is important not to tell the members of your triad how you actually do feel about the situation. Role-play for about 5 minutes.

Then do the same thing, but this time take a new situation; number 2 will be pro, and number 3 will be con. Number 1 will be the helper.

Finally, take a third situation and this time, number 3 will be pro; number 1 con; and number 2 will be the helper.

Situations

- Abortion
- Capital Punishment
- Opening an X-Rated bookstore in your neighborhood
- Increased Taxes
- Decreased military spending
- Affirmative action
- Increased tuition

Processing the exercise. In class, generate a list of reasons you couldn't at times effectively listen to the other person. For instance, someone might say, "I was so upset that I just wanted to tell the other person how *I* felt." The instructor can put a list of "hindrances" to effective listening on the board. In class, discuss the following:

1. Why is it difficult to hear someone who holds differing values than your own?

2. How can you learn to accept differing values?

3. What techniques can you use to listen more effectively to an individual who holds values that vary from your own?

4. Why is acceptance of diversity important when you are in the role of helper?

6. Ethical Issues

1. Generate a list of ethical issues you would want addressed by a professional association's code of ethics.

2. Bring your list to class and together generate a class list of items you would want addressed by a professional association's code of ethics.

3. As you read the book during the semester, see whether the items on the list you generated in class have been discussed in the ethics section of the chapters.

4. The instructor should have available a copy of the code of ethics of the APA, the ACA, NASW, and/or the NOHSE/CSHSE ethical guidelines listed in Appendix A. Examine those guidelines and compare those standards with the list generated in class.

2

The Human Service Profession: History and Current Issues

Why Look at History?

A Brief History of the Field
Psychology / Social Work / Counseling

The Human Services Today: Integrating Psychology, Social Work, and Counseling
The Human Service Field: Recent History / The Human Service Worker Today: A Generalist

Professional Issues for the Human Service Worker
What Is the Human Service Worker Trained to Do? / Professional Associations in the Social Service Professions / Credentialing: Registration, Certification, and Licensure

Ethical and Professional Issues
Competence and Qualifications as a Professional

The Developmentally Mature Human Service Worker: Professionally Committed, Ethically Assured

Summary

Experiential Exercises

There I was, finishing college as an idealistic, energetic young man trying to decide what to do next. Rather than work, I decided to go to graduate school (although a few years of work experience probably would have been good for me). I knew I wanted to stay in the helping professions, so I asked my psychology professors for advice. They suggested I pursue a doctoral degree in psychology. They offered no alternatives—there were no alternatives as far as they were concerned. I thought there must be some other options, so I went to the career center where I was given the same advice. In the early 70s, these advisors felt there was only one choice for men going into the helping professions—psychology. Now I realize that these good-intentioned advisors were likely sexist, uninformed, and perhaps a little elitist in their views about the helping professions. For them, men became psychologists and women went into social work. For those who couldn't make it into the few doctoral programs in psychology, well, they could become counselors. Unfortunately, some of these same views are still prevalent today. These views tend to originate from the history of the professions and the ways in which society uses sex-role and culturally based stereotypes in current definitions of careers. In this chapter, we will explore the history of the fields of psychology, social work, and counseling; examine some of the stereotypes that have emerged based on these histories; and look at how these three fields have greatly affected the beginnings of the human service profession.

Why Look at History?

Can you imagine a woman burned as a witch because she was mentally ill or placed in a straightjacket and thrown into a filthy, rat-infested cell for the remainder of her life? Can you envision a man placed in a bathtub filled with iron filings to cure him of mental illness or bled to rid him of demons and spirits that caused him to think in "demonic ways"? What about having a piece of your brain scraped out in order to change the way you feel? These examples are a part of the history of our profession.

Unfortunately, I've taught long enough to know that when history is approached it often is not as interesting as what you just read. In fact, my experience has been that half the class mentally steps out. Why is this? Learning names, dates, and a few facts is just plain boring for many people. If you're a student who is dreading this chapter, you may be asking yourself, "Why learn it?"

In 1962 T. S. Kuhn wrote a book called *The Structure of Scientific Revolutions*. This book had a profound effect on me because it helped put my ideas about knowledge and change in perspective. In particular, Kuhn's concept of the **paradigm shift** intrigued me. He said that knowledge builds upon itself and that new discoveries are based on the evolution of past knowledge. However, Kuhn went on to note that sometimes current knowledge does not adequately explain the way things work. It is at this time that circumstances are ripe for a change in our understanding of the world—ripe for a paradigm shift. For instance, for hundreds of years individuals were at ease with the concept that the earth is flat. However, the advent of new scientific equipment seemed to contradict this model of viewing the world. A new explanation was needed. Thus, it was explained that the earth must be round. Similarly, in the social sciences, past theories adequately worked—for a while. For instance, for many years psychoanalysis was the treatment of choice for mental illness. However, with research on the effectiveness of treatments and with the advent of new theories and new treatment procedures, it was found that psychoanalysis should not always be the treatment of choice. In other words, a paradigm shift took place in the mental-health field.

The human service field has had and will have paradigm shifts. By studying the history of the field and by gaining knowledge about its roots, perhaps you will be the person to develop the next paradigm shift!

A Brief History of the Field

As noted in Chapter 1, the human service field is relatively new and has its origins in many of the social service fields. Clubok notes that "the human service knowledge base is derived as much from psychology, guidance and counseling, nursing, etc., as it is from social work" (1984, p. 3).

The field of psychology has given us an understanding of the process of therapy and a rich appreciation for testing and research. The social work field brought us a deep caring for the underprivileged and an awareness of the power of social and family systems. The field of counseling brought to the human service profession a *holistic* and *wellness approach* that attempted to understand the individual within the context of his or her career, love relationships, and group interactions. Although today these fields share much in common, their somewhat divergent histories have made a strong impact on the human service worker. In the following sections, we will examine briefly these three fields, discuss how they affect today's human service worker, and then examine the recent history of the field itself.

Psychology

The field of psychology has a rich history founded in religion, philosophy, and science. Although much of this history has not directly affected the human service field, the history of psychology is a large part of the underpinnings of the social service field today. It is important to keep in mind that the brief history presented here just skims the surface.

Hippocrates (460–377 B.C.) was one of the first individuals in recorded history to reflect on the human condition. Whereas many of his contemporaries believed that possession by evil spirits was responsible for emotional ills, Hippocrates thought differently, and his suggestions for the treatment of the human condition might even be considered modern by today's standards. For instance, for melancholia he recommended sobriety, a regular and tranquil life, exercise short of fatigue, and bleeding, if necessary. For hysteria, he recommended marriage—an idea with which many in today's world might argue.

As with Hippocrates, one might think that some of Plato's (427–347 B.C.) ideas came right out of a text on modern psychoanalysis. He believed that introspection and reflection were the road to knowledge and to the understanding of reality and that dreams and fantasies were substitute satisfactions. In addition, he considered problems of the human condition to have physical, moral, and spiritual origins. Although Plato's views were enlightening, some consider his student Aristotle (384–322 B.C.) to be the first psychologist because he used objectivity and reason to study knowledge and his writings were psychological in nature (Wertheimer, 1978). He developed a systematic treatise on how people learn through association and the role that the senses play in learning.

Although individuals such as St. Augustine (A.D. 354–430) and St. Thomas Acquinas (A.D. 1225–1274) highlighted consciousness, self-examination, and inquiry as philosophies that dealt with the human condition, there was actually very little innovative thinking regarding the psychology of the mind during this 800 year period, sometimes called the Dark Ages. Partly this was the result of the rise of Christianity which renewed the focus on the supernatural and fostered a movement away from viewing the person in any objective sense as Aristotle did.

Following this dark period in the history of science, the Renaissance and the era of modern philosophy arose in Europe. Here was a rediscovery of the Greek philosophies and a renewed interest in questions regarding the nature of the human condition.

Soon following the Renaissance, we saw the beginnings of modern psychology. In the early to mid-1800s individuals like Wilhelm Wundt (1832–1920) and Sir Francis Galton (1822–1911), the first experimental psychologists, developed laboratories to examine physical differences among people for such things as height, head size, and reaction time. The natural outgrowth of this movement was the testing era. The rise of the testing movement saw individuals like Alfred Binet (1857–1911) develop the first individual intelligence test, which was used to help the French Department of Education separate those children who were "normal" from those who were "abnormal" (Hothersall, 1984). Later, ability tests such as school achievement tests and personality tests were developed. Today, tests are found everywhere and are often an important component to a deeper understanding of our clients.

The beginnings of the testing movement paralleled the rise of **psychoanalysis**, the first comprehensive approach to doing therapy. Developed by Sigmund Freud (1856–1939), psychoanalysis held the new view that an individual's problems may in part have psychological origins. Freud was greatly influenced by individuals like Anton Mesmer (1734–1815) (from whom the word *mesmerize* was derived) who were practicing a new phenomena called hypnosis. Up to this time, all mental illness was thought to be of a physical nature. However, when some individuals with certain kinds of physical illnesses were placed under a hypnotic trance, their ailments would disappear, suggesting the illness had psychological origins. Freud later gave up the use of hypnosis and developed a rather complex theory to understand the origins of human behavior. His new view on mental health and mental illness was revolutionary and continues to profoundly affect the ways in which we conceptualize client problems (Appignanesi, 1979).

Freud's theory, which tended to be somewhat pessimistic concerning the nature of the individual and the ability of people to change, emphasized instincts and early child-rearing patterns in understanding personality development. Partly in response to Freud's bleak views concerning the individual's development, contemporaries and students of his such as Alfred Adler (1963) and Erik Erikson (1963) developed theories that were more humanistically based and stressed the influences of social forces on the development of an individual's nature. Today, there are many approaches to psychotherapy, a good number of which are an outgrowth of or a reaction to Freud's psychoanalytic approach. (See Chapter 3 for a further discussion of Freud and psychoanalysis.)

The 20th century has seen a great expansion in the field of psychology. Today, we still find experimental psychologists working in laboratories trying to understand the psychophysiological causes of behavior and clinical psychologists working directly with clients doing therapy. In addition, we find other highly trained psychologists doing testing in schools, working for business and industry on organizational concerns, and working in many other areas.

The American Psychological Association (APA), which was founded in 1892 by G. Stanley Hall, started with an initial membership of 31 but now has approximately 70,000 members. The APA publishes numerous research journals through which an attempt is made to understand human behavior. Along with the American Psychiatric Association, the APA was instrumental in the development and continued refinement of the ***Diagnostic and Statistical Manual III–Revised (DSM III–R)*** (American Psychiatric Association, 1987). This manual is instrumental in helping the clinician understand the individual, and insurance companies use it for diagnosis when processing mental health claims.

Although in the beginning the field of psychology was dominated by white males, recently we have seen the emergence of women and minorities as prominent psychologists. Of all the mental-health professions, psychology has focused the most on trying to understand mental health and mental illness. Today, the field of psychology continues to lead the way in the development of new theories of working with the individual and of attempting to explain normal and abnormal behavior.

Psychology's impact on the human service field.   For the human service worker, the field of psychology has had many practical implications. From providing the theoretical underpinnings that help us understand the nature of the person, to assisting us to understand human behavior, and to helping us find better ways of working with our clients, the field of psychology has been a major force in the social sciences. Psychologists often may be our employers, our supervisors, or individuals with whom we consult. Acknowledging their relationship to our beginnings is important.

Social Work

The emergence of the social work field grew out of concern for the underprivileged and deprived in society. In contrast with the psychology field, which focused more on understanding the nature of the person, the field of social work originated in the desire to help the destitute.

In England, until the sixteenth century, providing relief to the poor was voluntary and usually overseen by the Church. However, given the dismal social conditions, the English government, under Henry VIII, established one of the first systems of social welfare (Schmolling, Youkeles, & Burger, 1993). The Poor Law of 1601 established local "overseers of the poor" within each parish. These individuals were responsible for finding work for the poor, aiding those who could not work, and providing shelter or **almshouses** for those who were incapable of taking care of themselves. Although crude in its initial establishment, this law became a model for social welfare programs. As a carryover from the English system, local governments in the United States during the colonial period enacted laws to help the poor. During this same time organized charities, usually affiliated with a religious group, arose in the United States.

The Beginnings of the Modern Mental Hospital

In 1773 the "Public Hospital for Persons of Insane and Disordered Minds" admitted its first patient in Williamsburg, Virginia. The hospital, which had 24 cells, took a rather bleak approach to working with the mentally ill. Although many of the employers of these first hospitals had their heart in the right place, their diagnostic and treatment procedures left much to be desired. For instance, some of the leading reasons that patients were admitted included masturbation, womb disease, religious fervor, intemperance, and domestic trouble—hardly reasons today for admission to a mental institution. Normal treatment procedures were to administer heavy dosages of drugs, to bleed or blister individuals, to immerse individuals in freezing water for long periods of time, and to confine people with straitjackets or manacles. Bleeding and blistering was thought to remove harmful fluids from the individual's system (Zwelling, 1990). It was believed important to cause fear in a person, and even individuals like Dr. Benjamin Rush, known for his innovative and relatively benign treatment of the mentally ill (Woodside & McClam, 1990), spoke of the importance of staring a person down:

The first object of a physician, when he enters the cell or chamber of his deranged patient, should be, to catch his EYE . . . The dread of the eye was early imposed upon every beast of the field. . . . Now a man deprived of his reason partakes so much of the nature of those animals, that he is for the most part terrified, or composed, by the eye of a man who possesses his reason. (Cited in Zwelling, 1990, p. 17).

Although many believed in these rather extreme procedures with the mentally ill, there were some who tried tirelessly to employ more humane methods. John Minson Galt II, who administrated the hospital from 1841 to 1862, believed that comfortable surroundings, social interaction, and job-related activities could help the mentally ill get better. Dorothea Dix also fought for humane treatment of the mentally ill and helped to establish 41 "modern" mental institutions.

In the 1800s, as populations in cities grew, an increasingly large underclass developed in the United States. Because the traditional charitable organizations could not meet the needs of these individuals, there was mounting pressure by politicians to create specialized institutions. Thus, reform schools, lunatic asylums, and other specialized institutions were established.

For the underprivileged who were not institutionalized, two major approaches arose to help them in their plight. **Charity organization societies** (COSs) maintained a list of volunteers who would enter the poorer districts of cities, become acquainted with the people, aid in educating the children, give economic advice, and generally assist in alleviating the conditions of poverty. Usually, the poor were not given money but were given advice, support, and, at times, a few "necessities." The volunteers, who were often called *friendly visitors*, also stressed moral judgment and religious values. Sometimes these friendly visitors would spend years assisting one family. The COSs are seen as the beginning of social casework. **Social casework** is that process by which the needs of a client are examined and a treatment plan is designed to facilitate client growth.

In contrast to the COSs, the **settlement movement** had staff who actually lived in the communities in which they sought to help the poor and immigrants:

In essence it was simply a residence for university men in a city slum. . . . These critics looked forward to a society that encouraged people's social responsibility, not self-interest, to create a life that was kindly, dignified, and beautiful, as well as progressive and prosperous. Some of these thinkers rejected capitalism in favor of an idealized medieval community. (Leiby, 1978, p. 129)

These idealistic young staff believed in community action and tried to persuade politicians to provide better services for the poor. One of the best-known settlement houses was Hull House, established by Jane Addams in 1899 in Chicago (Addams, 1910). Addams was a social activist known for her liberal views and progressive ideas.

Out of this involvement with the underprivileged came articles and books concerned with methods of adequately meeting the needs of the underclass. Following the development of these "casebooks," and spearheaded by Mary Richmond at the turn of the century, the first social work training program was established at Columbia University. By 1919 there were 17 such programs in the country. Over the next 30 years, the social work field grew in many different directions, with some of its main areas focusing on social casework, social group work, and community work.

Starting in the 1940s and continuing to the present, an increased emphasis on understanding social and family systems has emerged in this country. Because social workers had already been intimately working with social systems and with families, this increased emphasis on the functioning and dynamics of these systems became a natural focus for many social work programs. Such programs were the first to view the individual in a *contextual* or *systems* framework, as opposed

to seeing the individual in isolation as did many of the early philosophers and psychologists. One social worker in particular, Virginia Satir
(1967), was instrumental in reshaping some of the practices of the
mental-health profession by including a greater systems focus.

In 1955 a number of social work organizations combined to form
the National Association for Social Work (NASW). In 1965 NASW established the **Academy of Certified Social Workers** (ACSW), which
set standards of practice in the field for master's-level social workers.
Today, NASW has 138,000 members, of which 61,000 are certified social workers. Social workers can be found in a variety of social service
settings from hospitals, to mental-health centers, to homeless shelters—the roots of the social work profession. In addition, although
many social workers today do individual psychotherapy and family
therapy, some work in community settings doing advocacy work and
others administer social service organizations.

Because the social work field grew out of charity organizations and
volunteerism and because women in the 1800s did not work outside
the home, many women found their sense of meaning through these
charitable efforts. For many years the field had the reputation of being
a "woman's occupation." Recently, this has drastically changed as the
field and American values have transformed.

Social work's impact on the human service field.   The field of social
work brings much to the human service profession. The beginnings of
the social work field in many ways echo the essence of much of what
today's human service worker does. Like the early social worker,
today's human service worker helps the poor, the deprived, the underprivileged, and the mentally ill. And, like the early social worker, much
of the human service worker's major emphasis is on support, advocacy, and caretaking.

On a more practical level, the social work field has taught us casework approaches, how to work with systems, how to advocate for our
clients, and the importance of respect and caring for our clients. One
might say that the human service worker of today has taken on many
of the functions and roles that the social work field used to embrace.
Today, like psychologists, social workers are often our supervisors, administrators, or consultants. The human service field is clearly a second cousin to the social work profession.

Counseling

The Industrial Revolution, which began in the United States after the
Civil War, changed the social and economic structure of the country.
Many rural Americans, as well as immigrants—most of whom came

from Europe to escape oppression—were drawn to urban factory centers in search of a better life. By the turn of the century, we saw the spread of the use of tests. These events set the stage for the very beginning of the counseling profession, which at that time was focused on guidance. Teachers and administrators were soon using tests in the schools to help individuals understand their skills and abilities and to "guide" them to appropriate professions. One of the leaders of this guidance movement was Frank Parsons, often said to be the founder of vocational guidance (Isaacson, 1986). These events led to the founding in 1913 of the **National Vocational Guidance Association** (NVGA) considered to be the forerunner of the ACA. As early as 1911, Harvard offered the first graduate courses for guidance specialists, and soon after, in Boston and New York, counselors were certified (Gladding, 1992).

Up until the 1940s most "counselors" were still doing vocational guidance. But during this decade, Carl Rogers (1942, 1951) and his nondirective, **humanistic approach** greatly affected the field of counseling. This *client-centered* revolution dramatically changed the way counselors were working, and they soon were giving less advice, focusing more on the "here and now," doing less testing and evaluation, and doing more *facilitating*. The humanistic approach to counseling was in stark contrast to the psychoanalytic approach of Freud. World War II brought with it a need for counselors and psychologists to work with war veterans, and that was when counselors began working outside the schools, practicing this new humanistic approach to counseling.

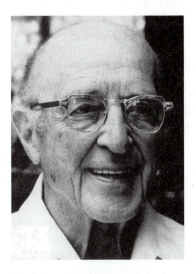

Carl Rogers, the founder of the humanistic approach to counseling, dramatically changed the ways in which many mental-health professionals work with clients.

Probably the decade that most affected the counseling field was the 1950s. The **National Defense Education Act** (NDEA) of 1958 was a direct response to the Soviet Union's launching of Sputnik and funded the expansion of school counseling programs to identify gifted students. As a result, school counselors at the middle and secondary levels proliferated. It was also during this decade that the **American Personnel and Guidance Association** (APGA) was founded. APGA was formed out of NVGA and other related counseling associations that were prevalent at the time.

In the 1960s, President Johnson's Great Society initiatives funded many social service programs. Partly in response to the greater need for counselors, the field diversified and counselors moved into mental health, rehabilitation, higher education, and other related disciplines. At the same time, APGA began to grow, and in the 1970s membership in APGA reached 40,000. It was in this decade that the **Association for Counselor Education and Supervision** (ACES), a division of APGA, delineated standards for a master's-level counseling program. It was also in this decade that differing types of group counseling expanded.

In the 1980s and into the 1990s, the counseling field has continued to expand. To reflect the greater emphasis on counseling and prevention, APGA changed its name to the **American Association for Counseling and Development** (AACD). More recently, AACD underwent another name change to the more streamlined American Counseling Association (ACA). Today, counselors can be found in almost any setting in which there are mental-health professionals. ACA now has nearly 60,000 members and 17 divisions that represent the specialty areas in counseling. Close to 600 graduate programs now train counselors (Hollis & Wantz, 1993). Also, in these decades, certification and state licensure expanded. Currently there are close to 20,000 nationally certified counselors, and 39 states have licensure for counselors. Counselors who are licensed in their states are generally called **licensed professional counselors** (LPCs).

Counseling's impact on the human service field.   The counseling field has had a major impact on the human service field. The humanistic approach to the individual, which tends to be the focus of most counseling programs, is also pervasive in human service education. The emphasis on support, education, and training can also be found in many human service programs. The concept that counseling skills or techniques can be taught in a systematic and focused manner originated in the counseling profession and has been adopted by many human service programs. Counseling programs and many human service programs have stressed the importance of career as a major life force. Finally, the focus on a preventive and developmental approach to clients is an often-used model in the human services.

The Human Services Today: Integrating Psychology, Social Work, and Counseling

The Human Service Field: Recent History

In the late 1940s Congress created the **National Institute of Mental Health** (NIMH). This was the first real effort by the federal government to examine mental-health issues, and it resulted in a systematic effort to do research and training in the mental-health field. On the heels of the creation of NIMH came the **Mental Health Study Act** of 1955, which was a broadly based effort to study the diagnosis and treatment of mental illness. On the basis of the research from this act, Congress passed the **Community Mental Health Centers Act** of 1963. This bill greatly changed the delivery of mental-health services in the United States by providing federal funds for the creation of comprehensive mental-health centers across the country. Although mental-health centers may seem commonplace in today's society, the concept of having treatment centers available to the general public for mental-health concerns is relatively new. Community mental-health centers have greatly changed the face of mental-health services across the country by supporting the use of paraprofessionals in the delivery of some services, by advocating for deinstitutionalization and the care of the chronically mentally ill within local municipalities, and by supporting the concept of *primary prevention*, which involves educating the public to mental-health problems *before* they arise. Today, community mental-health centers are a common place to find the human service worker.

The 1960s saw great upheaval in American society. There was unrest in the ghettos and a country in bitter turmoil over the Vietnam War. The civil rights movement was growing in momentum. Martin Luther King, Jr., and Robert Kennedy were advocating new directions for the country. They both were slain. It is often said that change cannot occur without pain. The death of some of our greatest leaders is perhaps a sad acknowledgment of this truth. For out of the turmoil of this decade came landmark civil rights and social change legislation. As a result of President Johnson's Great Society legislation, civil rights laws and economic and social laws were passed:

Service programs were intended to provide the resources and skills that would allow many poor and near poor individuals to compete for jobs effectively. Much of the emphasis was on youth and on education and training programs. Some of the key legislative changes included the Manpower Development and Training Act, Job Corps, Elementary and Secondary Education Act, Head Start, and the Work Incentive Program.

The effort at reshaping the environment extended to the social and economic fabric of the community as well as its physical contours. Various types of discrimination were outlawed. . . . Key legislative actions included the . . . Economic Opportunity Act of 1964, The Public Works and Economic Act of 1965, The Civil Rights Act of 1964, the Voting Rights Act of 1965, and the Model Cities Program of 1966. (Kaplan & Cuciti, 1986, p. 3)

During the 1980s and into the 1990s, there have been changes in the ways services have been delivered and attempts to cut back on some of the programs of the 1960s. During the Reagan administration some programs were eliminated or reduced and there was a move toward federal **block grants**. This allowed the states to decide which programs to fund and resulted in less money for some programs. In addition, the Reagan administration stressed volunteerism and suggested that business and industry address some of the social woes of the country. The efficacy of this move is in dispute. Despite these efforts by the Reagan administration to change social policy, many of the programs of the 1960s and 1970s have lasted. However, as is evidenced by the riots in Los Angeles associated with the Rodney King incident, the continued economic recession, the rise of violence in society, and the continued lack of or poor health care for a substantial number of citizens, deep social problems still exist.

Partly as a result of the social changes of the 1960s, the human service field emerged. The many federally funded programs and the increased focus on mental-health concerns resulted in a need for additional mental-health workers and other social service personnel. With this new focus on comprehensive mental health and the diversity of social service agencies, there was not only a need for the highly trained doctoral- and master's-level professionals but also a demand for associate's- and bachelor's-level human service professionals. Community colleges became popular. Around this time Dr. Harold McPheeters of the Southern Regional Education Board (SREB) applied for and received a grant from NIMH for the development of mental-health programs at community colleges in the Southern region of the country. This was the beginning of the associate's-level human service degree in the United States. Therefore, some consider Dr. McPheeters to be the "founder" of the human services field.

More recently, we have seen the rise of the bachelor's-level degree in human services (Clubok, 1984; Fullerton, 1990). These programs were a response to an increased need for professionalism as well as a desire to offer an additional educational path for associate's-level human service majors. With funding from NIMH and SREB, during the mid-1970s several workshops and conferences were offered throughout the country that explored the possibility of offering a bachelor's degree in human services—a degree that would offer professional training in the human services that borrowed from the knowledge base of the three main disciplines of psychology, counseling, and social work. Although these three fields all explored the possibility of offering a bachelor's-level degree in the mental-health professions, they have steadily moved toward training graduate-level professionals only, with the APA moving increasingly toward training only doctoral-level professionals and the ACA and NASW training mostly master's- and some doctoral-level professionals (Fullerton, 1990).

The establishment of the Council for Standards in Human Service Education (CSHSE) evolved out of the movement toward a bachelor's-

A Conversation with Dr. Harold McPheeters

Question: I think what is particularly interesting is that when the movement started it really was related to several factors that appeared to be unrelated.

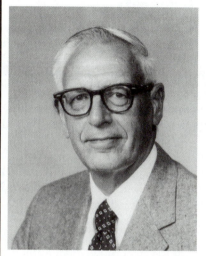

McPheeters: Well, there were several things that made it an opportune thing to do. There was rampant professionalism that said "It's got to be done this way or it won't be right." The "Great Society" with its pressure for more manpower was clearly in conflict with that approach. There were a lot of other things that also came together. The New Careers movement, the "hire now, train later" movement, was strong at that point. The movement was seen as a way for minorities and persons from deprived backgrounds to make it into human services. Otherwise, those groups tended to be excluded from the education programs and from the professions. There were civil rights issues that added to the pressure of the development of human services. (McClam & Woodside, 1989, pp. 3–4)

level degree in human services. Today, this council offers a variety of services for both associate's- and bachelor's-level human service programs. Although a detailed list of some of these services can be found in Appendix B, a summary of the major functions of this council includes the following:

- Approves undergraduate human service programs

- Provides directory of human service education programs

- Provides special reports and a monograph series in the human services

- Provides workshops and conferences for human service education

Today, CSHSE works hand-in-hand with NOHSE to set program standards, to offer workshops and conferences, to provide ethical guidelines, to offer professional journals and newsletters, and to provide an opportunity for networking and mentoring in the field. No doubt, both CSHSE and NOHSE have been setting the standards for professionalism in the human service field (Clubok, 1987).

The Human Service Worker Today: A Generalist

The human service worker today is seen as a generalist who draws from all the major mental-health fields. Thus, we see the curriculum of the typical human service major "borrowing" ideas from psychology, social work, and counseling in a defined and integrated manner. Because of the cross-training that occurs, the human service worker is probably well equipped to work side-by-side and consult with social workers, counselors, and psychologists, as well as other mental-health professionals.

The generalist worker as viewed by the human service profession was defined by McPheeters and King (1971) as one who "works with a limited number of clients or families in consultation with other professionals to provide 'across-the-board' human services as needed; is able to work in a variety of agencies and organizations that provide mental health services; is able to work cooperatively with all of the existing professions in the field rather than affiliating directly with any one; is familiar with a number of therapeutic services and techniques rather than specializing in one or two areas; and is a 'beginning professional' who is expected to continue to grow and learn (p.10)." (Clubok, 1984, p. 2)

The human service worker today is a professional and a specialist who has completed a defined curriculum of study at the associate's and/or bachelor's level. Drawing from psychology, social work, and counseling, the human service worker today has gained knowledge in an integrated fashion from all three fields. As a professional with a broad-based background, the human service worker is often the important link between the client and the more highly skilled social worker, counselor, or psychologist.

Professional Issues for the Human Service Worker

Commitment to professionalism is often shown through credentialing, membership in professional associations, attendance at professional workshops, and reading professional journals. It is also shown through knowing one's professional limitations and recognizing what one is trained to do and what one is *not* trained to do.

What Is the Human Service Worker Trained to Do?

Although the human service field has emerged out of the fields of psychology, social work, and counseling, there are differences in the roles and functions of professionals in the various fields. For instance, does the human service worker do counseling or psychotherapy? What about the social worker, counselor, or psychologist?

When I ask my students to make associations with the word *psychotherapy*, I usually get responses that include "long-term, deep personality change," "secrets unveiled," "unconscious," "focus on past." For the word *counseling*, the responses are usually "short-term," "conscious," "problem solving," "present focus." In actuality, although dictionary definitions may vary, if you pick up a text on "theories of counseling and psychotherapy" (for example, see Corey, 1992) you would see that whether you are doing counseling or psychotherapy, both rely on the same theoretical underpinnings (see Chapter 3 for a further discussion of theory). However, although the theories are the same, how practitioners implement them may vary. Therefore, individuals who see themselves as *doing* counseling may be applying a theory somewhat differently than individuals who sees themselves as *doing* psychotherapy. A rule of thumb may be that as you receive more education and training, you are able to move out of a supportive role and become capable of doing counseling and eventually psychotherapy.

Generally, it is agreed that human service workers do *not* do counseling or psychotherapy. However, what they do certainly may be therapeutic in that they assist the client in the change process. Usually, the work of the human service worker is focused around one or more of 13 roles and functions of human service workers as identified in 1969 by the SREB. These roles include the following:

- **Outreach worker** who might go into communities to work with clients

- **Broker** who helps clients find and use services

- **Advocate** who champions and defends clients' causes and rights

- **Evaluator** who assesses client programs and shows that agencies are accountable for services provided

- **Teacher/educator** who tutors, mentors, and models new behaviors for clients

- **Behavior changer** who uses intervention strategies and counseling skills to facilitate client change

- **Mobilizer** who organizes client and community support in order to provide needed services

- **Consultant** who seeks and offers knowledge and support to other professionals and meets with clients and community groups to discuss and solve problems

- **Community planner** who designs, implements, and organizes new programs to service client needs

- **Caregiver** who offers direct support, encouragement, and hope to clients

- **Data manager** who develops systems to gather facts and statistics as a means of evaluating programs

- **Administrator** who supervises community service programs

- **Assistant to specialist** who works closely with the highly trained professional as an aide and helper in servicing clients (Mandel & Schram, 1985)

In accomplishing any one of these 13 roles, how is the role of the human service worker different from the role of the counselor, social worker, or psychologist? Usually, the human service worker relies directly or indirectly on assisting the client with some specific task as opposed to facilitating personality reconstruction. Table 2-1 shows a visual representation of some of the differences between how a human service worker might approach working with a client as compared with the counselor, social worker, and psychologist.

Table 2-1   Various approaches to working with clients

	Human Service Worker	Counselor/ Social Worker	Psychologist
Directive	High	Moderate	
Problem-focused	High	Moderate	
Works with conscious	High	Moderate	
Focused on present	High	Moderate	
Supportive	High	Moderate	
Nondirective		Moderate	High
Insight-oriented		Moderate	High
Works with unconscious		Moderate	High
Focused on past		Moderate	High
Facilitative		Moderate	High

Professional Associations in the Social Service Professions

Human service workers can join a number of professional associations that serve a number of purposes including the following:

- Providing a political base (for example, lobbying efforts) which helps secure jobs for human service workers, and advocates political agendas relative to the profession (for example, client-rights issues).

- Offering conferences and workshops to foster innovative ideas in the areas of client services, teaching, and advocacy.

- Publishing newsletters and journals to keep members abreast of the latest innovations in the field.

- Providing a process that encourages networking and mentoring.

- Offering grants for special projects related to the field.

National Organization for Human Service Education (NOHSE).
Founded in 1975, NOHSE* is a relatively new association whose main purpose is . . . to provide a medium for cooperation and communication among human service organizations and individual practitioners; . . . to foster excellence in teaching, research, and curriculum development for improving the education of human service delivery personnel; . . . to encourage, support, and assist the development of local, state, and national organizations of human services; . . . to sponsor conferences, institutes, and symposia that foster creative approaches of meeting human service needs. (NOHSE, 1990, p. 72).

NOHSE has six regions as well as a student chapter. The six regions are the Mid-Atlantic, Midwest, Northeastern, Northwest, Southern, and Western. Each region has its own professional meetings, and they operate somewhat independently in offering workshops, conferences, and other professional activities.

If you are interested in becoming more involved professionally as a human service worker, NOHSE along with the region and/or student chapter are the associations to join. NOHSE is still in the building stages and provides an opportunity to get involved on the "ground floor" of an exciting organization.[†]

American Counseling Association (ACA).   This association of nearly 60,000 members was founded in 1952 to meet the professional needs of counseling and human development specialists in the schools,

---

*If you are interested in becoming a member of NOHSE, contact Douglas Whyte, NOHSE Membership Information, Community College of Philadelphia, 1700 Spring Garden St., Philadelphia, PA 19130–3991.

†If you are interested in becoming a member of any of the regions or the student chapter, contact Marriane Woodside, NOHSE Vice-President for Regional Development, University of Tennessee–Knoxville, Human Services Program, 137 Claxton Addition, Knoxville, TN 37919.

community agencies, rehabilitation settings, business, higher education, and private practice. The association maintains 17 divisions and publishes 16 journals in a variety of counseling specialty areas. The association has numerous conferences and workshops at the state, regional, and national level. Although the association is geared toward master's- and doctoral-level counselors and counselor trainees, undergraduates who are interested in the counseling field are welcomed.*

National Association of Social Workers (NASW).   This association of nearly 140,000 members was founded in 1955, and its current purpose is "to create professional standards for social work practice; advocate sound public social policies through political and legislative action; [and] provide a wide range of membership services, including continuing education opportunities and an extensive professional program" (*Encyclopedia of Associations*, 1993, p. 1366). The association publishes four journals and other professional publications. Only undergraduate and graduate students in social work are allowed to join this association.†

American Psychological Association (APA).   The main purpose of this association, which maintains a membership of 70,000, is "to advance psychology as a science, a profession, and as a means of promoting human welfare" (*Encyclopedia of Associations*, p. 1539). The association has 46 divisions in various psychology specialty areas and publishes numerous journals. Undergraduate human service workers are eligible to join APA as affiliate members.‡

Credentialing: Registration, Certification, and Licensure

The credentialing of a professional is one method of assuring minimum competence in a field. Three types of credentialing are registration, certification, and licensure. Generally regulated by state or national legislation, registration is less restrictive than certification, which is less restrictive than licensure. Although many states might register, certify, or license varying professional groups, requirements

---

*For more information write, ACA Membership Information, 5999 Stevenson Ave., Alexandria, VA 22304.

†For more information write, NASW Membership Information, 750 1st St., NE, Washington, D.C. 20002.

‡For more information write, APA Membership Information, 1200 17th St., NW, Washington, D.C. 20036

might differ from state to state. For example, whereas one state might license a psychologist who has 2 years of postdoctoral experience, another state might only require 1 year of postdoctoral experience. Although in most states human service workers are not registered, certified, or licensed, as the profession becomes more solidly defined, we will likely see the beginnings of such a process. In addition, on a state-to-state basis, opportunities may arise for human service workers to become certified or registered in related fields. For example, in Virginia, as in many other states, the human service worker can become a certified substance-abuse counselor if he or she meets the educational and supervisory experience requirements. (For a comprehensive examination of the types of credentialing, see Vroman & Bloom, 1991.)

Registration.   Registration is the most basic form of ensuring minimum competence for a profession. States will often set minimum education or training requirements and will require individuals to register in order to practice within the state.

Certification.   States or national organizations usually set the requirements for certification. Besides requiring minimum education or training as in registration, an exam is often mandatory. For example, to become a nationally certified counselor (NCC) or to become a member of the Academy of Certified Social Workers (ACSW) requires obtaining a master's degree in the respective field and passing a national exam.

Licensure.   States generally set the standards for this most rigorous form of credentialing, and it requires a minimum educational level, usually a state or national exam, and additional documentation of expertise such as evidence of posteducation supervision. States may vary considerably on their requirements for licensure. For example, the requirements as a professional counselor will vary from state to state, with some states requiring a national exam, a submission of a case report, and possibly an oral hearing, whereas other states require only an exam. Because of the idiosyncrasies in licensure from state to state, it is best to contact the licensing board of a particular state in order to determine its requirements.

In reference to registration and certification, McPheeters noted that, although CSHSE has in the past encouraged the registration of human service workers and at one point attempted to establish a national certification process, up to this time there has been little support for their efforts. However, as the human service profession becomes more established, no doubt registration, if not certification, will become an inevitability (cited in McClam & Woodside, 1989).

Ethical and Professional Issues

Competence and Qualifications as a Professional

Although human service workers have generally not obtained registry, certification, or licensure status nationally, the human service worker must be aware of his or her level of competence and training as a professional. The proposed ethical guidelines of NOHSE/CSHSE state that the human service workers should not misrepresent their qualifications, should not make grandiose statements concerning their expertise, should know the limitation of their training, and should know when to refer to appropriate sources if additional expertise is necessary (see Appendix A). The ACA (1988), APA (1989), and NASW (1990) codes of ethics make similar statements.

In a similar vein, the human service worker must keep abreast of current trends in the field. Therefore, it is my belief that the human service worker should become a member of his or her professional association(s), subscribe to and read the professional journals, and attend workshops and participate in other continuing education experiences. Excellence as a human service worker means commitment to educational competence.

The Developmentally Mature Human Service Worker: Professionally Committed, Ethically Assured

The developmentally mature human service worker is committed to his or her professional growth and competence. This commitment is not lip service; it is a deep-felt belief that to do one's best in the profession means embracing the field in a professional manner. The developmentally mature human service worker knows the roots of his or her profession and can work in a consultative and mature manner with related professions. The developmentally mature human service worker knows appropriate ethical conduct because he or she is familiar with the ethical guidelines. Although many ethical decisions are "judgment calls," the ethically assured human service worker makes "wise" judgment calls because he or she is familiar with the ethical guidelines and has kept abreast of the most recent trends in the field.

Summary

We examined the importance of "history as knowledge" in understanding paradigm shifts. We reviewed a brief history of psychology, social work, and counseling professions, which serve as the base for the human service profession. This was followed by a chronology of the more recent events that brought about the actual emergence of the human service field.

We also examined the roles and functions of the human service worker as compared with other mental-health professionals. Noting that the human service worker is trained as a generalist with a history that draws from all the major social service fields, we discussed what the human service worker is trained to do and what he or she is *not* trained to do within this context. We discussed the importance of credentialing as one way of ensuring competence in the roles and functions of professionals.

We discussed the importance of keeping abreast of changes in the field, and the significance of knowing one's limitations as they relate to the ethical issue of competence. Finally, we noted that the developmentally mature human service worker knows his or her roots, can work side-by-side with other professionals, is committed to the field, and has a strong sense of ethical correctness.

Experiential Exercises

1. Important Names and Places

In the space provided, write a brief statement that defines the term or name listed.

1. Paradigm shift _____

2. Hippocrates _____

3. Plato _____

4. Aristotle _____

5. St. Augustine _____

6. St. Thomas Acquinas _____

7. Wilhelm Wundt _____

8. Sir Francis Galton _____

9. Alfred Binet _____

10. Sigmund Freud _____

11. Anton Mesmer _____

12. G. Stanley Hall_____

13. American Psychological Association _____

14. *DSM III–R* _____

15. Poor laws_____

16. John Galt_____

17. Dorothea Dix _____

18. Charity organization society _____

19. Friendly visitors_____

20. Social casework_____

21. Settlement movement _____

22. Jane Addams _____

23. Hull House _____

24. Mary Richmond _____

25. National Association for Social Work _____

26. Academy of Certified Social Workers _____

27. Frank Parsons _____

28. National Vocational Guidance Association _____

29. Carl Rogers_____

30. National Defense Education Act_____

31. American Personnel and Guidance Association _____

32. Great Society _____

33. American Association for Counseling and Development _____

34. American Counseling Association _____

35. National Institute of Mental Health_____

36. Mental Health Study Act_____

37. Primary prevention_____

38. Block grants _____

39. Dr. Harold McPheeters _____

40. Southern Regional Education Board_____

41. National Organization for Human Service Education _____

42. Council for Standards in Human Service Education _____

43. Registration _____

44. Certification _____

45. Licensure_____

2.   Interviewing Professionals in the Field

First, using the following questions as a guideline, have one-fourth of the class interview a human service worker; one-fourth a social worker; one-fourth a psychologist; and the remainder, a counselor.

1. Why did he or she decide to enter the chosen profession?
2. What degree(s) was (were) obtained?
3. What is the "theoretical" orientation of the professional?
4. What are the job roles and functions as defined by the professional?
5. What was his or her entry-level salary?
6. What is his or her current salary?
7. What is his or her view on the differences between the four professions?

Then, with one student representing each of the disciplines, divide into groups of four. In your small groups, discuss the similarities and differences you find in the professions. Second, is there evidence that the history of the profession had an impact on the individual's current job functions?

3.   Are We Ready for Another Paradigm Shift?

Do you think the mental health professions are "primed" for another paradigm shift. If yes, in what direction do you think it would take? If no, why not?

4.   Visiting an Institution for the Mentally Ill

Make arrangements to visit a modern mental institution. How does the current mental hospital differ from early institutions as discussed in the text? What similarities do you think exist between today's institutions and the ones in the 1800s?

5.   Discussing the Problems of the Poor and Destitute

Have a discussion with a homeless street person, visit a shelter for the homeless, visit a storefront walk-in center for the underprivileged. Then, in class discuss the problems of the poor and destitute. What solutions do you think would work in today's society? How are your solutions similar to or different from the solutions of the charity organization societies and settlement houses of the 1800s?

6. **Discussing the Difference between Counseling and Psychotherapy**

In class, the instructor will put the words *counseling* and *psychotherapy* on the board. "Free-associate" to these words, and the instructor will note these associations on the board. Then, as a class, discuss the differences between the two terms. What do you think the counseling limitations are of the human service worker? Do you think the human service worker does counseling? Refer to Table 2-1 when discussing this question.

7. **Joining Professional Associations**

What professional association(s) do you want to join? Why might you join one association as compared with another?

8. **Registration, Certification, and Licensure**

What are the advantages of registration, certification, and licensure? Are there disadvantages? What might they be?

9. **Ethical Vignettes**

Discuss the following ethical vignettes in class. In your discussion, decide whether the human service worker acted ethically. If you think that he or she acted unethically, what action might you take?

Vignette 1. A bachelor's-level human service worker takes some workshops in how to do Gestalt therapy. He feels assured about his skills and decides to run a Gestalt therapy group. The state in which he works licenses counselors, psychologists, and social workers as therapists. Is it ethical (and legal) for the human service worker to run such a group?

Vignette 2. An associate's-level human service worker, who is planning to return to school to obtain his bachelor's and master's degrees, tells his colleagues that he is a "master's degree candidate" in human services. If this person is not yet enrolled in a graduate program, is he misrepresenting himself? Might clients be confused by the term "master's degree candidate"?

Vignette 3. You are working with a client who begins to share bizarre thoughts with you concerning the end of the world. You decide that this individual needs special attention, so you decide to spend extra time with him. Is this appropriate?

Vignette 4. A client tells you she is taking Prozac, an antidepressant, and it isn't having any effect. She asks advice regarding taking an increased dosage and you state "If the current dosage isn't working, perhaps you should consider taking a higher dosage." Is it appropriate for a human service worker to suggest changing dosage levels to clients?

Vignette 5. A human service worker who has received specialized training in running parenting workshops on communication skills decides to run a workshop at the local Holiday Inn. She rents a room and advertises in the local newspaper. The advertisement reads "Learn How to Talk to Your Kid—Rid Your Family of All Communication Problems." Should she do the workshop? Is this ad ethical?

Vignette 6. A human service worker of 20 years is your colleague. He does not belong to his professional associations. He never attends any continuing education workshops. He is not abreast of new information in the field. Is this ethical? Is this professional?

3

Theoretical Approaches to Human Service Work

I always thought of myself as a kind-hearted person. I remember that even as a young child I felt a little different from everyone else—a bit more sensitive, a bit more aware of other people's feelings. For instance, if I were playing ball at the park, I was always worried about the feelings of the kid who was picked last. Similarly, I was worried about the feelings of the kids in class who were overweight, or withdrawn, or "nerdy."

Later, when I was in college, I still was the "nice guy"—trying to do what was just and right and to be the caretaker in the crowd. When shifting my major to psychology, I truly believed that my caring attitude was in and of itself the sufficient tool I would need to be an effective helper. Therefore, I held an attitude that there was little I could learn that would actually benefit me as a helper. As I went on to graduate school, I continued to think I already had the natural skills that alone would make me an effective helper. Basically, I was going to school to get the degree. I believed this so strongly that no one dared tell me how to interact with a client—I knew it all. Just let me at those clients; I could help them. I didn't need any specific training. After all, wasn't I a caring person? Wasn't some caring and a little motivation enough?

Well, I do think having a caring attitude is one basic ingredient in being an effective helper. However, over the years I have found that often (if not usually) caring alone is not sufficient to be effective at what you do. Although our clients may appreciate our caring, it is often not enough to assist them in the change process. Even worse, my experience has been that many human service workers are burned out. Burnout leads to cynicism, and cynical people are not caring (Edelrich & Brodsy, 1980).

Individual versus Systems Approach to Clients

If caring alone is not enough, what does work? Over the years, a quiet debate has ensued over two theoretical approaches to helping the individual change. The *individual approach* assumes that we are each islands unto ourselves and that, although social forces might influence us, the change process should focus on how the individual can change his or her conditions in life. On the other hand, the *systems approach* assumes that our lives are the result of social conditions such as family dynamics, poverty, crime, racism, and sexism and that it is important to work with the system to effect any significant change in the person.

Supporting the individual approach, theorists like Viktor Frankl (1984) and William Glasser (1985) strongly make the case that our reality is a construction of internal messages and that we create our attitudes. As evidence of this, Frankl notes that despite the fact that he was a victim of a Nazi concentration camp, he was able to maintain a sense of hope and self-dignity while existing in this hell on earth. He therefore argues that we create our contentment through our search for meaning, and if we have no meaning, we have no contentment:

Once an individual's search for a meaning is successful, it not only renders him happy but also gives him the capability to cope with suffering. And what happens if one's groping for a meaning has been in vain? . . . In the concentration camps, [there were] those who one morning, at five, refused to get up and go to work and instead stayed in the hut, on the straw wet with urine and feces. Nothing—neither warnings nor threats—could induce them to change their minds. And then something typical occurred: they took out a cigarette from deep down in a pocket where they had hidden it and started smoking. At that moment we knew that for the next forty-eight hours or so we would watch them dying. Meaning orientation had subsided, and consequently the seeking of immediate pleasure had taken over. (Frankl, 1984, p. 141)

Others argue that, to a large degree, social forces determine the ways in which we respond to situations and we must respond to social concerns with socially oriented actions (Alinsky, 1971). Therefore, the individual who is besieged by poverty, surrounded by drug use, living in a crime-ridden slum, and/or has been abused has little chance for survival and little hope for the future. Advocates of the systems approach would argue that this person is unlikely to develop any sense of inner strength or hope.

Joshua

When Joshua was 5 years old, he lived with his mother, his 15-year-old half-brother, and his 20-year-old half-sister and her two children. Both of his half-sister's children had different fathers. There were no male role models except for periodic boyfriends of his mother and half-sister. The family lived in poverty in a three-room apartment in the poor section of town. Drugs and violence were common. Although his mother worked, her income barely made ends meet. Joshua's mother believed that discipline was taught through hitting. Although she might not be considered abusive, she noted that Joshua "got a good whipping when he needed one." She knew little about nutrition, and Joshua grew up on a diet high in fat and carbohydrates and low in protein. Also, it was discovered that the apartment they lived in had lead paint and lead water pipes (ingestion of lead can result in brain damage). When Joshua was older he became abusive toward his girlfriend, took drugs, and lived on the edge of a life of crime.

Has Joshua created this situation, or is he the result of situational influences? Is Joshua responsible for his life situation?

Perhaps the truth lies somewhere in between. Maybe the individual is affected both by his or her attitudes and by systems, and changing the individual *and* changing the system can be productive. In this chapter we will focus only on the individual approach to working with clients. We will take a look at the systems approach in Chapter 6.

Why Have a Theory?

According to Webster (1975), a theory is ". . . an exposition of the general or abstract principles of any science or humanity which have been derived from practice; a plan or system suggested as a method of action. . . ." Theory comes from practice, is a way of organizing our ideas, and leads to suggested plans of actions. Therefore, regardless of whether you adhere to an individual or systems approach, you must have a theoretical base with which to approach your clients. Otherwise, everyone would be just "doing their own thing" and there would be no rhyme or reason to client interventions. Or, as Hansen, Stevic, and Warner put it, "To try and function without theory is to operate in chaos, for without placing events in some order it is impossible to function in a meaningful manner" (1978, p. 16). All the current, well-known counseling theories have a long history, have gone through revisions, and have been supported to some degree by research.

Views of Human Nature

Although there are literally dozens of theories of counseling and psychotherapy, most of them can be placed into four major theoretical approaches: psychodynamic, behavioral, humanistic, and cognitive. A theory is placed in one of these categories because it shares some key concepts related to its *view of human nature.* Our view of human nature describes how we understand the reasons individuals are motivated to do the things they do.

Our lives would be much easier if we knew which of these approaches held "the answer"—that is, which was right. All the approaches, however, seem to have some validity, and all add something to our understanding of the individual. Having a theory that allows us to examine the motivations of individuals is the first step in developing techniques for working with an individual. For instance, if you think people are inherently evil, you certainly would not encourage your clients to "be all that they can be." Instead, you would be apt to encourage individuals to learn how to place restraints on certain aspects of their behavior—in other words, to help them find ways of controlling their behavior so their evil would not hurt the world. On the other hand, if you think people are born with innate goodness, you would want to allow them the opportunity to express this goodness in the world. You would want to help them get in touch with their goodness and allow it to blossom. Think about these two polarities in reference to a person like Charles Manson. If you believe people are inherently evil, you would want Manson to learn how to place restraints on his evil nature. You might view his past actions as a product of his evil nature taking over. You would probably also believe that we all have such an evil side. On the other hand, the individual who believes we are born with innate goodness would see Manson as a person who had lost touch with his innate loving side—probably through a series of horribly abusive experiences in childhood. You would therefore want him to get in touch once again with his caring and loving side, and you would offer him an environment that would allow him to do this.

Deterministic versus Antideterministic View of Human Nature

Such divergent views of human nature, as noted in the example, tend to lend themselves to either a deterministic or an antideterministic view of the individual. A **deterministic view** asserts that forces such as instincts and early childhood development are so great, there is little ability for the person to change. Those who take a deterministic view of human nature are often adherents to the **medical model,** in that they believe there is most likely a genetic/biological predisposition to mental illness. They postulate that temperament, character, and resulting emotional problems can be viewed as an "illness" and therefore can be diagnosed and managed much like a disease. Proponents of this approach will often use psychotropic medications (medications that affect psychological functioning) as an adjunct to therapy. On the other hand, those who take an **antideterministic view** use a **wellness approach** and tend to reject the notion that early childhood development and biological/genetic factors determine psychological problems. These theorists have a strong belief in the ability of the individual to change. In highlighting these differences, William Glasser, the founder of **reality therapy** and a strong proponent of the antideterministic approach, states that "while illness can be cured by removing the causative agent [for example, through the use of psychotropic medications, surgery, electroconvulsive shock therapy], weakness can be cured only by strengthening the existing body to cope with the stress of the world . . . [for example, through the use of therapy and behavior-change strategies]" (Glasser, 1965, p. 56).

Directive versus Nondirective Approach to Clients

Regardless of whether one is an adherent of the deterministic or wellness view of human nature, he or she may take a directive or nondirective stance in working with individuals. The helper who takes a

directive view believes that clients need direction or guidance in the change process. These individuals tend to teach about and direct the client toward healthier ways of living. On the other hand, the helper who takes a **nondirective view** has trust in the client's own ability to make change; therefore, he or she attempts to provide a safe, helping environment that enables the client to define his or her own strategies for change. Helpers who adhere to this approach generally rely on the use of empathic understanding and respect for the client's own change process in their *facilitation* of client growth.

Today, few helpers are strictly deterministic, antideterministic, directive, or nondirective. Instead, most take an eclectic, or integrative, approach toward working with clients. Such an approach requires helpers to reflect on their own views of human nature, with the resulting outcome being a view of human nature that borrows from the varying viewpoints. In this chapter, when you are examining the differing helping theories, think about whether you believe people are determined, whether they need to have problems dealt with from a medical model or wellness orientation, and whether you would have a tendency to be directive or nondirective. Then think about what aspects of the varying theories you like and how you might try to integrate the theories into your own eclectic, or integrative, approach.

Major Theoretical Orientations

Psychodynamic Approach

It is the latter part of the 19th century. A person walks into a physician's office complaining of melancholia and paralysis of the left arm. No apparent physical problems are found. What does the physician do?

Up until this time, these symptoms were thought to be organic in nature—that is, they were considered physical in origin. If the physical problem could not be immediately discovered, it was because science had not yet found the physical origins of the problems. Then, in the late 1800s, Sigmund Freud developed a comprehensive theory that he applied when doing therapy with individuals. Through the use of hypnosis, he discovered some amazing things. For instance, some patients who had lost the use of a limb or were blind were found not to have symptoms while under hypnosis. Freud had discovered that their illness was not physical but instead had psychological origins (**conversion disorder**). Freud spent years trying to understand the complex intricacies of the mind. Although he later gave up the use of hypnosis for other techniques, he felt strongly that there were **unconscious factors**—factors beyond our everyday awareness—that mediated our behavior. In other words, he thought that the reasons we do things are

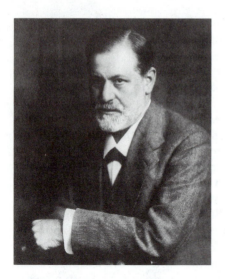

Sigmund Freud (1856–1939).

often beyond our understanding. Freud spent most of his life developing his psychoanalytic theory to explain the causes of human behavior. As the years have gone by, some of Freud's theory has been debunked, some has been changed, and some has been accepted as fact. In addition, a number of theorists have borrowed from Freud's original ideas and moved in innovative directions. Freudians and neo-Freudians are often subsumed under the heading psychodynamic theorists.

The psychodynamic view of human nature. Although individuals who adhere to a psychodynamic view vary considerably on many points, they do share some basic beliefs concerning their view of human nature. For instance, the **psychodynamic approach** has at its core a belief that drives motivate behavior and that these drives are at least somewhat unconscious. Whereas Freud thought that these drives are the instinctual drives of sex and aggression (Appignanesi, 1979; Freud, 1947), other theorists like Alfred Adler (1964) and Erik Erikson (1982) believed that people are motivated more by social drives. Still others like Heinz Kohut (1984) play down the effects of sex, aggression, and social forces but highlight the ways we attach and separate from important "others" in our lives. Regardless of which motivating force an individual believes is most important, psychodynamic-oriented individuals believe that our perceptions of our childhood—as well as the actual events that occurred when we were children—in combination with our drives, greatly affect our **psyche** and, consequently, our later adult development. Therefore, the purpose of psychodynamic therapy is to help the individual understand his or her early childhood experiences, and how those experiences, in combination with the individual's drives, motivate the person today.

Key concepts of the psychodynamic approach. Psychodynamic approaches tend to specify rather complex **developmental stages**. These stages describe psychological and physical tasks that must be accomplished throughout the life span. An individual who does not adequately master the tasks of one stage may become **fixated** in that stage; that is, he or she will not successfully pass through later stages because of unresolved issues in the earlier stage. This developmental framework is an important aspect of the psychodynamic approach and has major implications concerning how the human service worker may approach the individual or family. (See Chapter 5 for a more detailed examination of developmental theory as defined by psychodynamic theorists.)

Psychodynamic theorists believe that, as we pass through our developmental stages, **repression** (putting painful memories out of consciousness) may occur. Therefore, assisting the individual through the change process can be a difficult and long ordeal—a process of peeling back the layers of the person to get to the repressed memories. For instance, the adult who was abused as a child might have repressed early memories, might have learned dysfunctional ways of interacting, and might not be conscious of his or her maladaptive behaviors. One can readily see that "uncovering" the root causes of current behavior might take years. Usually, helpers who are psychodynamically oriented will begin the relationship in a nondirective fashion as they attempt to understand the early root causes of the client's behavior. However, at a later point in the counseling process, the helper will become more directive as he or she attempts to interpret the client's behavior and offer possible avenues for change.

Because of the belief that early childhood experiences together with our instincts affect us in unconscious ways, psychoanalysis was originally considered a deterministic approach, which often espoused a medical orientation toward working with clients. However, some of the more recent psychodynamic approaches have placed less emphasis on the long-term effects of early childhood and instincts and have focused more on the conscious process, social causes of behavior, and the ability of the individual to change (Dinkmeyer, Dinkmeyer, & Sperry, 1987). Despite some of these modifications, the psychodynamic approach still asserts that the change process can be formidable.

> Now the years are rolling by me
> They are rocking evenly
> I am older than I once was
> Younger than I'll be
> But that's not unusual
> No it isn't strange
> After changes upon changes
> We are more or less the same
> After changes we are more or less the same.
>   (Paul Simon, 1969)

Generally, psychodynamic theorists believe that patterns of behaviors learned in the first few years of life are repeated with our significant others—including the human service worker or therapist with whom the client is working. Therefore, in this context, the helper must understand that the behaviors the client exhibits had their origins in childhood and that the client may not fully understand why he or she behaves in particular ways. This concept is called **transference**. Adherents of the psychodynamic approach try to maintain an emotionally distant relationship with their clients—a relationship where the client expresses his or her feelings but little if any **self-disclosure** takes place on the part of the helper. This would allow the professional to separate clearly the client's issues from the therapist's issues.

The human service worker's use of the psychodynamic approach. Traditionally, the psychodynamic approach has been used mostly in the intensive psychotherapeutic setting. However, some aspects of this approach can be adapted for the human service worker to use. First, this approach offers us a developmental model by which we can understand the individual. Understanding that clients may be responding to deep-seated motivations that stem from early childhood and are mostly unconscious helps the human service worker have empathy and patience when working with very difficult clients. Second, this approach helps us particularly to understand deviant behavior. The notion that such behavior is the result of abusive or neglectful early childhood caretaking may help us understand that deviants, perpetrators, criminals, and abusers are also victims. Only with this knowledge can we begin to have deeper caring and understanding to work with such difficult populations.

Finally, the psychodynamic approach has given one other important contribution to the human service field: the concept of **countertransference**. Just as our clients might respond to individuals as if they were significant people from their past, mental-health professionals who have not resolved their past issues may do the same. It is important for human service workers to have worked through their own issues in order to avoid countertransference with their clients. Countertransference can have negative effects on your relationships with your clients because, due to your own unresolved issues, you may respond in unhealthy ways toward your clients.

Behavioral Approach

Around the turn of the century, the Russian scientist Ivan Pavlov (1848–1936) found that a hungry dog that salivated when shown food would learn to salivate to a tone if that tone had been repeatedly paired, or associated, with the food. In other words, eventually the dog would salivate when it heard the tone, whether food was present or not. Pavlov discovered what was later called **classical conditioning**.

In the 1920s psychologist B. F. Skinner showed that animals would learn specific behaviors if the target behavior was reinforced. His **operant conditioning** procedures demonstrated that if one presents a **positive reinforcement** (presentation of a stimulus that yields an increase in behavior) or a **negative reinforcement** (removal of a stimulus that yields an increase in behavior), one can successfully change behavior. Skinner became so good at changing behavior in animals that during World War II he used his techniques to reinforce pigeons to steer gliders toward enemy targets—gliders that had explosives attached (Skinner, 1960)! Despite great accuracy, the military decided not to use this technique. Significantly, Skinner's approach has also shown that punishing an individual (presenting an aversive stimulus) is a very poor means of changing behavior.

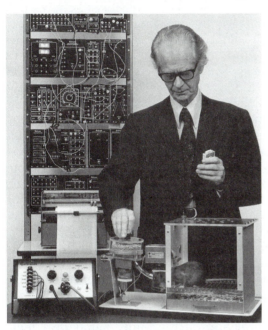

B. F. Skinner's views on operant conditioning showed how reinforcement can be used to change behaviors.

In the 1940s Albert Bandura discovered another behavioral approach. He had children view a film in which an adult acted aggressively toward a Bobo doll. Later, when placed in a room with a Bobo doll, those children acted more aggressively than did children who had not seen the film (Bandura, Ross, & Ross, 1963). This **social-learning**, or

A Very Bright Pigeon

I walk into a small store in New York's Chinatown, and I see a sign that says "As Seen on *That's Incredible,* Play Tic-Tac-Toe with the Pigeon." Being a wealthy man, I place a quarter in the slot, then another quarter, then another. I can't beat the pigeon. Well, I guess operant conditioning really does work—or maybe pigeons are brighter than I thought. On the other hand, maybe I'm not quite as smart as I might think.

modeling, approach has also shown that although we may not always act out behaviors we have viewed, if the behavior is needed at a later date, we have the capacity to act it out.

The three **behavioral approaches** of classical conditioning, operant conditioning, and modeling all share a common view of human nature and have been widely applied to the helping professions.

The behavioral view of human nature.   The behaviorist believes that all behavior is learned and that we are conditioned by reinforcers in our environment. This view does not stress the unconscious and does not place emphasis on gaining insight into our early childhood experiences. Instead, this approach assumes that we have *learned* our current behaviors and that we could learn new behaviors by applying the principles of behaviorism. Therefore, by using classical conditioning, operant conditioning, or modeling, in a scientific and **empirical** manner, we can explore with our clients the types of behaviors they wish to change and use these approaches to assist them in the change process. Although the past may have been important in conditioning our current behaviors, focusing on the past is not particularly important in the behavioral approach. In its early days, the behavioral approach was seen as a directive approach to working with a client in that the helpee's situation was examined and diagnosed and strategies for behavior change were made. However, establishing a relationship through such nondirective approaches as the use of empathy and modeling, prior to suggesting specific behavior changes, has recently become more important (Spiegler, 1983).

Applications of the behavioral approach.   Many behavioral techniques have been very successfully used in a variety of human service, educational, and therapeutic settings. For instance, the behavioral technique of establishing a **token economy** has been successfully used with the developmentally disabled. In this case, an individual is given a token for specific targeted behaviors that he or she is asked to exhibit. For example, a person might receive a token for successfully getting dressed in the morning, for exhibiting "appropriate" personal traits, for bathing himself or herself, and so forth. At the end of a specified amount of time, such as a day or a week, the individual can trade in his or her tokens for money or some other reinforcer such as candy or items in a gift shop. On which of the three behavioral approaches is the token economy based?

A second common use of behavioral approaches is in the treatment of phobias. One treatment for phobias includes teaching an individual a series of deep-relaxation exercises and then pairing the feeling of relaxation with the image of the feared object. For instance, suppose an individual had a debilitating fear of cats. A therapist might

The Power of Reinforcement

I had a friend who used to work at a residential home for the mentally retarded. One boy who lived there would clap loudly and smile broadly after he successfully urinated in the toilet bowl. For years human service workers would reinforce (applaud) him when he could successfully urinate in the toilet, and he was copying their behavior. On which of the three behavioral approaches is this example based?

teach the individual deep-relaxation techniques and then pair the image of a cat with the relaxation. At a later date, a live cat might be paired with the feeling of relaxation. Techniques like these generally take repeated trials to be successful, and there are often relapses, which are called **spontaneous recovery** of the symptom. On which of the three behavioral approaches is this treatment of phobias based?

One other use of behavioral approaches with which you might be familiar is in the learning of assertive behavior. In this case, individuals who have difficulty asserting themselves are shown effective and nonaggressive ways of stating how they feel and expressing their needs. Almost always the facilitator or trainer comes up with a situation in which he or she **role-plays** how to be assertive. Nonassertive individuals can then practice what they just watched. This type of training often works well in a group or workshop setting. On which of the three behavioral approaches is this type of training based?

The human service worker's use of the behavioral approach.   Unlike the psychodynamic approach, the behavioral approach has been widely applied outside the psychotherapeutic setting. Aside from the preceding examples, behavioral concepts are commonly used in a wide variety of human service settings. For example, reinforcement is used in schools, residential and rehabilitation settings, and day-treatment programs, whereas modeling via role-playing is commonly used at employment offices, in educational workshops, and in the training of human service workers.

Today, finding some behavioral techniques incorporated into the human service worker's repertoire of skills is not unusual. In fact, for some disabilities (for example, phobias, mental retardation), the use of behavioral techniques has been shown to be so powerful in facilitating the change process that it would be unethical for a human service professional not to use them or not to have the client referred to someone who is an expert with these kinds of techniques. Behavioral techniques are advantageous because, in collaboration with the client, the human service worker can identify client goals, apply specific techniques, and see results in relatively short periods of time. In residential settings, behavioral techniques are easily understood by clients and help give direction and focus for both staff and clients.

Humanistic Approach

During the 1940s the mental-health field underwent a revolution in its approach to working with people. Individuals like Carl Rogers, Rollo May, and Abraham Maslow, led a reaction against the deterministic flavor of the psychodynamic approach and the scientific reductionistic notions of the behavioral approach. This **humanistic approach** highlights the strengths and the positive aspects of the individual and rejects the concept that people are determined by early childhood experiences or reinforcers in the environment:

I think it is now possible to be able to delineate this view of human nature as a total, single, comprehensive system of psychology even though much of it has arisen as a reaction *against* the limitations (as philosophies of human nature) of the two most comprehensive psychologies now available—behaviorism (or associationism) and classical, Freudian psychoanalysis. . . . In the past I have called it the "holistic-dynamic." . . . (Maslow, 1968, p. 189)

The humanistic view of human nature.   Besides being a reaction to psychodynamic and behavioral theory, this humanistic approach had its origins in **existential philosophy** and **phenomenology**. Therefore, adherents of the humanistic approach believe that we all have choices and that we constantly are making choices that create our existence. Humanists generally think that there is no such thing as an *objective* reality; instead, they stress the *subjective* reality of the individual. Trying to understand how the individual constructs his or her reality and helping facilitate the individual's perception of his or her experience is the major goal of this approach. In addition, humanistic theorists generally agree that people are born with some type of **actualizing tendency**, or growth force. This means that individuals have the ability to transcend their current existence and move toward a more fulfilling and harmonious existence. Therefore, although the past may have been important in affecting how we act today, a counseling relationship does not have to focus on the past to help a person change and grow. Many approaches to counseling have taken the philosophy of the humanistic approach and applied it to educational, therapeutic, and human service environments. Although techniques might vary among these approaches, all believe in the basic philosophy of this approach.

Key concepts of the humanistic approach.   Probably, the humanistic approaches that have most affected the human service and mental-health fields have been the **person-centered approach** of Carl Rogers (1951) and the hierarchical approach of Abraham Maslow (Maslow, 1968, 1970). Maslow's theory stresses a **hierarchy of needs** in which he stated that a lower-order need would have to be satisfied before the next need on the hierarchy could be approached (see Figure 3-1). This concept has great implications for working with individuals. For instance, by examining Figure 3-1, we can see that an individual who is hungry or in need of shelter probably has little ability to focus on the needs of belonging or self-esteem. The highest need to be satisfied, is self-actualization. Some of the qualities that are embodied by the **self-actualized person** are spontaneity, the ability to be in touch with one's feelings, high self-worth, and the development of one's own sense of spirituality.

Although Rogers would agree with much of Maslow's philosophy, his approach focuses more on the actual counseling relationship. He

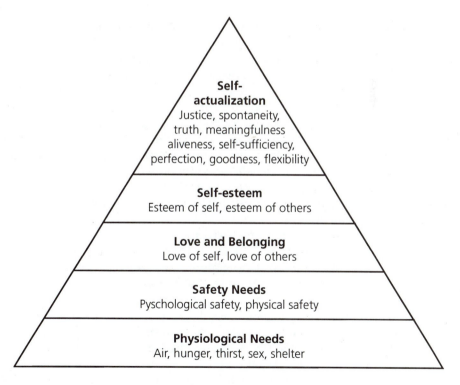

Figure 3-1   Maslow's hierarchy of needs

believed that the conditions of empathy, unconditional positive regard, and genuineness (see Chapter 1) are necessary and sufficient for the growth process of the person (Rogers, 1957). In other words, these personality characteristics alone are enough to facilitate change in the person. In referring to this nondirective approach, Rogers noted that:

> Nondirective counseling is based on the assumption that the client has the right to select his own life goals, even though these may be at variance with the goals the counselor might choose for him. There is also the belief that if the individual has a modicum of insight into himself and his problems, he will be likely to make this choice wisely. (1948, pp. 126–127)

As a humanist, Rogers believed that people are born good with an actualizing tendency. However, such a belief does not negate the fact that individuals do end up with emotional problems. In explaining this, he stated that because significant others in our lives would place expectations and conditions on us, we end up acting as they would have wanted us to be as opposed to how we actually are—we end up acting nongenuine or incongruent. Often, the individual is "out of touch" or not aware of his or her incongruence. Rogers thought that people could get in touch with the natural part of themselves if they were around people who are empathic and who show unconditional positive regard. He used the term **subception** for the professional's ability to perceive feelings and deeper meanings beyond what the individual actually experiences within himself or herself. Rogers would certainly have agreed that regardless of where on Maslow's hierarchy of needs we find the person, offering the client empathy, unconditional regard, and genuineness would assist the individual in his or her ability to move up the hierarchy. Later in Rogers's life, he stated that his theory was applicable to all individuals, not just to individuals in the helping professions (Rogers, 1980). He thought that people would live a more peaceful coexistence if they could embody some of the characteristics he deemed important.

The humanistic approach stresses the positive aspects of the individual and displays a belief that the person can change and grow. Unlike adherents of the psychoanalytic approach, proponents of the humanistic approach do not state that we are determined by our early experiences and do not stress the role of instincts in our lives. The role of the unconscious is also deemphasized in the humanistic approach; most humanistically oriented professionals stress the ability to increase awareness. Finally, whereas proponents of the psychodynamic approach stress emotional distance and little use of self-disclosure on the part of the helper, and adherents of the behavioral approach stress the ability of the professional to use techniques in a scientific, objective manner, advocates of the humanistic approach stress the personal

Can a Behaviorist Be a Humanist?

During the defense of my doctoral dissertation, my advisor, who was a behaviorist, asked me if "a behaviorist can be a humanist." I went on to give what I thought at the time to be a rather esoteric response, noting that the basic orientations of the approaches were philosophically different and therefore incompatible with each other. A few years later, I had the opportunity to hear Skinner talk at a church in New Hampshire. Following his talk, I asked him, "Can a behaviorist be a humanist?" Waiting a moment, he turned to me and, with a deeply reflective look, said, "Well, I don't know about that, but he can surely be humane."

qualities of the professional in the change process. Helpers using this nondirective approach believe that these qualities alone are the key to client growth.

The human service worker's use of the humanistic approach. Maslow's hierarchy of needs has become an established method of recognizing how to approach the individual initially. In this model, the human service worker who is spending the majority of time attempting to raise an individual's self-esteem when that individual is homeless and cold would be doing the client a disservice.

Today, the personal characteristics of empathy, being nonjudgmental, and being genuine have become the essential qualities for mental-health professionals to embrace. Along these same lines, stressing the importance of the relationship between the helper and the client has become a key ingredient in the helping relationship. Today, whether the human service worker views himself or herself as psychodynamically, behaviorally, or cognitively oriented, the ability to embody the humanistic personality characteristics and to form a strong relationship has become essential. When the human service worker does not show these qualities, it is very often an indication of burnout and that it's time for the human service worker to take a self-inventory.

Cognitive Approach

Another approach to working with the individual has gained some prominence. The **cognitive approach** stresses how the individual thinks, particularly how *cognitions* affect our behaviors and how we feel. Although Albert Ellis (Ellis, 1988; Ellis & Harper, 1961) popularized this approach in the 1960s, more recently Aaron Beck's research and treatment applications have gained much prominence (Beck, 1976). However, the concept that our thinking process is the root of our personhood can be traced back to early philosophers:

. . . if you have right opinions, you will fare well; if they are false, you will fare ill. For to every man the cause of his acting is opinion. . . . (Epictetus)

The cognitive view of human nature.   Cognitive-oriented professionals tend to believe that the individual's thinking is conditioned, starting in early childhood, that our ways of thinking are reinforced throughout our lives, and that these ways of thinking are directly related to how we act and how we feel. They believe that we are not born with innate goodness or evil, as rational or irrational beings, or as individuals who are depressed, happy, angry, or content. Adherents to the cognitive approach propose that our thinking can be changed through **counterconditioning**—that is, we can reinforce new, healthier ways of thinking. Therefore, what had been learned in childhood can be relearned. They believe that although it might be interesting to understand *why* we behave the way we do, such understanding is not crucial, and perhaps not even important, in making changes in the way we think. Such changes in our thinking, they believe, will ultimately help us cope with our daily living and will change dysfunctional behavior patterns.

Key concepts of the cognitive approach.   The cognitive approach can be used with many different client populations. As a teaching approach, it places less emphasis on the qualities of the relationship between the client and the helper and more emphasis on how clients learn about changing the ways in which they think. Proponents of this approach stress the importance of continually evaluating the thinking process and of trying to extinguish past destructive ways of thinking while practicing new, positive ways of thinking. The intent of the cognitive approach, however, is not to *change* the core values of the individual but to *examine* how the client's thinking is negatively affecting his or her ability to function in the world. Those who adhere to this approach will usually carefully analyze the way a client thinks in order to try to understand how a client's thinking is resulting in negative feelings. Once patterns of thinking are identified, clients are challenged to change their thinking and therefore adopt new behaviors and more positive feelings. Some therapists have combined many of the techniques from the behavioral approach with the cognitive approach.

The human service worker's use of the cognitive approach.   Although human service workers have not widely adopted the cognitive approach, professionals in most settings can readily use its basic concepts. Helping clients understand the connection between thinking, behaving, and feeling can dramatically impact how they interact in the world. Understanding that at least to some degree our thinking creates our feelings and actions can give clients hope regarding their future. Perhaps one challenge for human service workers today is to understand and embrace cognitive theory more fully so they can better help clients take responsibility for their thinking, feeling, and acting.

Eclectism: An Integrative Approach

When using an **eclectic** approach, mental-health professionals draw from a number of different orientations to develop an approach to working with their clients. Professionals using this approach, however, must not "shoot from the hip"; instead, they must carefully reflect on their views of human nature and draw techniques that fit their ways of viewing the world. Unfortunately, my experience has been that many individuals who call themselves eclectic use a hodgepodge of techniques, which may end up being confusing to a client. How many mental-health professionals are eclectic? One study of psychologists (Smith, 1982) reports that 41% stated they were eclectic, whereas another study of counselors shows that 34% saw themselves as eclectic (Neukrug & Williams, 1993). Before you borrow techniques from the differing orientations, you must carefully examine your view of human nature. Once you have established your belief about the nature of the individual, use the techniques that will fit that view. In the exercises at the end of this chapter, you will have an opportunity to examine your view of human nature.

Ethical and Professional Issues

The Importance of Supervision for the Human Service Worker

To become a better human service worker, it is important to constantly examine your view of human nature, your theoretical approach, and, ultimately, your effectiveness with your clients. One way of accomplishing this is through the supervisory relationship. Supervision should start during one's training program, to "serve as a unique link between preparation and skilled service" (Cogan & O'Connell, 1982, p. 12), and should continue as long as one is working with clients in the human service field. There is nothing better than a good supervisory relationship that is based on trust, mutual respect, and understanding to help us take a good look at what we are doing (Sadow, Ryder, Stein, & Geller, 1987).

Unfortunately, all too often I have seen professionals avoid supervision because of fears about their own adequacy. These fears can create an atmosphere of isolation for the human service worker, an isolation that leads to rigidity and an inability to examine varying methods of working with clients. It is important that we as professionals face our own vulnerable spots—to look at what we do not do well. A good supervisory relationship can help us look at issues such as when to break confidentiality or when we might be losing our objectivity because of a dual relationship.

Confidentiality and the Helping Relationship

Regardless of the theoretical approach to which one adheres, keeping client information confidential is one of the most important ingredients in building a trusting relationship. However, is confidentiality always guaranteed or warranted? For instance, suppose you encounter the following situation:

A 17-year-old client tells you that she is pregnant. Do you need to tell her parents? What if the client was 15 or 12? What if she was drinking while pregnant, or using cocaine, or. . . . What if she tells you she wants an abortion? What if she tells you she is suicidal because of the pregnancy?

Although most of us would agree that confidentiality is an important ingredient to the helping relationship, it may not always be best to keep things confidential. Although all ethical decisions are to some degree a judgment call, we can follow some general guidelines when making a decision to break confidentiality (always check local laws, however, to see if there are variations). You can break confidentiality:

1. If a client is in danger of harming himself or herself or someone else

2. If a child is a minor and the law states that parents have a right to information about their child

3. If a client asks you to break confidentiality (for example, your testimony is needed in court)

4. If you are bound by the law to break confidentiality (for example, a local law that requires human service workers to report the selling of drugs)

5. To reveal information about your client to your supervisor in order to benefit the client

6. When you have a written agreement from your client to reveal information to specified sources (for example, other social service agencies that are working with the same client)

Now that we have looked at when it is all right to break confidentiality, let's examine times when it is not permissible:

1. When you're frustrated with a client and you talk to a friend or colleague about the case just to "let off steam"

2. When a helping professional requests information about your client and you have not received written permission

3. When a friend asks you to tell him or her something interesting about a client with whom you are working

4. When breaking confidentiality will clearly cause harm to your client and does not fall into one of the categories listed above

Confidentiality is an ethical guideline, not a legal right. The legal term that ensures the right of professionals not to reveal information about their clients is **privileged communication**. In many states, lawyers, priests, physicians, and licensed therapists have the legal right to privileged communication. Generally, this means that, if called to court, these professionals do not have to reveal information. Because human service workers are *not* protected by privileged communication, they cannot ensure confidentiality under these circumstances.

The ethical guidelines of ACA, APA, and NASW, as well as the proposed ethical guidelines of NOHSE/CSHSE, ensure the right of confidentiality, usually with some limitations as listed above (see Appendix A). More specifically, the proposed guidelines state that

The client has a right to confidentiality except when such confidentiality would cause harm to the client or to others, when agency guidelines state otherwise, or under other stated conditions (e.g., local, state, or federal laws). Clients should be informed of the limits of confidentiality prior to the onset of the helping relationship.

Dual Relationships and the Human Service Worker

Is it all right to have as a client a friend, relative, or lover? Some professional groups like the American Counseling Association (ACA) and the American Psychological Association (APA) have taken clear stands that state this is *not* ethical: ". . . Dual relationships with clients that might impair the member's objectivity and professional judgment (e.g., as with close friends or relatives), must be avoided. . . ." (ACA, 1988, p. 2).

Similarly, the proposed ethical guidelines of NOHSE/CSHSE prohibit dual relationships with clients that may hinder the effectiveness of the helping relationship: "Human service workers should avoid any dual relationship that might negatively impact on the helping relationship with the client. During the course of the helping relationship, sexual relationships with clients are unethical and prohibited" (see Appendix A).

Because human service workers are not involved in intensive psychotherapeutic relationships, the relationship with their clients differs from those of counselors and psychologists. I believe, however, that it is the responsibility of each human service worker to decide whether his or her objectivity and professional judgment are impaired by having a dual relationship with a client. Generally, it is not wise to have a dual relationship, especially because, in almost every case, another human service worker can help that individual.

The Developmentally Mature Human Service Worker: Committed to a Counseling Approach and Willing to Change

Remember Perry and the concept of commitment with relativism (Chapter 1)? Well, effective human service workers have reflected on the various approaches to counseling and have made a commitment to that approach. This commitment includes learning more about the approach, reading current research about that and other approaches, being open to the supervisory process, and, most important, changing the approach if evidence indicates that it is ineffective. Committed-in-relativism human service workers are willing and eager to explore new theories and to adapt their theories as evidence accrues that a newer approach is more effective. These are human service workers who are truly dedicated to the field, to the self, and to their clients.

Summary

We explored the psychodynamic, behavioral, humanistic, cognitive, and eclectic approaches to working with the individual. Each approach is distinguished by its unique view of human nature, which emphasizes beliefs about the nature of the person. We learned that the psychodynamic approach stresses unconscious factors, early childhood development, and instincts, whereas the behavioral approach focuses on how the individual was conditioned and what types of models were prominent in an individual's life. Whereas both approaches were originally considered to be deterministic, modern versions focus more on the ability of the individual to change. We learned that the humanistic approach was originally a reaction to the deterministic views of the psychodynamic and behavioral approaches and that this approach, along with the cognitive approach, has a strong belief in the ability of the individual to make choices that can positively affect the individual's functioning in the world. Whereas the humanistic approach stresses the importance of increased awareness for the client in making effective choices, the cognitive approach stresses being able to alter our thinking process in making changes in our lives. In addition, the eclectic approach is seen *not* as a hodgepodge of techniques but as the ability of the human service worker to develop a comprehensive way of working with clients based on a well-thought-out view of human nature.

Finally, we examined the ethical and professional issues of supervision, confidentiality, and dual relationships. The supervisory relationship is particularly important, especially because that relationship can help us understand how we interact with our clients, provide feedback when we might be losing objectivity, or help us make difficult decisions related to breaking confidentiality.

Experiential Exercises

1. What Is Your Theoretical Approach?

What is your view of human nature? To the left of each statement, place the appropriate number. When you have finished, turn to the back of this chapter to find which theoretical approach most closely matches the statement. Write the initials of that approach in the space following the statement; then examine the ratings for the various statements and look for any patterns; that is, are there certain theoretical statements in which you consistently score high or low? This will give you an approximation of the approach with which you most identify.

1. I very strongly believe this is true.

2. I strongly believe this is true.

3. I mildly believe this is true.

4. I mildly do *not* believe this is true.

5. I strongly do *not* believe this is true.

6. I very strongly do *not* believe this is true.

_____ 1. People can go beyond their early childhood experiences and make major personality changes in their lives. _____

_____ 2. People are born with an innate goodness, but due to experiences they may lose touch with their goodness. If placed in a nurturing environment, however, a tendency for their goodness will re-emerge. _____

_____ 3. Reinforcements in the environment greatly affect how we act. _____

_____ 4. We are born with drives that greatly affect how we live our lives. These drives are often out of our consciousness; that is, we behave in ways to meet our drives, yet we don't realize that this is the underlying reason why we're doing what we're doing. _____

_____ 5. My sexual urges greatly affect my behavior in mysterious and un-known ways. _____

_____ 6. My thinking affects my feelings. _____

_____ 7. My behaviors affect my feelings. _____

_____ 8. My feelings affect my behaviors. _____

_____ 9. I have a number of instincts that may affect my behavior in myste-rious and unknown ways. _____

_____ 10. If placed in a loving and nurturing environment, I would be able to get in touch with my "true" self. _____

_____ 11. Although some change is possible, much of my life is predestined due to my early childhood experiences. _____

_____ 12. I know that if I can change the way I perceive the world and the way I think, I can live a well-adjusted life. _____

_____ 13. Determining a client's diagnosis is probably the most crucial fac-tor in helping a client manage his or her problems. _____

_____ 14. My early childhood may have affected me greatly, but it does not determine my present-day behavior. _____

_____ 15. My early childhood affected me greatly and continues to affect how I live, and I have only a limited amount of control to change my life. _____

_____ 16. The environment has little effect on my behaviors; I control the way I am. _____

_____ 17. Because there are predictable stages of development occurring in early childhood, if we could understand the types of parenting that occurred during these stages, we can understand the problem of living faced by individuals later in life. _____

_____ 18. We have the ability to control the environment for a person and therefore allow the person to feel good about who he or she is. _____

_____ 19. It is not events that cause me to feel bad; it is what I believe about those events. _____

_____ 20. The bottom line is that things outside of me greatly control my life; I have little ability to change how I feel about myself if events around me are horrible. _____

_____ 21. How I think is the major force in creating my mental health. _____

_____ 22. How I act is the major force in creating my mental health. _____

_____ 23. How I feel is the major force in creating my mental health. _____

_____ 24. My feelings affect my thinking. _____

_____ 25. My behavior affects my thinking. _____

_____ 26. I believe that before achieving higher-order needs, one has to satisfy his or her lower-order needs. _____

_____ 27. I am in conscious control of most of my behaviors. _____

_____ 28. My unconscious mind controls most of my behaviors. _____

_____ 29. My early childhood probably affected my way of thinking, but I can change the way I think and live a healthier life. _____

_____ 30. A positive attitude toward life and belief in the ability of people to change is the most crucial aspect in helping a client work through his or her problems. _____

2.   Understanding Your View of Human Nature

Circle the items that best describe your view of the person. When you are finished, use all the circled items and write a paragraph describing your view of human nature. For each statement, circle as many items as apply.

1. At birth, I believe people are born
   a. Good
   b. Bad
   c. Neutral
   d. With original sin
   e. With a growth force that allows them to change throughout life
   f. Restricted by their genetics
   g. Capable of being anything they want to be

2. The aspects of the person that most affect an individual's mental health are

   a. Feelings

   b. The way the person thinks

   c. Behaviors

   d. Genetics

   e. Learning

   f. Early childhood environment

   g. "Brainwashing" by parents and other significant individuals

3. As people grow older, I believe they are

   a. Capable of major changes in their personality

   b. Capable of moderate changes in their personality

   c. Capable of minor changes in their personality

   d. Incapable of changing their personality

   e. Determined by their early childhood experiences

   f. Determined by their genetics

   g. Determined by how they were conditioned and reinforced

   h. Able to transcend, or go beyond, early childhood experiences

4. Most of our behaviors are determined by our

   a. Conscious mind

   b. Unconscious mind

   c. Early childhood experiences

   d. Genetics

   e. Instincts

   f. Conscious choices we make

3. Differing Theoretical Orientations to Working with Clients

Read the description of each of the following clients, and think about how each theoretical orientation listed in this chapter would describe the origins of this person's current situation. Then discuss how you might apply each orientation.

The story of Jill. Jill is a 32-year-old married mother of two children, ages 7 and 2. She states that, prior to getting married 6 years ago, she used to drink heavily, smoke pot, and "hang out with bikers and sleep with a lot of guys." She has settled down since then but has started hanging out with her neighbor Steven, drinking again, and is thinking about having an affair with him. She says that she loves her husband, but he has not been paying attention to her lately. She is angry at him but reports that she and her husband rarely talk about their feelings. Although she maintained average grades in school, she never completed high school and would like to obtain her GED. She reports having frequent anxiety attacks and rarely leaves her house other than to go to her part-time job in a factory.

Jill, the second child in a family of four, states that her father was verbally abusive, drank a lot, and generally didn't pay attention to her. Since he stopped drinking a few years ago, however, he has become closer to her. She reports her childhood as being chaotic because she never knew whether her father would blow up at her or at other members of her family when he was drunk. No one in her family has ever received a high school diploma.

The story of Harley. Harley was recently released from the state mental hospital where he has spent most of his adolescence. Harley has a history of being psychotic; that is, he has periodically been out of touch with reality. His parents abandoned him when he was 9 years old, and he has lived in foster homes and at state hospitals since that time. He just turned 18 years old.

Harley is currently taking antipsychotic and antianxiety medications and is in the day-treatment program at the local community mental-health center. At day treatment, he spends the day attending support groups, doing vocational skills training, and socializing. He has little memory of his childhood, but what he can remember is very painful. For instance, he does have vague memories of verbal and sexual abuse, and he thinks there were older siblings in his home. Harley's lifelong dream is to own a motorcycle, and he seems to talk about a motorcycle as if it were his lover. Confidentially, he reports having had sexual feelings toward a motorcycle. Harley has few friends and has an impulsive temper; that is, he periodically just blows up. Although he generally does not act out physically toward people, on rare occasions he has been known to attack someone in an impulsive rage. His medication seems to help him with his outbursts.

**4.   The Human Service Worker's Implementation
       of Varying Theoretical Approaches**

Describe how a human service worker in each of the occupations listed below might apply the theoretical orientations listed in this chapter.

1. A human service worker who helps at a shelter for the homeless

2. A human service worker who helps the mentally retarded at a residential home

3. A human service worker who helps the mentally ill at a day-treatment program in a mental health center

4. A human service worker assisting poor women at a problem-pregnancy counseling center

5. A human service worker who helps the poor at an unemployment office

5.   Ethical and Professional Issues—Supervision

1. Discuss the qualities you would want in a supervisor.

2. Have one person role-play a supervisor and one person role-play a human service worker and then discuss the case of Harley or Jill in Exercise 3.

   a. What theoretical approach do you think would work best with your client? Discuss with your "supervisor" what you think you might want to do to assist your client.

   b. Did the "supervisor" offer a supervisory environment that is conducive to you talking about your client? What supervisory qualities were helpful? Unhelpful?

**6.   Ethical and Professional Issues—Confidentiality
       and Dual Relationships**

Refer to Harley and Jill in Exercise 3 to discuss the following vignettes.

1. While helping Jill find study classes for the GED exam, she reveals that sometimes when she's drinking she takes the belt out and "whacks my kids good—they just won't shut up." Do you break confidentiality and tell child protective services?

2. While driving to work one day, your car breaks down. Harley sees you and says "I'm good with mechanical things, let me help for a small fee—besides I could use a little money for buying my bike."

You want to get your car fixed, and you want Harley to have his bike. Do you let him help you?

3. One day Jill tells you she is pregnant by Steven. She's going to have an abortion. Your state has a law requiring women to tell their spouses if they're to have an abortion. She refuses. What do you do?

4. Jill's husband shows up at your office demanding information about his wife. You tell him things are confidential. He tells you that he'll sue you and the rest of this "fleabag" operation. What do you do?

5. You've been encouraging Jill for months to get involved in more social activities—to get out of the house more. One day in your art class, Jill shows up saying that she signed up for the same class. What do you do?

6. Jill tells you that from time to time, usually when she's drinking, she gets severely depressed and thinks about killing herself. You ask her if she has a plan, and she says "Well, sometimes I think about just doing it with that gun my husband has." One day she calls you; she's been drinking, and she tells you she's depressed. She hangs up saying "I don't know what I might do." What do you do?

7. Harley stops taking his medication, stops by your office, and seems pretty angry. He says "That cheating Harley dealer, he's trying to rip me off. He told me I could have that bike at discount and went back on his word." You try to talk with Harley, but he storms out of your office saying "I'm going get that man!" What do you do?

Answers to Exercise 1
(P = Psychodynamic, H = Humanistic, B = Behavioral, C = Cognitive)

1. H, B, C	11. P	21. C
2. H	12. C	22. B
3. B	13. P	23. H
4. P	14. C, B, H	24. H
5. P	15. P	25. B
6. C	16. C, H	26. H
7. B	17. P	27. C, B
8. H	18. B	28. P
9. P	19. C	29. C
10. H	20. P, C	30. H

4

The Counseling Interview: Skills, Case Management, and Record Keeping

The first time I did counseling I was a volunteer at the drug crisis clinic at my college. I had no training, but somehow I instinctively knew that it was probably best to listen a lot and be kind. Having been a psychology major, I never had a course in counseling theories or counseling methods. I knew little about the "correct" way to respond to a drop-in at the center. I hope I did more good than harm as I tried to help students who had overdosed or were "bumming" from doing hallucinogens.

Immediately following my receipt of a bachelor's degree, I went on to obtain my master's degree in counseling. I then spent a few months painstakingly looking for employment. I obtained my first real job at "The Rap House." A drug-and-alcohol government-funded agency, this storefront drop-in and crisis center was the place where many of the street alcoholics could stop in, get a cup a coffee, and, if need be, talk to a counselor or get a referral to a detox center. These were my first clients.

Now that I had a graduate degree, I at least had some training in appropriate ways to respond to a client. At that time my "theoretical approach" was humanistically based, and I felt it was good if people could express their feelings and "let things out." Although my counseling approach had become somewhat focused, my old untrained self, which sometimes would get very advice oriented, periodically raised its ugly head.

From these experiences, I have come to learn that one is not born with an ability to counsel. Counseling skills can be learned. However, one need not have an advanced degree to become a fairly effective counselor (Danish, D'Augelli, Brock, Conter, & Meyer, 1978; Neukrug, 1987). What is important is learning the skills and practicing them. Much like riding a bicycle or putting on roller blades for the first time, learning counseling skills feels awkward at first. However, you will find that the more you practice, the more natural and at ease you feel. In my own life, I now approach the learning and refinement of my skills as a never-ending process. One never "gets there"; instead, we hope to get better as we learn new and more effective ways of working with our clients. Some of us are lucky because we had good modeling from our parents or other significant people and thus we have a head start in learning skills. Unfortunately, I have found that most of us have not been so blessed, so practicing tried-and-true techniques becomes extremely important.

More than any other area in the human services, I have found that learning skills is the most sensitive and awkward area for many students. This part of the curriculum is where students often feel that they are putting themselves "out there," showing their capabilities to their peers. Unfortunately, because students often feel so vulnerable in front of their peers, I find many protect themselves and partially shut out this important learning experience. If you are scared, that's normal.

However, if you find that this fear prevents you from taking an active role in learning these important skills, then reflect on what you are doing and see whether you can take a more open approach.

In this chapter, we will examine some of the techniques that over the years have been shown to be effective in working with a wide range of clients, regardless of the theoretical approach of the client. This chapter only presents a quick overview of these skills, but you will spend more time on understanding and learning these techniques in other classes.

In addition to responding effectively to your clients, good case management, along with good record keeping, is crucial to successful work with clients. Therefore, in this chapter, we will explore account-ability, ethical, and legal issues as they relate to these important matters.

Creating the Helping Environment

Office Environment

I'm sure you've had the experience of walking into someone's office and feeling as if it is a cold place. How we set up our office environ-ment gives a first message to our clients about whether they are wel-comed. Although all human service workers may not have an office of their own, *wherever* we meet our clients, we should attempt to make the environment as conducive as possible to a positive working rela-tionship. If we are lucky enough to have an office, simple things like nonglare lighting, comfortable seating, and not having obstructions (for example, large desks) between ourselves and our clients can be helpful to creating a comfortable helping environment.

Personal Characteristics of the Helper

As a human service worker, you often will not have the luxury of a one-to-one counseling relationship within an office. However, when-ever you are with your clients, you can help create a helping relation-ship that is facilitative. Therefore, it is important that we bring with us some of the attitudes noted in Chapter 1, that we are genuine, nondogmatic, and accepting of our clients, willing to examine our-selves in the relationship with our clients, and willing to do our home-work to discover the best ways to assist our clients. It is only with these characteristics that our clients will feel a sense of safety and trust with us. If you find a client who is particularly nasty or angry, first examine your attitudes to see how you bring yourself to the session. If you are *not* embodying the characteristics of the effective helper, per-haps it is your attitude that feeds the client's anger.

Importance of Nonverbal Behavior

> Yet when humans communicate, as much as eighty percent of the meaning of their messages is derived from nonverbal language. The implication is disturbing. As far as communication is concerned, human beings spend most of their time studying the wrong thing. (Thompson, 1973, p. 1)

The importance of our nonverbal interactions with clients is vastly underrated. How we present ourselves nonverbally can greatly add or detract to our overall relationship with our clients. Posture or tone of voice that says "don't open up to me" will obviously affect our clients in very different ways from the helper who is nonverbally conveying, "I'm open to hearing what you have to say." We tell our clients that we are there for them through an open body posture, in our ability to make eye contact, and in the types of verbal responses we make. In the next section, Listening Skills, you have an opportunity to do some **role playing.** As you do this, give one another feedback on how your body language is or is not facilitative for the other person.

Counseling Techniques

Listening Skills

> . . . First there is the hearing with the ear, which we all know; and the hearing with the non-ear, which is a state like that of a tranquil pond, a lake that is completely quiet and when you drop a stone into it, it makes little waves that disappear. I think that [insight] is the hearing with the non-ear, a state where there is absolute quietness of the mind; and when the question is put into the mind, the response is the wave, the little wave. (Krishnamurti, cited in Jayakar, 1986, p. 325)

Assuming we have created an environment conducive to a positive client/helper relationship, we are now ready to assess the client situation. Usually, our first step is to understand the issues our clients bring with them. This means being able to hear our clients—good listening.

Webster (1975) defines *listen* as "to give close attention in order to hear, to give ear; to hear and attend to." Whenever I have taught listening skills, I like to stress that good listening involves keeping one's mouth shut. Although these definitions seem basic, I have found that too many people confuse listening with advice giving. It's almost as if we have learned that if someone is in distress or has a problem, we should tell them what to do. Although advice giving has its place (we will talk more about this later), my experience has been that, more often than not, most people want to be heard as opposed to being given advice.

When I ask you to listen to me and you start giving me advice, you have not done what I asked.

When I ask you to listen to me and you begin to tell me why I shouldn't feel that way, you are trampling on my feelings.

When I ask you to listen to me and you feel you have to do something to solve my problem, you have failed me, strange as that may seem.

Listen: All that I ask is that you listen, not talk or do—just hear me.

When you do something for me that I can and need do for myself, you contribute to my fear and inadequacy.

But when you accept as a simple fact that I do feel what I feel, no matter how irrational, then I can quit trying to convince you and get about this business of understanding what's behind them.

So, please listen and just hear me.

And, if you want to talk, wait a minute for your turn—and I'll listen to you. (Author Unknown)

Hindrances to listening.   Even when we know how to listen, we are often blocked in our ability to do so. Our own prejudices and issues tend to interfere with our ability to hear the other person. Therefore, to effectively hear another person, we need to be aware of the unique prejudices or blocks that we might have to opening our inner selves to the helpee. Activity 4-1 helps point this out.

Knowing the blocks and prejudices you hold is crucial to effective listening. However, it is also helpful to have some useful techniques:

Stop talking. You cannot listen while you are talking.

Don't interrupt. Give the speaker time to finish what he or she is saying.

Show interest. With your body language and tone of voice, show the person you're interested in what he or she is saying.

Don't jump to conclusions. Take in all of what the person says and don't assume you understand the person more than he or she understands himself or herself.

Concentrate on what is said. Actively listen. Many people do not realize that listening is an active process that takes deep concentration. If your mind is wandering, you are not listening.

Concentrate on feelings. Listen, identify, and acknowledge the person's feelings to him or her.

Concentrate on content. Listen, identify, and acknowledge *what* the person is saying.

Activity 4-1   Hindrances to Effective Listening

In class, break into triads (groups of three). Within your group, each person takes the number 1, 2, or 3. With the three topics listed below (or other topics of the instructor's choice), have the instructor assign one of the topics to persons 1 and 2. Number 1, you be "pro" the situation, and, number 2, you be "con" the situation. Now, one of you start debating the situation while the other "listens." When the first person is finished, the second person should repeat back *verbatim* what he or she heard. Then, debate back-and-forth, taking turns listening and repeating verbatim until the instructor tells you to stop. Number 3, you are an objective helper, to give feedback if needed. As the objective person, don't forget also to give feedback concerning each person's body language. When you have finished this first situation, have numbers 2 and 3 do the second situation, and then numbers 3 and 1 do the third situation with the third person being the objective helper.

When you have finished, the instructor will ask for feedback concerning what things prevented you from hearing the other person. Make a list on the board, and in particular make sure you discuss some of the following items: preoccupation, defensiveness, emotional blocks, and distractions.

Situations:

Abortion

National health insurance

Capitol punishment

Empathy: A Special Kind of Listening

Many of the early Greek philosophers noted the importance of listening to another person from a deep inner perspective (Gompertz, 1960). In the 20th century, Lipps (1935) is given the credit for coining the word *empathy* from the German word *Einfuhlung*, "to feel within," but probably the person who had most impact on our modern-day understanding and usage of empathy was Carl Rogers: "The state of empathy, or being empathic, is to perceive the internal frame of reference of another with accuracy and with the emotional components and meanings which pertain thereto as if one were the person, but without ever losing the 'as if' condition" (Rogers, 1959, pp. 210–211).

Since Rogers originally defined empathy, others have attempted to **operationalize** the concept. This means that they have taken Rogers's definition and developed a means to measure one's ability to make empathic responses. Carkhuff (1969) developed a 5-point scale to measure empathy. He notes that level 1 and level 2 responses in some ways detract from what the person is saying (for example, advice giving, not accurately reflecting feeling, not including content), with a level 1 response being way off the mark and a level 2 only slightly off. For instance, suppose a client said "I've had it with my Dad, he never does anything with me. He's always working, drinking, or playing with my little sister." A level 1 response might be "Well, why don't you do something to change the situation—like tell him what an idiot he is" (advice giving and being judgmental). A level 2 response might be "You seem to think your Dad spends too much time with your sister" (does not reflect feeling and misses some important content).

On the other hand, a level 3 response accurately reflects the affect and meaning of what the helpee has said. Using the same example, you might say, "Well, it sounds as if you're pretty upset at your Dad for not spending time with you."

Level 4 and level 5 responses reflect feelings and meaning beyond what the person is outwardly saying and adds to the meaning of the person's outward expression. For instance, in the example a level 4 response might be "It sounds like you're pretty hurt because your father seems to ignore you" (expresses new feeling—hurt, which client did not outwardly state). Level 5 responses are usually made in long-term therapeutic relationships by expert therapists. They express to the helpee a deep understanding of the pain he or she feels as well as a recognition of the complexity of the situation. Usually, human service workers are not involved in the intensity of work that leads to a level 5 response.

Usually, in the training of helpers, it is suggested that they attempt to make level 3 responses because such responses have been shown to be effective for clients (Carkhuff, 1983). Using the Carkhuff (1969) operational definition of empathy, an enormous body of evidence indicates that making good empathic responses (level 3 or above) can be taught in a relatively short amount of time and that such responses by both paraprofessionals and professionals are beneficial to clients (Carkhuff, 1983; Neukrug, 1980).

Over the years, good empathic responses have been sometimes confused with *active listening* or *reflection of feeling*. Although Rogers was instrumental in encouraging the use of empathy, he warned against a mechanistic and wooden response to clients:

Although I am partially responsible for the use of this term [reflection of feelings] to describe a certain type of therapist response, I have, over the years, become very unhappy with it. A major reason is that "reflection of feelings" has not been infrequently taught as a technique, and sometimes a very wooden technique at that. . . . Such training has very little to do with an effective therapeutic relationship. (Rogers, 1986, p. 375)

As Rogers alluded to, although it is important to learn this new skill of empathy, sometimes making such responses will feel stilted and mechanistic. With practice your responses to clients will become naturally empathic. Activity 4-2 gives you an opportunity to practice this important skill of empathy.

Activity 4-2   Making Empathic Responses

In class, break up into triads. Two students role-play a helping relationship, trying to make Carkhuff level 3 responses, while the other student tries to rate the responses of the helper. Then switch roles, giving each student the opportunity to be the helper. After a few minutes, give one another feedback concerning your nonverbal behavior and the ability to make Carkhuff level 3 responses. Then discuss the level of comfort (or discomfort) you felt with this activity. Do you feel natural in your ability to making empathic responses? If you don't, how can you work to make it more natural?

Encouragement, Affirmation, and Self-Esteem Building

The need for supporting core self-esteem doesn't end in childhood. Adults still need "unconditional" love from family, friends, life partners, animals, perhaps even an all-forgiving deity. Love that says: "no matter how the world may judge you, I love you for yourself." (Steinem, 1992, p. 66)

Many of the clients with whom you will be working are coming in with hurts from the past that continue to infiltrate their lives. These hurts create depression and anger that seem to have lost their origins. Such hurts create negativity and at times an "attitude" toward the world. But worst of all, they create a sense of low self-esteem in the individual. These individuals are some of the most difficult clients with whom we will work because they come in with such negative attitudes toward the world. Sometimes our inclination may be to tell the person to "cut it out" or "pick yourself up off your duff"; this is the last thing in the world these individuals need. They are so used to being abused and put down that, unconsciously, they expect this attitude from everyone, even the human service worker. Carrying around

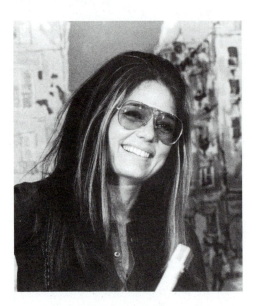

Gloria Steinem believes that our need for high self-esteem continues through adulthood. Fulfilling that need starts with our ability to love ourselves.

this attitude in life rarely, if ever, brings them what they really need—affirmation of self and an attitude that says "you can do it."

Human service workers must be able to see beyond the hurts, the depression, the anger, and the attitude. They need to believe that clients have potential—can "do it." Human service workers can express this positive attitude toward clients through encouragement and affirmations. For instance, when a client does something positive, telling him or her "good job" or "I knew you could do it" assists in the affirmation of the client. Saying things like "I know you are lovable and capable" or "you are a good person inside" helps the client feel supported and worthwhile. Ultimately, clients need to **internalize**, or believe that they possess these feelings on their own. This encouragement and affirmation process can be a first step in helping the client integrate a more positive attitude toward life.

Modeling and Self-Disclosure

It is not uncommon for our clients to look up to us, even idealize who we are. Therefore, if we are sharing personal information about our own lives or modeling behaviors we hope our clients will adapt, we must keep in mind how powerfully our actions may be received by our clients. **Self-disclosure** and **modeling** are two kinds of behaviors that, if used properly, can dramatically affect our clients in their change process (Perry & Furukawa, 1986).

We are constantly modeling for our clients. If we are empathic, then they may learn how to listen to loved ones more effectively. If we are assertive, they may learn how to positively confront someone in their lives. And, if we can show them that we can resolve conflict, then they may learn new ways of dealing with conflict in their lives.

We often model behaviors very subtly, just by being who we are. Other times, through self-disclosure of our own life events, we may show our clients other, more effective ways of coping. For example, one time I was asked to talk to a large family reunion about the importance of education. School always came easy for me, but I knew that this was not the case for the audience to whom I was giving my talk. For them, finishing high school was *very* difficult and going on to college was usually never an option considered. I decided instead to self-disclose—not about my various degrees but about the time I ran the New York Marathon. I was never very athletic, and running the marathon was more difficult than obtaining my doctorate. I worked and trained hard. It took perseverance, and I used this self-disclosure as an analogy for the importance of working hard for something you really want.

Self-disclosure must be done gingerly, at the right time, and only as a means for client growth—not to satisfy our needs: "A good interviewer discloses . . . if it appears that it will help the client" (Evans, Hearn, Uhlemann, & Ivey, 1993, p. 156). A former student once shared with me that her psychiatrist had recently committed suicide. She told me that for the couple of months prior to his suicide, during her sessions *he* was revealing more and more about himself and listening to her less. *She* now was feeling guilty about *his* death, thinking that she should have been attending to his needs. What a terrible legacy to leave her! We are *helpers*, care*givers*. We are not in this business to take—to have our needs met. Therefore, keeping a check on when and why we are self-disclosing is extremely important. One general rule of thumb I have is, if it feels good to self-disclose, don't. Probably you're meeting more of your needs than the needs of your client.

Use of Questions

In his classic book *The Helping Interview* (1981) Benjamin notes that the there is much that can be detrimental in the use of questions. He states that the overuse of questions can set up an atmosphere in which "the interviewee submits to this humiliating treatment only because he expects you to come up with a solution to his problem or because he feels that this is the only way you have of helping him" (p. 72).

Generally, asking a question is not as facilitative to a client as making an empathic response. This is because a good empathic response is empowering—it allows the client to feel as if he or she is discovering answers on his or her own. The fact of the matter is that most questions that are asked come from a "hunch" and could easily be turned around and made into an empathic response. For instance, suppose the client said the following:

Client: You know, I'm a bit disturbed that my parents never taught me how to be more in charge of my life.

A human service worker could respond by saying something like this:

HSW: Do you feel angry at your parents for not teaching you how to take charge?

However, probably a more effective response would be:

HSW: I get a sense that you're angry at your parents for not teaching you how to take charge.

The empathic response is more focused and to the point, and the client can respond in the affirmative if you are on target or deny your response if you are off the mark.

However, sometimes it may be important to ask questions. Obviously, if you need to know specific information like medical history or employment history, you will probably need to ask specific questions. Questions are also useful if you want to probe more deeply into a specific area.

Open versus closed questions. If you ask a question, an open question is more facilitative than a closed question. An open question such as "How do you feel?" allows a wide variety of responses on the part of the client. A closed question such as "Did you feel angry or sad?" may elicit a yes or no response. This type of question clearly lessens the likelihood of the client disclosing something other than the choices you gave.

Direct versus indirect questions. Benjamin (1981) notes that a question can be made even more open if it is asked indirectly. For instance, a helper can ask an open question directly:

HSW: How did you feel about your parents divorcing?

To make the question even more palpable to the client, however, you might ask it in the following manner:

HSW: I would guess you had a lot of feelings about your parents divorcing.

The indirect question is hardly a question at all; it clearly borders on being an empathic response. Open questions that are indirect tend to "sit well" with clients. They are easier to hear and therefore easier to respond to in an open way.

Use of why questions.   Generally, asking a why question is not rec-ommended. Although, ideally, asking why seems to make sense, people often feel interrogated and put on guard when asked why they felt or did something. Usually, what or how questions are more palpable for clients. For instance, compare the following why and what questions:

HSW: Why did you feel depressed and angry at your parents' divorce?

In this case, it is almost as if the interviewer is challenging the helpee about how he or she felt. Look at the following question, but this time starting the question with *what*:

HSW: What was it about your parents' divorce that made you feel de-pressed and angry?

In this case the helpee is *not* being put on the defensive.

Although much more can be said about the different uses of ques-tions in the interviewing process, one should always be careful when-ever questions are being used. Keeping this in mind, Benjamin (1981) suggests the following when asking questions:

- Are you aware of the fact that you are asking a question?

- Have you weighed carefully the desirability of asking specific ques-tions and have you challenged their usage?

- Have you examined the types of questions available to you and the types of questions you personally tend to use?

- Have you considered alternatives to the asking of questions?

- Are you sensitive to the questions the interviewee is asking, whether he or she is asking them outright or not?

- Will the question you are about to ask inhibit the flow of the inter-view?

Giving Information, Advice, and Offering Alternatives

Sometimes we may have some valuable objective information to offer our clients. For instance, suppose a client is eligible for Social Security disability and you have information on how he or she might apply for it. Obviously, you would not want to just sit there and reflect back the client's feelings—you would want your client to know about the infor-mation. Information should be given when you have some vital objec-tive piece of knowledge that you believe will help the client in some manner. Information giving, however, is *very* different from advice giving: "Presenting information is not the same as giving advice, suggestions, or directives; it is not value-laden material, but rather objective and accurate factual material about people, places, or things" (Doyle, 1992, p. 194).

Have you ever been in a situation where you have had someone try to give you advice and you felt like telling them to mind their own business? Unfortunately, I have seen this happen all too often. Most of us want to be (or at least feel) independent in our decision making, and when someone tries to tell us how to live our life, we may get defensive—sometimes even if their advice is good. Therefore, like confrontation, advice should only be given once you have established a relationship; even then, some better ways of facilitating change for the client might be available. For instance, offering alternatives might make more sense.

Usually, providing clients with a few options to consider is better than just offering advice or one suggestion. This helps clients feel empowered because they can choose the alternative rather than feeling as if you told them what to do. Don't be surprised, however, if the client has already thought about some of the alternatives you offer.

Confrontation: Challenge with Support

When hearing the word *confrontation,* many people often think of someone yelling at another or telling another person how to live his or her life. Along these lines, I have found that some clients "hook" me, and I start to argue with them about how to live life. This is rarely if ever helpful to the client and is almost always a result of some unfinished business of my own. In fact, trying to get another person to change if they are not "there yet" is nearly impossible. Confrontation that is facilitative is usually very different from this.

Confronting Sally

One time I worked with a client who was making close to $50,000 a year, was in an abusive relationship, had no major bills, and was insistent that she could not leave the relationship because she could not afford to live on $50,000. Clearly, her verbal statement that she could not leave the relationship did not match the reality that one could live on this amount (certainly, most of us would be happy to live on this amount). After building a relationship using empathy, I gently challenged this perception. This allowed her to examine the real reasons she was not leaving—reasons that had more to do with low self-esteem and fears of being alone.

If you have built a solid relationship with a person and gently challenge him or her, the individual will more likely hear what you are saying and will consider your suggestions. To build this kind of relationship, spend some time trying to understand the life circumstances of the client. The best way to do this is to make sure you have listened and have used empathy. Once you have this supportive base, confrontation becomes much easier.

One way of gently confronting a client is to make a higher-level empathic response, such as a level 4 response. These responses reflect back feelings that you sense from the person, feelings of which he or she is not quite aware—yet. Therefore, when you tell the client that you hear some deeper feelings underlying what he or she is saying and if you have that base of caring, the client might better be able to hear this feedback.

Another way of gently confronting a client is to suggest alternatives. Offering alternatives challenges the client to look at new ways of

A Scenario

You work at a problem-pregnancy clinic and a 17-year-old woman comes in seeking information about birth control. She has been sexually active for 2 years, has not used any birth control, and knows little about sexually transmitted diseases (STDs). When she comes into your office, you affirm her decision to come to the clinic. You then listen carefully and try to understand her situation. After you spend some time listening, you tell her about the various types of birth control, suggest that she may not want to have unprotected sex, and give her information about AIDS and other STDs. You also suggest that she might want to consider being tested for STDs. You then ask her if she has any thoughts about what she would like to do. She thinks a while and then says that she will try to use condoms but also thinks it might be smart if she is on the pill. She thinks she would like to be tested for STDs but would like more information on the testing process. After you explain the testing process to her, she agrees to come back to the clinic for the tests. You then thank her for coming in and schedule another appointment.

In this short scenario, one can easily see how a human service worker can be affirming, empathic, an information giver, an advice giver, a person who offers alternatives, and a problem solver. What do you think would be most effective for this 17-year-old? How might you work with her fears of having an STD? Are there other techniques that we have talked about that might be helpful for this young woman?

viewing the world. Like the case of high-level empathy, such a confrontation should only be done if there is a base of caring; otherwise, the client may respond defensively.

Pointing out discrepancies is a third way of confronting the client. In this case, you carefully highlight the fact that the there is some type of incongruence in what the client is saying. The key to effectively pointing out a discrepancy to a client is having built a trusting relationship and the client's ability to let you challenge his or her perception of the world. Try to do this too early, and the client will walk out on you. For instance, I have seen numerous clients who drink heavily, perhaps the equivalent of five or more beers a night, yet state they do not have a drinking problem. I have learned that unless I have an alliance with these clients, have built a relationship, they will not be able to examine the discrepancy between how much they drink and the statement about not having a drinking problem.

Whether you use higher-level empathic responses, the offering of alternatives, or pointing out discrepancies, using confrontation can be a very powerful technique in the counseling relationship.

Problem Solving and the Structure of the Interview

An effective human service worker has learned to integrate listening skills, empathic responses, questioning, confronting, probing, advice giving and offering alternatives, information giving, and self-esteem building to help problem solve for the client. Although all these techniques may be used during the various parts of an interview with a client, some of these techniques are more or less practiced at various times during the interview. Therefore, understanding the structure of a helping interview is essential.

Because the roles and functions of the human service worker can vary considerably, many different types of interviewing can occur. Some human service workers may do more information gathering, others may do more supportive work, and others may be doing counseling. Some may be seeing clients for 15 minutes, others for a couple of hours. Regardless of the kind of interviewing you're doing, be cognizant of a general outline or process of the interview. Although the outline that follows may not be applicable to the roles and functions of all human service workers, it does give a general framework.

Opening the Interview

When beginning an interview, you must inform the client about some of the basic issues related to the helping relationship. These issues include the limits of confidentiality, the length of the interview, the purpose of the interview, your credentials, the limits of the relationship, your theoretical orientation to the helping relationship, legal concerns to you and your client, any fees for services, and agency rules that might affect your client (for example, the reporting of a client's use of illegal drugs). This can usually be accomplished through a brief verbal statement at the beginning of the interview. Some authors, however, suggest the use of a **professional disclosure statement**, which is a written statement describing the preceding items (Corey, Corey, & Callanan, 1993). The agency itself can develop professional disclosure statement, but if your place of employment does not have such a statement, develop your own and/or encourage your agency to adopt such statements.

Following an explanation of these basic issues, building a facilitative helping relationship is particularly important. You can accomplish this by using your listening skills and empathy. These skills allow you to build trust and helps the client get oriented to the interview.

Information-Gathering Stage

After trust has been built, making sure that you have all the information needed to assist you in the planning phase of the interview is important. Therefore, if empathy and listening alone has not been enough to help you gather all the necessary information, then use your questioning techniques at this time. Sometimes, it is important to have a series of standard questions to ask the client. In fact, many agencies have developed standard questionnaires that help them in this information-gathering phase. This reduces the possibility of not obtaining important information from the client that could effect the goals that are set.

Goal-Setting Stage

After you have gathered information, you and your client can set some general and/or specific goals. These should be based on the information gained thus far in the interview and should be a **collaborative process**; that is, you alone are not setting goals for your client. Instead, it is a joint effort in which you and your client determine what goals would best meet his or her needs. This may be the time when you are giving information to the client, offering suggestions, using mild confrontation (for example, higher-level empathy), or offering advice. Effective listening is also important during this stage because it allows the client to feel empowered as he or she decides which goals to set. Although self-esteem building can be done at any stage, affirming the client's ability to meet his or her goals is particularly important in this stage.

Closure Stage

After you and your client have determined goals, review the goals to make sure he or she is clear about what they are. Then, summarizing what you did during the interview is often advisable. This can be done by reflecting the highlights of the interview. It is then important to determine whether you are going to meet again and, if you are, when the meeting will take place. If goals have been set, make sure the client is aware of his or her homework, or what goals he or she is supposed to accomplish before the next meeting. Make sure you say good-bye to each other and that there are no "loose ends." If this is the only time you will meet with the client, some kind of follow-up would be helpful in order to evaluate the success of your meeting.

Case Management and Record Keeping

Problems associated with writing and reading mental health records are well worth our attention. Large and ever-increasing numbers of people are going to be affected by the writing and reading of these records sometime during their lifetimes. As we approach the twenty-first century, more and more people are entering in an increasing number of mental health care delivery systems. At the same time, growing numbers of problems are coming to be defined as mental disorders. Consequently, an increasing number of people are writing and reading mental health records for an increasing number of purposes. (Reynolds, Mair, & Fischer, 1992, p. 1)

What Is Case Management?

Managing a caseload of clients can be tedious and time-consuming. The ways you help a client develop goals, how you manage client contact hours, how you monitor client progress toward goals, the way you keep records, and how you evaluate client progress are all part of **case management**. Case management therefore requires good organizational ability, good time-management skills, and adequate charting of client progress. Recently, due to an increased emphasis on accountability in the mental-health professions, these issues have become ever-more important.

The Extent of Record Keeping

When I first started in the human service field, record keeping was deemed important, but it was not necessarily an essential part of the process of working with a client. However, with the changing times has come a greater emphasis on the importance of accurate record keeping. Personally, I think that this sometimes goes to extremes; however, there is no question that good record keeping can reduce liability concerns, help track client progress, be a means of self-evaluation of professional skills, and in this age of accountability through the gathering of statistical information, even be a determining factor in which agencies will receive funding. With this in mind and although record-keeping procedures vary greatly from agency to agency, accurate record keeping relative to client progress is surely an essential part of the work of the human service worker.

Objectivity in Record Keeping

Again, keeping in mind that agency requirements will vary, probably the minimum information that should be included in records are the name of the client, the date, major facts noted during contact, progress made toward achieving client goals, and your signature. Whenever you write down any information about your client, it needs to be objective. Keep in mind that what you write could be subpoenaed to court and you may be held liable for your statements. Therefore, writing from an objective, dispassionate point of view is essential when keeping case notes. Generally, only the third person should be used in referring to the client. For example,

> POOR: I collected family information from Jim.

> BETTER: Family information was gathered from Jim.

Any subjective information that is gathered from the client should be noted as such. To assist in this, begin subjective statements with the following types of phrases:

> It seems that . . .
>
> Jim noted that . . .
>
> It appears that . . .
>
> Jim reported that . . .
>
> Claire related that . . .
>
> Claire recounted that . . .

In your writing style, be careful not to portray sexist attitudes or value-laden statements (unless, of course, the statements are paraphrasing what the client has said to you). Also, try to avoid any significant amounts of psychological jargon and write the report in a way that if other mental-health professionals would read it, it would be readily understandable. Beginning mental-health professionals will often want to "side" with their clients; take care not to do this when writing your report. Finally, use good grammar, of course.

Types of Record Keeping

Although almost all agencies today require case notes, how they are kept may vary. If you are lucky, your agency may use dictaphones, and you will have a secretary who will type your dictation. Today, we find that some agencies use computers, and you might be asked to know word processing and type your notes directly into the computer (Tiedeman, 1983). In fact, computers have become so important that computer literacy is being suggested by some as a crucial skill for today's professional (Nurius & Hudson, 1989a, 1989b). However, if you are not lucky enough to be using a dictaphone or a computer, more than likely you'll be asked to keep notes in the tried-and-true fashion of writing them out. Although some may find this laborious, writing notes can be useful because it helps organize your thoughts about your client.

Security of Record Keeping

The security of your records is vital because clients have the right to have information they share with others be kept confidential. Therefore, information obtained both verbally and in writing must be kept confidential and secured and not shared with others without client permission. There are some exceptions to this rule: if your employer requests information from you concerning your client, if you share client information with a supervisor as a means of assisting you in your work with a client, or if the court subpoenas your records. If you are going to share information with other agencies who might also be working with your client, obtaining written permission from your client is essential. This ensures your client's right to privacy and protects you legally.

Written client records need to be kept in secured places such as locked file cabinets. If records are kept on computer disks, then access to those computer files must be limited to you, your supervisor, and possibly your employer. Explain to clerical help the importance of confidentiality when working with records. In fact, some agencies have nonclinical staff who might have access to client information sign statements acknowledging that they understand the importance of confidentiality and that they will not discuss client issues outside the office. Obviously, the importance of hiring nonclinical staff whom you can trust with client information is paramount.

How Secure Are Records?

When I worked as an outpatient therapist at a comprehensive mental-health center, a client of another therapist had apparently appropriated his records that had been left "lying around." Because his records tended to be written in "psychologese" using diagnostic language, he was understandably quite upset by what he found. He would periodically call the emergency services at night and read his records over the phone to the emergency worker while making fun of the language used in the records.

Another time, when I was in my doctoral program, we were reviewing an intellectual test assessment of an adolescent that had been done a number of years earlier. Suddenly, one of the students in the class yelled out, "That's me!" Apparently, although there was no identifying name on the report, he recognized it as describing him (he had been give a copy of the report previously).

These two examples show the importance of keeping client information confidential and secure.

Ethical and Professional Issues

Primary Obligation: Client, Agency, or Society?

Think about the following scenario:

In building your relationship with a 17-year-old client, you discover that she is using crack cocaine, possibly selling drugs to friends, and involved in gang violence including looting. Your agency has a policy to report any illegal acts to the "proper authorities."

What is your responsibility to this client? What are the limits of confidentiality with her? If you are primarily responsible to your client, what are the implications of being required to report her to the proper authorities? If you do not report her to the proper authorities as you are suppose to do, what implications might this have on your employment? What responsibility do you have to protect society from the illegal activities in which she is involved? What liability concerns do you have if you do not report the illegal acts in which she is participating? These are some of the tough ethical and professional questions human service workers sometimes have to face.

If this were a dualistic world, there would be an easy answer to these tough ethical and professional dilemmas. The world is fortunately (unfortunately?) more complex than this. Although most ethical

The Tarasoff Case

The case of *Tarasoff* v. *Board of Regents of University of California* (1976) set a precedent for the responsibility that mental-health professionals have regarding maintaining confidentiality and acting to prevent a client from harming self or others. This case involved a client who was seeing a psychologist at the University of California–Berkeley health services. The client told the psychologist that he intended to kill Tatiana Tarasoff, his former girlfriend. After the psychologist consulted with his supervisor, the supervisor suggested that he call the campus police. Campus security subsequently questioned the client and released him. The client refused to see the psychologist any longer, and 2 months later he killed Tarasoff. The parents of Tatiana sued and won, with the California Supreme Court stating that the psychologist did not do all that he could to protect Tatiana.

Although state laws vary on how to handle confidentiality, this case generally is seen as signifying to mental-health professionals that it is their responsibility to protect the public if serious threats are made.

guidelines (for example, ACA, 1988; APA; 1989; NASW, 1990) will state that the mental-health professional's primarily responsibility is to the client, all of us must acknowledge legal and moral responsibility toward others. Therefore, ethical guidelines usually include a statement that requires the mental-health professional to take responsible action if a client's behavior is perceived as potentially harmful to self or others. The current proposed ethical standards of NOHSE/CSHSE (see Appendix A) have such a statement *and* require that the human service worker seek out supervision if a client's actions might harm self or others. The same standards also require that the human service worker follow agency guidelines as well as local, state, and federal laws. With these guidelines in mind, being clear about the limitations of the helping relationship *prior* to starting your work with clients is prudent. Probably the best way to do this is through the use of a professional disclosure statement.

Who Owns Your Case Notes? Ethical and Legal Concerns

One should expect that clients might request to see their records. Keep this in mind when you are writing case notes. Legally, although it seems to be a gray area, clients probably have a right to view their

Extent of Confidentiality of Communications between Helpers and Clients

Generally, the communications between human service workers and their clients are not protected under the law. This is because human service workers do not have the legal protection afforded to licensed professionals under **privileged communication** (see Chapter 3). Such privilege is determined state-by-state, although there often are similarities among states concerning how the laws are written. Licensed professionals who hold privileged communication may have limits placed on them. Listed below is an excerpt from Virginia's privileged communication law. You can see that there are many exceptions to confidentiality based on the discretion of the court.

Except at the request of, or with the consent of, the patient, no duly licensed practitioner of any branch of the healing arts shall be required to testify in any civil action, respecting any information which he may have acquired in attending, examining or treating the patient in a professional capacity if such information was necessary to enable him to furnish professional care to the patient; provided, however, that when the physical or mental condition of the patient is at issue in such action, or when a court, in the exercise of sound discretion, deems such disclosure necessary to the proper administration of justice, no fact communicated to, or otherwise learned by, such practitioner in connection with such attendance, examination or treatment shall be privileged and disclosure may be required. (Code of Virginia, 1950)

records; along these same lines, parents probably have the right to view records of their children. You should be aware of any specific local or state laws that might set standards for access to client records.

In terms of federal law, the **Freedom of Information Act** of 1974 allows individuals to have access to any records maintained by a federal agency that contain personal information about the individual. Similarly, the **Buckley Amendment** of 1974, otherwise known as the **Family Education Rights and Privacy Act**, grants parents the right to access their children's educational records (Committee on Government Operations, 1991). Of course, any records not protected by privileged communication (see Chapter 3) can be subpoenaed by a court.

On a more practical level, a client rarely asks to see his or her records. However, if a client did make such a request, I would first attempt to talk with the client about what is written in the records. If this was not satisfactory to the client, I would suggest that I might write a summary of the records. However, if a client steadfastly states a desire to view his or her records, I believe that this is his or her right.

"A final point should be made regarding the *confidentiality* of written reports. Increasingly, clients are exercising their right to reports which are kept on file in schools, hospitals and clinics. The writer should realize this fact before developing a report" (Wicks, 1977, p. 107).

The Developmentally Mature Human Service Worker: Looking for Feedback from Others

Developmentally mature human service workers are open to hearing both positive and negative feedback about their counseling skills. These individuals want to "stretch" and are willing to take a critical look at how they interact with clients. These individuals want to try out new approaches to working with clients and are willing to feel vulnerable to the learning process. These individuals actively seek out supervision and consultation from experts in the field. They view the learning of counseling skills as a process in which one continually grows and adapts his or her approach.

Summary

We examined the basic counseling skills used for working effectively with clients. Related to this, we noted the importance of having a conducive environment for the helping relationship, which includes the physical comfort of the surroundings, appropriate nonverbal behaviors, and positive personality characteristics of the human service worker. This was followed by a discussion concerning the foundations of good counseling skills, effective listening and use of empathy, and how to intersperse modeling and self-disclosure in an effective helping relationship. We examined how to use the additional skills of confrontation, information giving, advice giving, offering alternatives, asking questions, and self-esteem building as the process of the helping relationship unravels.

We also examined case management and the importance of writing good case notes. We reviewed the relevance of writing objective case notes in terms of monitoring client progress, as a means of evaluating your skills, and as one aspect of accountability. We discussed ethical and legal issues related to case notes and the responsibility to client, agency, and society. Finally, we noted that developmentally mature human service workers are those who see their counseling skills as continually in process; that is, mature human service workers are always willing to adapt their skills in order to become better helpers.

Experiential Exercises

1. Listening Quiz

Place an *X* next to each item based on how you *usually* listen to someone and place an *O* next to each item based on how you think you *should* listen to another. Look at the end of this chapter for the optimal answers. Discuss the answers in class and see whether you agree or disagree with the answers I present.

	Usually	**Sometimes**	**Seldom**
1. I try to determine what should be talked about during the interview.			
2. When listening to someone, I prepare myself physically by sitting in a way that I can make sure that I hear what is being said.			
3. I try to be in charge of the conversation.			
4. I usually clear my mind and take on a nonjudgmental attitude when listening to another.			
5. When listening to another, I try to tell the other my opinion of what he or she is doing.			
6. I try to decide from the other's *appearance* whether what he or she is saying is worthwhile.			
7. I attempt to ask questions if I need further clarification.			
8. I try to judge from the opening statement what is going to be said.			

	Usually	Sometimes	Seldom

9. I try to listen intently to feelings.

10. I try to listen intently to content.

11. I try to tell the other person what is right about what he or she is saying.

12. I try to analyze the situation and give interpretations.

13. I try to use *my* experiences to best understand the other person's feelings.

14. I try to convince the other person the correct way to view the situation.

15. I try to have the last word.

2.   Self-Esteem Building

On the left side of the page, write a list of childhood experiences that detracted from your self-esteem. On the right side of the page, write those things you can do today to counteract these early experiences.

Negative Behaviors   **Current Actions**

3.   Making Empathic Responses

A good empathic response accurately reflects to the client the feelings and the meaning of what the client has said (Carkhuff's level 3 response). For the following situations, write in the spaces provided the feeling followed by the meaning of what the client has said. Follow this by writing another statement that again reflects the feelings and meaning of the client, but this time in your own words.

In small groups in class, share some of your responses and get feedback from others about the accuracy of what you wrote. For example, wife to human service worker:

Client: I don't know what's wrong with my husband. Since he lost his job, he just sits around all day and does nothing, doesn't look for a job, doesn't cook, just does nothing. He seems worthless.

Next is an example of feeling followed by meaning in response to the preceding client statement:

HSW: You feel <u>angry</u> because <u>your husband doesn't do anything all day long.</u>

The following is an example of a response to the same client, but this time in your own words, again reflecting feeling and meaning:

HSW: <u>I guess I hear you're disappointed and upset at your husband for not taking charge of his life.</u>

Respond to the following scenarios:

1. Teenager to human service worker:

   Client: Why should I use condoms? I'm not going to get AIDS or nothing like that. Only fags get AIDS. Don't you agree?

   HSW: You feel _____ because _____

   _____ .

   HSW: _____

   _____ .

2. Abused wife to human service worker:

   Client: I don't know why I keep going back to him. He just keeps beating on me. But afterward, he always tells me he loves me. I think he loves me, but he just drinks too much sometimes.

HSW: You feel _____ because _____

_____ .

HSW: _____

_____ .

3. Pregnant teenager to human service worker:

   Client: I want this baby; I don't care what my parents say about an abortion. I can bring this baby up by myself. I'll quit school and get a job and bring the baby to work with me.

   HSW: You feel _____ because _____

   _____ .

   HSW: _____

   _____ .

4. Disabled enlisted person to human service worker:

   Client: Even though I lost my leg, I have lots to live for. I have a good family, and I know I'm employable. I just hope I can get through rehab quickly.

   HSW: You feel _____ because _____

   _____ .

   HSW: _____

   _____ .

5. Older person to human service worker:

   Client: Since I moved to this retirement home, I have nothing to live for. I can't drive anymore, and I know nobody here.

   HSW: You feel _____ because _____

   _____ .

   HSW: _____

   _____ .

6. Minority person to human service worker:

   Client: I think I'm getting the shaft with my realtor. I keep telling her I want to move to this one community, and she can't find *anything* for sale there. I don't believe it!

HSW: You feel _____ because _____

_____ .

HSW: _____

_____ .

7. Pro-life person to human service worker:

    Client: I refuse to let any more babies die. I'll do anything to close down those murdering abortion clinics.

    HSW: You feel _____ because _____

    _____ .

    HSW: _____

    _____ .

8. Pro-choice person to human service worker:

    Client: I believe a woman has a right to choose what to do with her body, and I'm sick and tired of these pro-lifers interfering with other people's right to choose!

    HSW: You feel _____ because _____

    _____ .

    HSW: _____

    _____ .

9. Estranged husband to human service worker:

    Client: So I wasn't faithful to my wife. So what? I loved her. She didn't have to leave me. I still was good to her despite my failings. I miss her so much!

    HSW: You feel _____ because _____

    _____ .

    HSW: _____

    _____ .

10. Estranged wife to human service worker:

    Client: I loved my husband, but I couldn't put up with his unfaithfulness any longer. He just couldn't give me the love I needed in a relationship. I'm sorry he is so depressed now, but I can't go back to him.

HSW: You feel _____ because _____

_____ .

HSW: _____

_____ .

4.   An Interview with a Client

The following is an interview between a client and human service worker who is employed at an employee assistance program for a large business. Go through the interview and identify the type of response being made by the helper (empathy, advice giving, information giving, offering alternatives, confrontation, self-disclosure, modeling, open questions, closed questions, self-esteem building, referral, and/or summarizing). Each response may have more than one answer. Check the end of this chapter for the answers.

1. **Client/employee:** I woke up this morning feeling depressed. My life is out of sorts, and I'm not sure why. Do you think this is something that will pass?

   HSW: So, it seems as if your depression just came out of nowhere, and you're not sure what's causing it.

2. **Client:** Well, yeah. I guess I haven't been real happy at work lately. I've been at this same job for twenty years, and it seems like I never get promoted. All my friends get promoted, and I just make my little yearly salary increases but never move up. Maybe I'm just no good.

   HSW: Well, I hear how you're not feeling real good about *you* and it seems to be at least partly related to the fact that things haven't worked out at your job as you thought they might.

3. **Client:** That's true. You know, maybe I should take some courses, and that would help me do better at work. What do you think?

   HSW: I'm not sure. But it seems as if you've had some ideas about how to change your life.

4. **Client:** Yeah, I've thought about going back to school, quitting my job, looking for another job, and even just storming into my boss's office and telling her what I think.

   HSW: What do *you* think about all these different options?

5. **Client:** Well, I guess I have thought about at least talking to my

boss and asking her what she thinks I might do. That would be at least a beginning.

HSW: Do you feel good or bad about your relationship with your boss?

6. **Client:** Well, I don't know if it's either. Perhaps more neutral. I don't really know her real well. She is not approachable, but on the other hand, maybe I'm not either.

    HSW: So on one hand it might be difficult to talk with her, but on the other hand, you also see that maybe you haven't made it easy for her to approach you.

7. **Client:** Kind of. Maybe I need to talk with her to see what the different options are for me.

    HSW: When you say "options," I'm unclear what you mean. Can you explain that to me?

8. **Client:** Well, I guess I mean whether I should take a course for credit, do some in-house workshops, or maybe something else . . . like, like talk to my supervisor more and get feedback from her, or become more active in the employees' association, or something.

    HSW: Well, it seems as if you have a lot of ideas that you can approach your boss with.

9. **Client:** Yeah, I guess I do. I hope I can do it. You know, I get pretty nervous talking to her.

    HSW: I *know* you can do it if you want to. I know you're capable of lots!

10. **Client:** Yes! I can do it. But you know, this fear I feel with her, that's something I feel with a lot of people in positions of authority. Like, take my church. You know, I've been on this fund-raising committee now for a number of years and I've had a lot of ideas, but I never tell them to the chair because I think he's going to put me down.

    HSW: So, you see this as a pattern in your life; that is, this fear you have expressing yourself with people in positions of authority.

11. **Client:** Yeah, I think it goes back to the fact that my parents, particularly my father, were really strict and always *told* me how to live my life. I get so scared sometimes around authority figures that I just don't know what to say or do.

    HSW: Well, you're bringing up some really important issues for yourself. What are your thoughts about seeking out counseling for this?

12. **Client:** It had crossed my mind. Especially because I believe this issue is something that prevents me from getting ahead in my life. What do you think?

    HSW: I know of some good counselors, and I know of an assertiveness-training group. I think considering some counseling might be really good for you.

13. **Client:** Yes, I think so.

    HSW: I admire your wanting to work on this issue. Here, let me give you the names of some counselors and a couple of groups. [HSW gives the names.]

14. **Client:** I really appreciate this. Sometimes I think I'm never going to get through this problem I have. I guess I think that change is really not possible.

    HSW: You know, I had some problems once in my life that were really difficult for me, and I saw a counselor. It really helped me get through it, and I feel much better about me now.

15. **Client:** Really?

    HSW: Yeah, it was really helpful. I know you can move on in your life in a positive way and feel good about you. You have all the ingredients in you to make this work.

16. **Client:** I hope so. I think this is a really good start. Can I talk about one other thing?

    HSW: Sure.

17. **Client:** I notice that on some nights, not all nights mind you, I seem to drink a lot. I wake up in the morning feeling terrible. I wonder if this affects my work performance. I've been thinking about maybe trying out an AA meeting. What do you think?

    HSW: I hear your concern about your drinking and the fact that you have been giving some serious thought to doing something about it.

18. **Client:** To be honest, sometimes I really think I go overboard with my drinking.

    HSW: Well, it sounds to me as if you might have a problem with alcohol and perhaps you should do something about it.

19. **Client:** Do you know of any AA meetings?

    HSW: Yep, let me give you a list I have right here. You know AA meetings usually last a couple of hours and one's anonymity is ensured. I have heard that people who go to AA meetings are usually accepting of one another.

20. **Client:** Well, you've been helpful. I appreciate all of what you've done for me.

HSW: Well, thanks. I hear that *you* are ready to do some important things for you. For instance, today you talked about some concerns you were having at work relative to getting promoted as well as how this might relate to both issues with authority figures and your drinking. You've gotten some referrals from me, and it sounds as if you're seriously thinking about following up on them. I think that it's great that you're so motivated. Maybe next week you can touch base with me to let me now what you've done to follow up.

5. Writing Case Notes

Using the interview in Exercise 4 and following the guidelines in this chapter, write case notes that have the following information:

1. Reason for referral

2. Summary of contact with client

3. Recommendations for client

6. Writing Case Reports

Meet with someone in class and have each student role-play a problem situation. Then write a two- to three-page case report that addresses the following categories:

1. Client Information

    Name

    Address

    Date of birth

    Date of interview

2. Reason for interview

3. Background information about person that is relevant to interview (for example, family background, educational background, work background)

4. Assessment of client problem

5. Summary and recommendations

6. Signature with credentials

7. Ethical and Professional Issues

For the following vignettes, write some possible solutions and be prepared to discuss them in class.

Case note security

1. A client who is coming to your agency demands to see her case notes. In them, you have noted that you suspect she may be lying about her Social Security eligibility and that you also suspect she might be paranoid. What do you do?

2. A client you have been seeing at a crisis center comes in and asks to see all records pertaining to him. These include crisis logs that have information in them about other clients, as well as case notes you have made concerning his contacts. What do you do?

Confidentiality and primary obligation: client, agency, or society?

1. You're working for social services, and in the course of a conversation with a client, you discover that she has been using heroine. An agency dictate states that any client suspected of using illegal drugs must be immediately referred to rehabilitation, and if he or she refuses, you can no longer see the client at your agency. You explain this to her, she gets angry, walks out, and states she'll "blow this place up." What do you do?

2. In your conversation with a client at the homeless shelter, you discover that he is drinking and taking Quaaludes in amounts that you believe could kill him. You mention this to him, but he tells you to mind your own business. What do you do?

3. In the course of working with a client, she expresses her concern about her grandmother who, she states, lives by herself, is depressed, has stopped eating, and has lost a considerable amount of weight. You contact her, but she refuses services. What do you do?

4. While talking with a 15-year-old male client, he informs you that on a recent vacation he was sexually molested by an uncle. He asks you not to tell his parents. What do you do?

5. A 15-year-old client tells you he is having sexual relations with his 14-year-old stepsister. What do you do?

6. An adult client informs you that he wants to kill his ex-girlfriend and her new boyfriend. He denies that he actually will act on these feelings but that he just "thinks about it a lot." What do you do?

Answers to Exercise 1: Usually: 2, 4, 9, 10. Sometimes: 7, 13. Seldom: 1, 3, 5, 6, 8, 11, 12, 14, 15.

Answers to Exercise 4: (1) empathy; (2) empathy; (3) empathy; (4) open question; (5) closed question; (6) empathy; (7) open question; (8) empathy, self-esteem building; (9) self-esteem building; (10) empathy; (11) empathy, open question, referral; (12) offering alternatives, advice giving, referral; (13) referral, self-esteem building; (14) modeling, self-disclosure; (15) self-esteem building; (16) not ratable; (17) empathy; (18) confrontation; (19) referrals, information giving; (20) summarizing, self-esteem building.

5

The Development of the Person

With each passage from one stage of human growth to the next we, too, must shed a protective structure. We are left exposed and vulnerable—but also yeast and embryonic again, capable of stretching in ways we hadn't known before. These sheddings may take several years or more. Coming out of each passage, though, we enter a longer and more stable period in which we can expect relative tranquillity and a sense of equilibrium regained. (Sheehy, 1976, p. 29)

In my senior year in college, I was staying with my college girlfriend, and in the middle of the night I began to have what I now would call a panic attack. I walked the campus the rest of the night trying to calm myself down. I thought I had lost it. The next day I went to the college counseling service and saw a psychologist who reassured me that I was not "crazy." I was soon referred to a group at the center for what became my first therapeutic experience. Subsequently, I have participated in different groups and in individual counseling. Through these experiences, I have had the opportunity to examine some of my life events that have dramatically affected my development. Some of these experiences, such as a childhood heart disorder and the death of my father, might be considered situational, in that they were unexpected events in my life that had a dramatic effect on me. Other experiences, however, such as developing a sense of my own values or belief system, going through puberty, entering the world of work, and dealing with how I create intimacy in my life are considered developmental, in that they are issues we all deal with at around the same times in our lives.

Although the counseling skills we examined in Chapter 4 can be used when dealing with both situational and developmental concerns, knowledge of developmental stages can assist the human service worker when applying those skills in an attempt to understand a client's predicament. For instance, knowing that our clients will pass through expected stages of development can prepare the human service worker to anticipate areas of potential concern for our clients. In addition, preventive educational programs can be developed for clients because we can expect them to be dealing with developmental milestones at predictable times in their lives. Finally, when clients present us with crises that are of a developmental nature, we can reassure them that these are issues most people will face at some point in their lives.

As noted in Chapter 1, developmental theories tend to be *sequential* and *hierarchical*; that is, there is a predictable pattern of movement from the first to the latter stages, and these latter stages build on what has already been experienced and integrated into our lives. Many theories of human development have been identified over the years. For instance, some developmental approaches have helped us understand the unique problems of students as they pass through school (for example, Havighurst, 1972; Neukrug, Barr, Hoffman, & Kaplan, 1993), the lifelong process involved in choosing and maintaining contentment in one's career (for example, Super, 1957; Super & Hall, 1978), the maturation of faith experiences over the life span (for example, Fowler, 1991) and the process toward self-actualization (for example, Maslow, 1968). An in-depth examination of developmental theories would require a separate course. Therefore, in this chapter, we will focus only on some of the more prevalent theories of child development, personality development, and life-span development. In addition, we will also examine how the human service worker might apply knowledge of human development. Finally, we will explore issues related to what is considered normal and abnormal development.

Child Development

The developing child offers many challenges for the human service worker. As the child grows, understanding his or her physical, cognitive, and moral development is crucial to our successful work with young people.

Physical Development of the Growing Child

As the child develops, major physiological changes take place. Although the rate of children's physical development is fairly consistent, the scope of a specific child's development is based on the genetic predisposition of the child in interaction with the environment. For instance, although most children will be ready to learn multiplication in third grade, the rate and depth of learning will vary based on genetics and environment. Along these lines, a brilliant child is at a major disadvantage if he or she is brought up in a home that has leaded paint and lead in the water or in an environment that does not nurture the child's innate intelligence. On the other hand, a child who is less able can shine if placed in a stimulating and nurturing environment.

The importance of a nurturing environment can be seen through the success of the **Head Start Program**. This federally funded program, which was started in the 1970s, places disadvantaged preschool children in intellectually stimulating and nurturing environments prior to entering public school. On average, these children have done noticeably better academically and socially than have children of a similar background who have not received such an opportunity (Lee, Brooks-Gunn, Schnur, & Liaw, 1990).

Because the vast majority of children will develop at fairly predictable rates, if a child specialist is aware of the expected physiological timetable that is *normed* for the majority of children, he or she can determine whether a child is on target for his or her physiological development. Sometimes, lagging behind in physical development can be a first indication of a physiological, emotional, or intellectual impairment. For instance, a friend of mine has a daughter who could not crawl at age 1. Because the majority of children are beginning to walk at this time, there was concern that this might be an indication of a developmental disability. Fortunately, the child had a rare but harmless form of hypertrophy of the muscles and was walking within a few months of being tested. However, if tests had revealed a developmental disability, early diagnosis could have been crucial to optimizing the skills that the child does possess.

Typically, child specialists will examine age-appropriate milestones in the areas of motor development, speech development, sensory development, and the development of secondary sex characteristics (breast development, pubic hair, and so on) in determining what may be considered normal as opposed to what may be a deviation from the norm (Sprinthall & Sprinthall, 1990). A course on human growth and development will help familiarize human service workers with many of these expected developmental milestones.

Cognitive Development: Jean Piaget

Probably the person who most helped us understand the intellectual or cognitive development of children has been Jean Piaget (Flavell, 1963). Piaget stated that as the child grows, he or she takes new information into an already existing view of the world. Known as **assimilation**, this process refers to incorporating new information within the framework that the child already has for understanding the world. For instance, when a friend's daughter, Courtney, was 3 years old, she asked me to give her something to eat. I made a piece of toast with jam. She said that she wanted more to eat than one piece of toast. I cut the toast in half; she looked at me and said, "Thanks, Ed." This child had not yet learned the concept of *conservation*, or the "notion that liquids and solids can be transformed in shape without changing their volume or mass" (Mussen, Conger, & Kagan, 1969, p. 452). Courtney did not understand that if you cut something in half, you

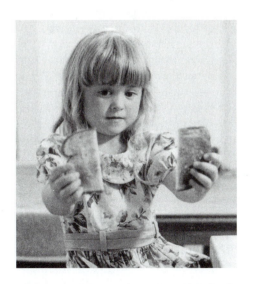

Now that Courtney is 5 years old, she is beginning to understand that one piece of toast cut in half is not more than one whole piece of toast, thus supporting Piaget's theory on conservation.

do not have twice as much. As Courtney grows older, she will eventually comprehend that cutting a piece of toast in half is not the same as having two full-size pieces. As she learns the concept behind this, she will **accommodate** to this way of knowing. In other words, she will change her previous way of understanding the world and adapt a new method. Piaget stated that in accommodating to the world, certain **schemata** or new cognitive structures (new ways of thinking), are formed that allow an individual to adapt and change his or her view of the world. This process of assimilation, forming new schemata, and eventual accommodation occurs throughout the life span.

Through his research on child cognitive development, Piaget determined that as children grow they pass through predictable periods, which he called the sensorimotor, preoperational, concrete-operational, and formal-operational stages. The **sensorimotor stage**, birth through 2 years, is when the infant responds totally to physical and sensory experiences. Because the child hasn't acquired full language ability, he or she cannot maintain mental images and responds only to the here and now of experience. Thus, trying to have a rational conversation with a child at this age would make little sense because he or she is cannot maintain such principles. For instance, imagine a parent saying to a 2-year-old child who just reached out for candy at a checkout counter "Let's sit down and talk about this when we get home so you'll understand why you shouldn't take candy without asking." Unfortunately, some parents try to make children understand this logic.

As the child moves into the **preoperational stage** (ages 2–7 years), he or she is developing language ability and can maintain mental images. This *intuitive* way of being in the world is when the child responds to what seems immediately obvious as opposed to the child having the ability to think logically. When this child sees a tall glass of water, he or she assumes that it has more volume than a smaller but wider glass of water (or the piece of toast cut in two is more than the one piece of toast). Because children at this age have not adopted logical thinking, trying to explain such logical principles would be difficult, if not impossible (unless the child is on the verge of entering the concrete-operational stage). Imagine trying to explain to 3-year-old Courtney why one piece of toast cut in half is not more than the original piece of toast. She just won't get it!

From age 7 through 11 years, the child enters the **concrete-operational stage** in which he or she can begin to "figure things out" through a series of logical tasks. Children in this stage often are very adamant about their logical way of viewing the world. For instance, when helping a friend's son figure out a math addition problem, I suggested to him a new way of doing it. However, because my method did not follow his "logical" way, he became very angry and told me I was wrong, even though the answer was the same. I was wrong because I didn't do it the way he learned, and he did not yet have the flexibility to examine other ways of problem solving. Children in this stage will have difficulty with metaphors or proverbs because they have not developed the capacity to think abstractly. However, when children move into the Piaget's final **formal-operational stage** (ages 11–16), they can begin to think abstractly and apply more complex levels of knowing to their understanding of the world. A child in this stage can understand how objects might have symbolic meaning (for example, the Liberty Bell is more than just a bell), test hypotheses, understand proverbs, and consider more than one aspect of a problem at one time.

Piaget's research on child development has greatly helped us understand how children learn and the limitations on their abilities based on their age and developmental stage. Such knowledge has greatly affected styles of teaching, ways to parent effectively, and methods of counseling children.

Moral Development: Lawrence Kohlberg and Carol Gilligan

Lawrence Kohlberg.   By having children respond to **moral dilemmas** (problems of a moral nature that have no clear-cut answer), Lawrence Kohlberg (1969) discovered that moral understanding and reasoning develop in a predictable pattern. He identified three levels of development, each containing two stages. The first level, **preconventional** (roughly ages 2–7 years), is based on the notion that children make moral decisions out of fear of being punished or out of desire for reward. In stage 1 of this level, moral decision making is based on perceived power that others hold over them and to avoid punishment from these individuals in authority. In stage 2, decisions are made with an egocentric/hedonistic desire to satisfy one's own needs and in hopes of gaining personal rewards. Imagine a 6-year-old wanting to watch her favorite video during dinner. A parent might say "No, you can't watch that now, but after dinner we'll make special time to do whatever you want." A child might initially say "Sure mom" (not wanting to get punished for doing the wrong thing), but then, when mom is not watching, secretly put the video in the VCR.

In Kohlberg's **conventional level**, moral decisions are based initially on social conformity and mutualism; later the accent is on adhering to rule-governed behavior—rules we are given to live by. In this level, children respond less to punishment or reward and more to avoid displeasing others and out of a sense of right and wrong as defined by rules of law and order. In stage 3 of this level, the child responds to what he or she believes friends would view as morally correct in hopes of avoiding their disapproval and of gaining their acceptance. Most children will reach stage 3 by age 13 (Zimbardo,

1988). An 8-year-old in this stage might decide to steal candy because his friends are encouraging him to do so and to avoid displeasing them.

In stage 4 of the conventional level, children will emphasize a system of laws and rules as a means of maintaining a sense of order in their lives. Here, some 10-year-olds will reason that it is not right to steal the candy because it is against the rules we are given to live by. Others might steal candy, yet know that their actions are wrong (know that it is against the rules we live by). In both cases, however, the 10-year-olds are reasoning from a stage 4 position; that is, both are using the rules as a basis for thinking about the act of stealing.

Kohlberg noted that many individuals will never reach the final **postconventional level** of moral development. If postconventional thinking comes at all, it comes only from age 13 and above. It is based on acceptance of a social contract that is related to democratically recognized universal truths (stage 5) and on individual conscience based on universal principles and moral values that are not necessarily principles or values held by others (stage 6).

In stage 5 of the postconventional level, the individual views laws as governed by social principles that can be examined, interpreted, and discussed. Such laws are seen as potentially changeable and are guides to help the individual make moral decisions. In this stage, an individual would probably not steal because there are governing moral principles and societal rules that prohibit stealing—principles that the individual considers important to the healthy functioning of society. However, a person in this stage would reflect on such a law to consider whether it makes sense at all times and might attempt to change the law when the law did not seem justified (for example, perhaps stealing would be allowed if it meant the survival of a child—if the parent of a starving child stole food for the child).

In stage 6, the final stage of the postconventional level, moral decisions are based on a sense of universal truths, personal conscience, individual decision making, and respect of human rights and dignity (Rice, 1992). Here an individual would consider moral truths in his or her decision-making process and, after deep reflection, might choose to break a law, deciding that such an action is taken out of respect for the dignity of people and for the betterment of society (Sprinthall & Sprinthall, 1990). For instance, during the civil rights movement of the 1960s, some individuals broke laws to advance the cause of civil rights for all people.

Carol Gilligan.   In 1982 Carol Gilligan wrote *In a Different Voice*, a book that questioned some of Kohlberg's assumptions. Gilligan, who had worked with Kohlberg, notes that most of his research had been done on a small group of boys and proposes that moral reasoning for

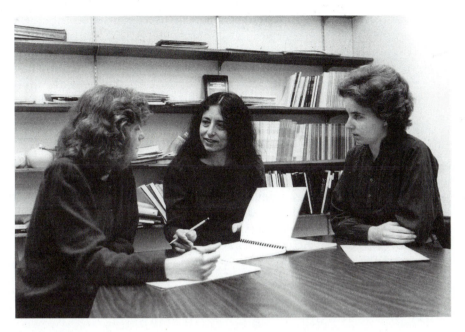

Carol Gilligan, center, states that women's moral development is different from men's in that women tend to stress interdependence as opposed to autonomy.

females might be based on a different way of knowing or understanding the world. She notes that Kohlberg's theory stresses the notion that high-stage individuals make choices autonomously, whereas her research seems to indicate that women value connectedness and interdependence and view the relationship as primary when making moral decisions. In describing the differences between men and women, Gilligan notes the responses of one of Kohlberg's subjects and compares him to a woman she interviewed: "Thus while Kohlberg's subject worries about people interfering with each other's rights, this woman worries about 'the possibility of omission, of your not helping others when you could help them'" (1982, p. 21).

Gilligan states that in the development of moral reasoning, especially in stages 3 and above, women will emphasize a "standard of caring" as they move toward self-realization. Also, she notes that women are more likely to be concerned about the effect their choices have on others, whereas men are more concerned about a sense of justice being maintained (Zimbardo, 1988). Noting these male and female differences, Gilligan states, "Given the differences in women's conceptions of self and morality, women bring to the life cycle a different point of view and order human experience in terms of different priorities" (1982, p. 22).

In thinking about the examples given to clarify Kohlberg's theory, you might consider how a woman's decisions might differ from a man's if her decision-making process takes into account how a person's decisions affect others and the interconnectedness of people. Gilligan has added a unique perspective to the concept of moral development and may be bringing to the forefront major differences that men and women hold toward moral reasoning. Understanding such differences are crucial in helping us comprehend why the different sexes make certain choices.

Although there is not a direct relationship between cognitive development and moral development, it is clear that one cannot be at the upper levels of moral development if he or she cannot think abstractly. Also, evidence indicates that our actions are not always in sync with how we think, in that most individuals prefer the reasoning of a moral development stage one level above where they actually are.

Knowledge of Child Development: Applications for the Human Service Worker

Although the human service worker is not necessarily an expert in child development, knowledge of such development can help the human service worker understand whether the child is developing within normal rates. If the human service worker can recognize physical problems or delays in social, cognitive, or moral reasoning, then appropriate referrals can be made to medical, psychological, or educational sources that can assist the child in his or her development. Early identification of such problems can greatly help to ameliorate these concerns.

Personality Development

How are our personalities formed? This question has intrigued philosophers for centuries. In the last 100 years, psychologists have attempted to answer this question through a number of theories that seek to explain the personality development of the individual. Paralleling the counseling theories discussed in Chapter 3, theories of personality development, based on views of human nature of the major counseling theories, describe a system for the developing person and explain the underlying beliefs that result in a specific counseling approach.

Although many theories of personality development have been developed over the years, we will examine Freud's theory of psychosexual development, learning theorists' views on development, and Rogers's humanistic understanding of growth and development. These represent three of the more prevalent views concerning personality development of the individual.

Sigmund Freud's Psychosexual Model of Development

Sigmund Freud viewed individual personality as forming within the first 5 years of life. As noted in Chapter 3, he believed that we are born with sexual and aggressive instincts that are regulated as a function of parenting received in early childhood. Freud stated that the child is born all **id**; that is, he or she responds only to instincts in an effort to satisfy his or her needs. As the child develops, the type of parenting he or she receives greatly affects the formation of the **ego**, or the ways in which the child deals with reality. As the ego is developing, the formation of the **superego**, which represents the formation of the child's morality and values, is greatly affected by the values of parents and society. Freud thought that the ways in which the id, ego, and superego are formed are dependent on the types of parenting we received in the first 5 years of life. He stated that the individual passes through five **psychosexual stages of development**, each of which affects the formation of these **structures of personality** (Appignanesi, 1979; Corey, 1992).

Stating that sexual satisfaction and resulting psychosexual development is centered on *erogenous zones*, Freud presented a unique view of the developing individual. During the **oral stage**, the first stage of psychosexual development, the infant receives pleasure through feeding. The major developmental task of this stage, which occurs between birth and age 1 1/2 years, is how the child becomes attached to the mother (or the major caretaker). Therefore, the relationship between caretaker and infant is extremely important. Clearly, a child who goes hungry or is physically abused will have difficulty successfully passing through this stage. Invariably, Freud stated, this child would develop trust problems as an adult.

During the **anal stage**, the child receives pleasure from bowel movements. During this stage, which occurs between ages 1 1/2 and 3 years, the child becomes physiologically ready to be toilet trained. How parents assist with the child's newfound ability to control his or her bodily functions greatly affects the child's ability to be independent, feel powerful, and express negative feelings. Think about the parent who demands the child "sit on the potty" versus the parent who encourages and supports the child's newfound control of his or her bodily functions. These two different types of parenting will affect the child's sense of autonomy very differently.

In the third stage of development, the **phallic stage**, which occurs between ages 3 and 5 years, the child becomes aware of his or her genitals as well as of the genitals of the opposite sex. Now the child receives pleasure from self-stimulation. The kinds of permission giving that parents afford the child in this stage can greatly affect the child's attitudes and values. The parent who consistently tells his or her child that it is sinful to touch the genitals will affect the child's values very differently than the parent who allows the child to feel good about his or her body within culturally acceptable standards.

The **latency stage**, occurring between age 5 years through puberty, is a period of relative relaxation for the child, in which he or she replaces earlier sexual feelings with a focus on socialization. Here the child becomes more aware of peers, and increased attention is placed on peer-related activities. Freud's final stage of development is the **genital stage**, which begins at puberty and continues through the life span of the individual. Here we see the unresolved issues that were raised in the first three stages of development emerge, and sexual energy is focused on social activities with peers and on love relationships.

Fixation in a stage may occur because of poor parenting. Because the child has not successfully completed the developmental tasks of a specific stage, dysfunctional patterns of functioning will develop throughout the lifetime. Many of our dysfunctional ways of relating, Freud stated, occur *unconsciously* or out of our awareness. This means that we respond to situations in ways for which we have no deep understanding. For instance, the child who is sexually abused at age 5 years might have repressed these memories; yet, Freud would say that the abuse still would affect the child's behaviors in unconscious ways. Therefore, it is not uncommon to see an adult who was sexually abused find ways to avoid dealing with his or her sexuality (for example, becoming obese, becoming a workaholic, or, in an extreme case, taking on multiple personalities).

Typically, to avoid and protect the individual from the anxiety that unresolved issues might arouse, the individual develops **defense mechanisms**. For instance, the sexually abused child might develop defenses as an adult to protect the ego that became so fragile as a function of the abuse. Although there are many defense mechanisms, some of the more common ones are: **repression**, pushing out of awareness threatening or painful memories; **denial**, distorting reality in order to deny perceived threats to the person; **projection**, viewing others as having unacceptable qualities that the individual himself or herself actually has; **rationalization**, explaining away a bruised or hurt ego; and **regression**, reverting to behavior from an earlier stage of development which has less demanding ways of responding to anxiety (for example, sucking one's thumb).

Freud's psychoanalytic model of personality development has added much to our understanding of the complexity of the individual and why there is such a variety of ways in which people respond. His stage theory and the concepts of the structures of personality, the unconscious, and defense mechanisms represented the first comprehensive approach to our understanding of the development of personality.

Learning Theory and the Development of the Person

B. F. Skinner and other learning theorists hold the belief that individuals are born a blank slate, or **tabula rasa**, and that personality development is based on the types of conditioning that have affected us throughout our lifetime (Bandura, Ross, & Ross 1963; Skinner, 1971) . Drastically differing with Freud's notion on instincts, Skinner believed that "the most important causes of behavior are environmental and [that] it only confuses the matter to talk about inner drives" (Nye, 1986, p. 82).

As noted in Chapter 3, individuals can learn behaviors through **operant** or **classical conditioning** or **modeling** (social learning). Learning theorists do not view personality development related to changes that occur through developmental stages as in the psychoanalytic model. Although behaviorists do not deny that a person's genetics or biology can affect behavior, they emphasize how positive or negative reinforcement, social learning, and the pairing of an unconditioned stimulus with a conditioned stimulus affect our personality development.

Learning theorists believe that personality development is generally shaped by the significant people in one's life. Skinner and other learning theorists believe that reinforcements from significant others could occur very subtly, often in ways that we do not immediately recognize (Nye, 1986; Skinner, 1971; Wolpe, 1969). Therefore, changes in voice intonation, subtle glances, or body language could subliminally affect one's personality development. Learning theorists note that if a situation is examined closely enough, one could attain an understanding of the types of **reinforcement contingencies**, or modeling, that were instrumental in shaping behavior.

Because the reinforcement contingencies are so powerful, these behaviors are generalized to other situations. This is why an individual's behavior will be relatively consistent from situation to situation. Extinguishing behaviors that have been continually reinforced is difficult; however, the major task of helpers who work with maladaptive personality formation is to use **counterconditioning** (conditioning new adaptive behaviors) so the individual can learn more effective ways of living in the world. Counterconditioning is not an easy task because the original behaviors are often the results of years of conditioning.

Learning theory has had great impact on our ability to change maladaptive behaviors (see Chapter 3). We owe much to Skinner and his colleagues for adding this important dimension to our understanding of personality development.

The Humanistic Understanding of Personality Development

As noted in previous chapters, Carl Rogers greatly affected our understanding of the person. His thoughts on personality development are in stark contrast to the views of Freud and Skinner. Although representing just one of the many humanistic approaches to understanding personality development, Rogers's ideas embody many of the key concepts put forth by the humanistic theorists.

Rogers believed that individuals are born good and have a natural tendency to actualize and obtain fulfillment if placed in a nurturing environment that includes *empathy, congruence*, and *positive regard* (see Chapters 1 and 3). As opposed to Freud, Rogers did not emphasize the importance of instincts, the unconscious, or developmental stages in the formation of personality development. As opposed to Skinner, Rogers did not place much value on reinforcement contingencies as creating the personality of the individual. Instead, he viewed the relationship between the child and his or her major caretakers as the most significant factor in personality development (Rogers, 1951, 1957, 1980).

Rogers believed that we all have a need to be loved. He stated that significant people in our lives often set up **conditions of worth** or ways we should act in order to receive their love. Therefore, as children we will sometimes act in ways to please others in order to obtain a sense of acceptance—even if the pleasing self is not our real self. At this point the child has learned that if he or she practices **incongruity**, or not being real, he or she will receive acceptance. This nongenuine way of living then becomes our way of relating to the world and prevents us from becoming self-actualized—becoming our true self. Often this is seen through our **introjection** (swallowing whole) of the values of others without ever giving ourselves the opportunity to reflect and decide whether these are values to which we truly adhere. This is when our self-actualizing tendency is squashed. The helper who works with an individual who is incongruent attempts to set up an environment in which the client feels safe enough to get in touch with his or her true self. It is only when one realizes his or her true self that one can become self-actualized, as noted by Abraham Maslow in his hierarchy (see Chapter 3).

The Story of Ellen West

This story, so eloquently told by Rogers (1961), describes the history of a famous psychotherapy client (a client Rogers knew about but never saw himself). Rogers described the estrangement of this person from her feelings—how she felt as if she had to follow her father's wishes and not marry the man she loved, how she disengaged herself from her feelings by overeating, how a few years later she again fell in love but married a distant cousin according to her parents' wishes. Following this marriage, she became anorexic, taking 60 laxative pills a day, again as an apparent attempt to divorce herself from her feelings. She saw numerous doctors, who gave her differing diagnoses, treated her dispassionately, and generally denied her humanness. Eventually, disenchanted with her life, Ellen West committed suicide.

This story, Rogers noted, gives a poignant view of what it is like to lose touch with self—to be incongruent. Because Ellen West felt she needed to gain the conditional love of her parents, she gave up the most valuable part of self—her real self. Losing touch with self led to a life filled with self-hate and a sense of being out of touch. Eventually, she was viewed by therapists as being mentally ill, which Rogers implied might have added to her feelings of estrangement and her eventual suicide.

The humanistic approach to personality development represents a departure from the deterministic views of Freud and the reductionistic ideas of the learning theorists. The humanists' stress on the importance of significant relationships has added an important dimension to our understanding of personality development.

Knowledge of Personality Development: Applications for the Human Service Worker

When we initially meet clients, we are sometimes bewildered by their actions. Why does a rapist rape? Why does a parent abuse his or her child? Why does an adult who seemingly has everything live in a state of depression? Why does an able-bodied, intelligent person end up on the streets as a homeless person? Understanding the personality development of the individual can give us insight into the world of the client. Such insights into the developing world of the person as offered to us by psychoanalysts, humanists, and learning theorists can assist

A Psychotic Relative

When I was about 10 years old, I had a favorite relative named Joyce with whom I loved to play. Suddenly, she no longer came to visit. I heard rumors that Joyce's father, David, had had a "nervous breakdown" and that his wife had divorced him. The families became estranged at that point. David, who was college-educated, never seemed the same after his nervous breakdown. He rarely bathed, wore dilapidated clothes, and often would come up with rather grandiose ideas about life. When I was older, I was told that David had an acute psychotic episode. He had lost touch with reality, was paranoid, and had been hospitalized in a large, city psychiatric hospital. Since his hospitalization, he would often stay in sleazy apartments and at times was a homeless "Bowery bum." What had happened to David?

Recently, when I asked my mother about David, she stated that he had at times seemed different, even before the hospitalization. I often wonder about David's personality development. What kinds of early childhood development affected his personality? What kind of parenting did he receive? Were there genetic and/or biological factors that affected his mental health. Unfortunately, much of David's life is masked in mystery. Perhaps with early intervention and knowledge of personality development, the tragedy that befell him and his family would never have occurred.

us in our ability to empathize with our clients, help us in treatment planning for our clients, and give us the base knowledge to help us make appropriate referrals. If we did not have this basic understanding of personality development, we could be left without a clue to the makeup of the person or how to work with the individual.

Life-Span Development Theories

Some models of understanding the development of the person have taken a life-span approach; those who adhere to this approach believe that, the individual continues to grow over the life span, with development *not* suddenly ending in childhood. One of the more prevalent models of life-span development has been Erik Erikson's stages of **psychosocial development**. More recently, Robert Kegan's **interpersonal model** has gained some prominence. In Chapter 1 we viewed the adult stages of Kegan's model; here we will view the whole model, from birth through adulthood.

Erik Erikson's Stages of Psychosocial Development

Although Erikson started out studying Freud's psychoanalytic approach, he later developed a model that rejected many of Freud's original tenets. Contrary to Freud, Erikson believed that the individual is not determined by instincts, early childhood development, and the unconscious but instead believes that psychosocial forces are major motivators in the development of the individual over the life span. As opposed to Freud's deterministic philosophy, Erikson had faith in the ability of the individual to overcome many of his or her problems. Erikson believed that as the individual passes through life, he or she has specific age-related developmental life tasks to overcome. If the individual successfully masters these developmental milestones, a strong ego is formed, a positive identity is created, and the individual is ready to move on to the next level. On the other hand, if the individual cannot cope with the developmental tasks, then he or she develops a low self-image and bruised ego and carries these dysfunctions into the next levels, making it difficult to successfully complete later developmental tasks. Erikson's eight life-span stages offer a means of helping us understand the typical developmental tasks of the individual (Erikson, 1968, 1982).

> *Trust versus mistrust (ages birth–1 year).* During this first year of life, the infant develops a sense of trust or mistrust based on the type of caretaking received from significant individuals in his or her life.

> *Autonomy versus shame and doubt (ages 1–3 years).* During these years the child begins to explore the environment and the ways in which significant caretakers promote (or inhibit) autonomy. The child who is not allowed to explore may feel ashamed and/or doubtful of self.

> *Initiative versus guilt (ages 3–5 years).* As the child continues to explore the environment and gain an increased sense of independence, how caretakers encourage exploration can greatly affect the child's sense of self.

> *Industry versus inferiority (ages 6–12 years).* In this stage the child begins to examine what he or she does well. The testing ground for this stage is often with peers at school where the child begins to compare his or her skills with those of others. The ability of the child to feel a sense of self-worth through his or her interaction with others is crucial in this stage.

> *Identity versus role confusion (adolescence).* As adolescents begin to identify the temperament, values, interests, and abilities they hold, they are able to recognize the specific attributes that determine

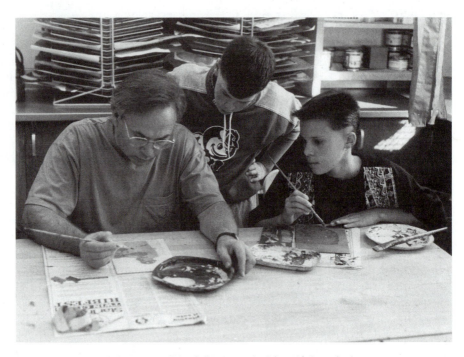

Positive role models can assist adolescents in identifying their temperaments, values, interests, and abilities.

their personality makeup. Significant others such as caretakers, peers, teachers, and school counselors can assist in such development. Lack of role models and lack of experiences that encourage such self-understanding can lead to a lack of identity and confusion about self.

Intimacy versus isolation (early adulthood/adulthood). Once the young adult has achieved a sense of self, he or she is ready to develop relationships that lend themselves toward intimacy with others. Lack of self-understanding leads to isolation from others and/or an inability to have mutually supporting relationships that encourage individuality with interdependency.

Generativity versus stagnation (middle/late adulthood). The healthy adult in this stage is concerned about others and about future generations. This individual has a life that is productive and responsible and can find meaningfulness through such activities as work, volunteerism, parenting, and/or community activities.

Integrity versus despair (later life). In this last stage of development, the older person examines his or her life and may feel a sense of fulfillment or despair. Successfully mastering the preceding developmental tasks will lead to a sense of integrity for the individual.

The Case of Miles

I once saw a 32-year-old client who was having trouble with intimacy. Miles was engaged despite the fact that he had rarely dated, had very poor interpersonal skills, and was quite fearful of having a sexual relationship. He was a virgin when he eventually married, and he soon found that he could not maintain an erection and have intercourse with his wife. Although he was dealing directly with Erikson's intimacy-versus-isolation stage, it became evident that he had never successfully passed through earlier stages. He had been verbally abused as a child, which resulted in his having difficulty building trust and being fearful of the world. This gave him an inferiority complex, which made him want to hide from people. He therefore was unable to interact successfully with his peers and generally felt lost in the world. He never discovered what he was good at, what he liked, or what he valued. Clearly, he had a very poor identity formation. His problems with intimacy seemed closely related to not successfully completing earlier stages of development.

As Miles and I worked on his concerns related to intimacy, we also spent much time examining issues related to earlier stages of development. As he reflected on his life and as he worked through his issues, he eventually was able to have a closer, more intimate relationship with his wife. This eventually also led to their having a satisfactory sexual relationship.

Erikson's life-span model is often used as a cornerstone for helping individuals understand expected crises through which they may pass. Such understanding can sometimes help normalize problems that may feel unbearable in the moment.

Robert Kegan's Constructive Model of Development

As opposed to Freud's deterministic early childhood model, Kegan believes that our understanding of the world is based on the ways in which we construct reality as we pass through life. His **subject/object** theory states that individuals pass through specific developmental stages that reflect a meaning-making system. Movement from a lower to a higher stage necessitates a letting go of the earlier stage. This is not done easily, and Kegan (1982) suggests that movement occurs most successfully if there is challenge to one's existing view of the world within a supportive environment.

Being born into the **incorporative stage**, Kegan states that the self-absorbed infant is all reflexive and has no sense of self as separate from the outside world. However, as very young children begin to experience the world, reflexes are no longer the primary focus; instead children attempt to have their needs met through attainment of objects outside of self: "In disembedding herself from her reflexes the two-year-old comes to have reflexes rather than be them, and the new self is embedded in that which coordinates the reflexes, namely, the 'perceptions' and the 'impulses'" (Kegan, 1982, p. 85). In this **impulsive stage** children have limited control over their actions and act spontaneously to have needs met. No wonder the second year of life is often called the "terrible twos."

As children gain control over their impulses, they move into the **imperial stage** where needs, interests, and wishes become primary and impulses can begin to be controlled. For instance, children begin to recognize what they want, can begin to reflect on such needs, and can control impulses to meet the needs. The child who wants a new toy, perceives the toy, and recognizes the desire for it now has some control over how to obtain the toy.

Garrett: Responding from the Imperial Stage

Garrett is a 12-year-old son of a friend. Recently, when wanting to spend time with a friend of his, he was told that this friend had already made plans to spend time with another boy. Garrett felt rejected and left out. If Garrett had still been in the impulsive stage, he might have thrown a temper tantrum. Instead, having passed into the imperial stage, he had control over his impulses and devised a way to have his needs met. He manipulated a way to spend time with both of them, disregarding their need to be with each other. In the imperial stage, one can control impulses and develop plans to have one's needs met. However, in this stage, there is little empathy for other people's desires. Therefore, Garrett did not yet have the ability to talk over his feelings with his friends. Hopefully, when he is a little older, he will be able to share his feelings of being left out and understand his friends' desire to be with each other.

When his father was explaining this situation to me, he said that at first he was going to try to talk to his son about the other boys' feelings, but then he realized that Garrett just could not hear that yet. If someone is in the imperial stage and not yet ready to give it up, there is little you can do to make that person move to the interpersonal stage.

The last three stages occur primarily in adulthood and were noted in Chapter 1. Briefly, during the **interpersonal stage**, the individual is embedded in relationships; relationships become primary, and needs and wishes are met through the relationship. In this stage, there is a beginning awareness of other people's feelings. This is manifested by the ability of individuals to show empathy because it helps them understand the other with whom they are embedded. The stage 3 need for relationships is highlighted by many of the songs of this and past generations, songs that say, "Without you, I can't go on living."

As the individual moves out of embeddedness in other, he or she moves into the **institutional stage** where a sense of autonomy and self-authorship of life is acquired. Relationships in this stage are still important but no longer seem to be the essential ingredient for living. In this stage, the individual's understanding of his or her values and interests becomes important. Here the individual may *choose* a partner because he or she shares similar values; however, the person in this stage does not *need* the partner as he or she does in the interpersonal stage.

Kegan's final stage, the **interindividual stage**, highlights mutuality in relationships; that is, the individual can share with others and learn from others in a nonembedded, nondependent way. Here there is a sharing of selves without a giving up of self. In this stage, differentness is tolerated and even encouraged at times.

Kegan's model offers an important departure from the other life-span developmental models in that it stresses the interpersonal nature of development. Growth is based on our ability to interact with others and to let go of past, less effective types of relating. Although Kegan gives some general timelines for when movement into higher levels could occur, it is not unusual to find older adults who have not moved out of the interpersonal and sometimes even the imperial stages. Knowing the developmental stage of a person can help human service workers provide an environment that is conducive to the personal growth of the client.

Knowledge of Life-Span Development: Applications for the Human Service Worker

Whereas knowledge of child development and personality development can be crucial to understanding the person, these views tend to stress early development instead of changes in the individual *throughout* the life span. On the other hand, the life-span approach acknowledges that growth and struggles continue after puberty and on through older age in a predictable manner. Knowledge of some of the life-span stages can help the human service worker facilitate the expected transitions through which the individual will pass. Therefore, the human service worker is better able to make appropriate referrals, counsel adequately, and provide educational materials to help the client.

Counseling across the Life Span

Life-span development is more than linear growth over time. We do not just move through a series of events in our lives. Our early individual and family experiences remain with us. The manner in which we have connected with others in the past provides us with resources as we move toward autonomy and individuation. (Ivey, 1991, p. 120)

Allen Ivey (1991) developed a process for helping professionals use their knowledge of human development in the helping process. He states that understanding the developmental level of the client is crucial to working effectively toward client goals. Therefore, key components to Ivey's approach include assessing developmental level, devising developmental-based strategies to working with the client, and supporting yet challenging the client toward growth. Ivey believes that it makes no sense to try to assist a client toward growth if we cannot meet the immediate needs of the client. For instance, it would make no sense to be working on a client's sense of self-esteem if he or she is hungry. Feed the client first, then later worry about sense of self. Therefore, Ivey's model necessitates knowledge of the different developmental levels in order for the helper to aid the client.

Human service programs are now acknowledging the importance of the developmental perspective for their students (Petrie, 1984). As ways of infusing human development theory into human service programs become more common, we hopefully will see new means of applying such knowledge to the work with our clients (Petrie, 1987).

Comparison of Developmental Models

The varying models of development discussed in this chapter offer differing dimensions to our understanding of the person. Figure 5-1 outlines the varying stages of the theories we examined. Keep in mind that many individuals become fixated in stages. This will hinder their passage through the later stages.

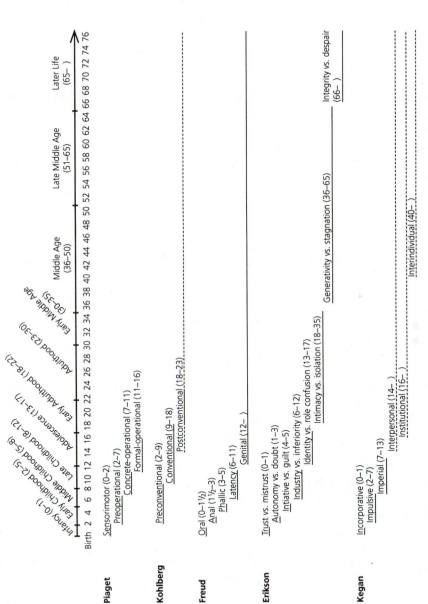

Piaget

Sensorimotor (0–2)
Preoperational (2–7)
Concrete-operational (7–11)
Formal-operational (11–16)

Kohlberg

Preconventional (2–9)
Conventional (9–18)
Postconventional (18–23)

Freud

Oral (0–1½)
Anal (1½–3)
Phallic (3–5)
Latency (6–11)
Genital (12–)

Erikson

Trust vs. mistrust (0–1)
Autonomy vs. doubt (1–3)
Intiative vs. guilt (4–5)
Industry vs. inferiority (6–12)
Identity vs. role confusion (13–17)
Intimacy vs. isolation (18–35)
Generativity vs. stagnation (36–65)
Integrity vs. despair (66–)

Kegan

Incorporative (0–1)
Impulsive (2–7)
Imperial (7–13)
Interpersonal (14–)
Institutional (16–)
Interindividual (40–)

Birth 2 4 6 8 10 12 14 16 18 20 22 24 26 28 30 32 34 36 38 40 42 44 46 48 50 52 54 56 58 60 62 64 66 68 70 72 74 76

Infancy (0–1)
Early Childhood (2–5)
Middle Childhood (5–8)
Late Childhood (8–12)
Adolescence (13–17)
Early Adulthood (18–22)
Adulthood (23–30)
Early Middle Age (30–35)
Middle Age (36–50)
Late Middle Age (51–65)
Later Life (65–)

Note: The onset of certain stages can vary by several months in childhood and several years in adulthood. In fact, Kegan and Kohlberg state that individuals may never reach the later stages of possible development. A dashed line represents the age range in which an individual could *potentially* attain a particular stage. A solid line represents the age range in which an individual is more *likely* to attain a particular stage. *Remember:* Attainment of a particular age may *not* mean attainment of a particular stage.

Figure 5-1   A comparison of developmental models

Normal and Abnormal Development

While employed as an outpatient therapist at a mental-health center, I was working with a 35-year-old married woman who had a history of several **acute psychotic episodes**. This meant that for short periods of time she had lost touch with reality, she had auditory hallucinations, and her thinking process had become disorganized, or not clear. I saw her for a few months and she seemed rather coherent, warm, and relatively normal. One day I received a call from her panicked husband who stated his wife was "out of control." He brought her to the mental-health center, and I was startled to see a woman I hardly recognized. She thought she was possessed by the devil, was in a panicked state, and was screaming about some unusual sexual acts in which she stated she had participated. It was difficult to follow her line of reasoning. In fact, little of what she said seemed to make sense. This once warm, coherent, lucid woman seemed like a different person. She was placed on medication to calm her and to help her regain stability and lucidity.

As a young therapist, I wondered how much of what she stated was real, how much was fantasy, how did a seemingly "together" person suddenly lose it, and what could I do to help her get back in touch with reality. This woman was *very scared* and desperately wanted help. To this day, this woman represents to me the difference between what we call "normal" and "abnormal," as well as how fragile that line can sometimes be.

Mental-health professionals have for years struggled with the concepts of normal and abnormal. When do people cross the line to abnormality? Some individuals like Thomas Szaz, William Glasser, and R. D. Laing do not believe in the traditional views on mental illness and abnormal behavior. For instance, Szaz believes that abnormal behavior is a function of **power dynamics** in relationships. He believes that individuals, institutions, and/or society places undue demands on some individuals, and it is these demands that push an individual into stressful behaviors that many people call abnormal (Szaz, 1961, 1990). Glasser (1961) believes that abnormal behavior is a function of irresponsible behavior, and if you can help identify and change such behaviors, the person can then show responsible or normal behaviors. Laing (1967) viewed mental illness or abnormal behavior as a normal response to a stressful situation. In fact, he even encouraged people to get in touch with their own psychosis as a means of letting go of these stressors in their lives. Laing developed hospitals in England where individuals could go to become schizophrenic, and he would periodically "allow" himself to "become" schizophrenic.

Today, there is growing evidence that biological and genetic factors may affect personality development. For instance, it is now pretty much taken for granted that alcoholism runs in families and probably has genetic links. Growing evidence indicates that **schizophrenia**, and perhaps even **major depression**, have genetic links. Most developmental models that examine psychopathology and abnormal behavior have room for genetic and biological ties to such behaviors.

The various types of developmental models we examined in this chapter approach the understanding of abnormal behavior differently. For instance, psychoanalytic theorists state that psychopathology is a result of dysfunctional parenting in the first 5 years of life. Such early patterning of one's personality is represented through the development of the individual's id, ego, and superego. These theorists also believe that the earlier the dysfunction, the more serious the pathology and the more difficult it is to change.

On the other hand, although not dismissing possible biological and genetic determinants of behavior, the humanistic and learning theorist state that change can occur at any point in one's lifetime and that, although pathology may be a function of learning or parenting styles early in life, new ways of learning can occur throughout one's lifetime.

Finally, the life-span developmental theorists view behavior as being affected throughout the life span and as a function of specific predictable developmental tasks. Not dismissing biological or genetic determinants of behavior, these theorists also believe that problems in any one of these stages can seriously affect healthy functioning.

As our understanding of development becomes clearer, many individuals now believe that the psychoanalysts, humanists, learning theorists, and life-span development theorists all offer some bits of truth to our understanding of normal and abnormal behavior.

Diagnosis and Abnormal Behavior: What Is the *DSM III–R*?

The American Psychiatric Association in consultation with the American Psychological Association has over the years developed a manual to help in the diagnosis of mental disorders. In its third edition, revised (the fourth edition is soon to be released), it offers a full range of descriptive behaviors that epitomize different types of mental illnesses and emotional problems. The ***Diagnostic and Statistical Manual III– Revised*** (*DSM III–R*) (American Psychiatric Association, 1987) is a complex manual that can be of great assistance in our understanding, diagnosis, and treatment of individuals. This manual has also become extremely important for the payment of mental-health benefits because most health insurance companies will not pay for mental-health counseling unless there is an appropriate diagnosis from a duly licensed clinician.

The *DSM III–R* also has its critics. Some say that it is to reductionistic—that is, it tries to reduce mental illness and emotional problems into very neat categories, categories that some believe do not really exist. Others say a diagnosis tends to be a self-fulfilling prophecy in that once a client is given a diagnosis, others tend to see the client in that light and will tend to reinforce those behaviors in the person.

Despite its critics, the *DSM III–R* seems to offer us a means of understanding emotional problems and is an important step to our treatment of various mental-health concerns.

Ethical and Professional Issues

Abnormal Behavior and Mental Illness—Myth or Fact?

Over the years, I have seen individuals argue over whether there is such a thing as mental illness. I have seen some vehemently state that mental illness is a disease, genetically and/or biologically caused, and should be treated as such. Others have just as strongly expressed the view that mental illness is the result of societal or family pressures or irresponsible behavior. Where lies the truth? Despite making great strides in the fields of personality development and its effect on mental illness, as well as giant leaps in our understanding of the **psychobiology** of mental illness, there is still much to be known. It appears to me that to come to any conclusions at this date about the **etiology**, or origins, of various forms of mental illness would be a mistake. Most important, the human service worker needs to be well-read concerning the most recent literature in this area. Current knowledge along with an open mind can help the human service worker make important decisions when working with those who have severe emotional problems. These decisions may very well affect our clients for the rest of their lives.

When working with the mentally ill, we must ask ourselves what are the wisest decisions we can make to protect the welfare of our clients. Because there still seems to be much for us to find out about the etiology of mental illness, it seems that the wisest decisions for us to make would be to gather the data and keep an open mind before assisting our clients in treatment planning. Whatever decisions are made, they should be made with the welfare of our clients in mind.

The integrity and welfare of the client by the human service worker must be respected at all times; each client should be treated with humaneness and unconditional regard in a non-manipulative fashion. (NOHSE/CSHSE proposed ethical guidelines; see Appendix A)

The Developmentally Mature Human Service Worker: Willing to Understand His or Her Own Development

What is it about my development that I have lived 42 years, never married, yet now so want a family? Why did I end up in the field of human services and teaching? Why do I sometimes feel an emptiness inside that seems insatiable and at other times feel so totally filled with joy and excitement that I wonder how I could ever feel empty? How does my personal developmental history affect the ways in which I interact with people, especially my clients? Clearly, knowledge of my own developmental history can greatly help me in my understanding of self as well as the ways in which I work with my clients. It seems to me that *not* trying to understand one's own developmental history can negatively affect our work with our clients through countertransference. It is our responsibility to put ourselves in situations that help expand awareness of self. Such vehicles as counseling, self-help groups, meditation, and reading literature on personal development are just a few of the many ways in which we can better understand self.

Summary

This chapter presented an overview of human growth and development from birth through old age. Briefly examining the physical development of the child, Piaget's child cognitive-developmental model, and moral development as presented by Kohlberg and Gilligan gave us insight in our understanding of the growth of the child and adolescent. Exploring personality development as presented by Freud, Rogers, and the learning theorists helped us understand the many and interesting ways in which people behave. Finally, viewing development as a life-span model as presented by Erikson and Kegan gave us insight into how development is a never-ending process that continues until our death.

We also explored the differences between normal and abnormal development and the ways we have tried to understand psychopathology. We discussed major differences in understanding abnormal behavior, along with one attempt to classify mental illness and emotional maladjustment as presented in the *DSM III–R*.

Finally, we noted the importance of understanding our own development and how it can affect our work with our clients, and the significance of finding activities that can assist us in our own personal developmental history.

Experiential Exercises

1.   Reflecting on Your Personality Development

Refer to the personality theories of Freud, Rogers, and the learning theorists, and then reflect on your personality development as it might be described from each of these perspectives.

1. How does each perspective explain characteristics of your personality?

2. In explaining your personality development from the differing perspectives, what commonalities do you see between the varying theories?

3. In explaining your personality development from the differing perspectives, what differences do you see between the varying theories?

2.   Examining the Development of an Adult with a Developmental Disability

The following is the story of Gloria. From a developmental perspective, describe Gloria from a

1. Child development viewpoint

2. Personality development viewpoint

3. Life-span development perspective

Gloria's life story. Gloria, a 53-year-old developmentally disabled adult, was born mildly mentally retarded and with cerebral palsy. Soon after her birth, her parents hospitalized her in an institution for the developmentally disabled. She lived in this institution until she was 31, at which time she was placed in a group home for the mentally retarded.

As a child, Gloria's language development was delayed. She could not speak in sentences until she was 4 years old. She was not toilet trained until age 7. Although her parents would visit her periodically, her main caretakers were the social service workers at the institution. Gloria was schooled at the institution where she acquired the equivalent of a second-grade education. Gloria had few friends in the institution and was considered a loner. Despite working on socialization skills while in the institution, Gloria still prefers to be alone and spends much of her time painting. She has become a rather good artist, and many of her paintings are found in the institution and in the group home. Visitors often comment on the paintings and are generally surprised that a developmentally disabled person can paint so well. Gloria has a part-time job at a local art-supply company where she generally does menial work.

Although Gloria does have some friends at the group home and at the art-supply store, generally, when she spends much time with someone, she ends up having a temper tantrum. When this happens she will usually withdraw—often to her painting. Gloria generally blames other people for her anger.

Gloria is a rules follower. She feels very strongly about the list of rules on the bulletin board at her group home. She methodically reports people who break the rules. She always feels extremely guilty after having a temper tantrum because she sees herself as breaking the rule "talk things out rather than get into a fight." In a similar vein, Gloria feels that laws in the country "are there for a purpose." For instance, at street crossings she always stops at red lights and waits for the light to change.

Gloria has no sense of her future. She lives from day to day and, despite periods of depression, generally functions fairly adequately. She states she wants to get married, but her lack of socialization skills prevents her from having any meaningful relationships with men.

Overall, the human service workers who have contact with Gloria describe her as a rigid, conscientious, talented person who has trouble maintaining relationships. They note that, despite being in individual counseling and in a socialization support group, she has made little progress in maintaining satisfying relationships. Their feeling is that she probably will maintain her current level of functioning, and they see little hope for change.

3. Examining the Development of a Gifted Child

The following is the story of Joe. From a developmental perspective, explain Joe's development from a

1. Child development viewpoint

2. Personality development viewpoint

3. Life-span development perspective

Joe's life story.   Joe is 13 years old and is the only child, grandchild, and niece or nephew on his mother's side of the family. Joe's parents separated when his mother was 5 months' pregnant with him. His parents, both of whom are highly educated, went through a tumultuous separation and divorce but now have a cordial relationship. Following his birth, his mother was distraught over the breakup of her marriage but subsequently has maintained a strong sense of self and high self-esteem. Following Joe's birth, his mother, who works full-time, was fortunately able to afford a live-in Nanny. This woman still lives with them and has been a significant help for the family and an additional source of comfort for Joe.

Joe's mother remarried when Joe was 10 years old and his father has been involved in a long-term relationship. Joe lives with his mother but spends every other weekend, some weekdays, and extended periods of time during the summer and holidays with his father. He seems to have a good relationship with both parents, his stepfather, and his father's girlfriend.

Joe, who has always done well in school, currently attends a private school. He maintains very high grades and has a high IQ. Joe is at ease in relationships, as evidenced by his many friends and his ability to relate to people of all ages. He has many skills and is just beginning to examine those things that he is best at. He is just entering puberty, and girls are becoming more important to him. Overall, most people would describe Joe as a bright, personable, and thoughtful young man who is at ease with himself.

Although sometimes he may appear a little "spoiled," he generally is thoughtful and can recognize other people's feelings. He can think abstractly, and it would not be difficult to have a conversation with him concerning such philosophical matters as death and the existence of God.

4.   Counseling Gloria

If you were to counsel Gloria, how would your knowledge of her development help you in the strategies you used?

5.   Counseling Joe

If you were to counsel Joe, how would your knowledge of his development help you in the strategies you used?

6.   Understanding Defense Mechanisms

Provide an example of each of the following defense mechanisms:

1. Repression _____

_____

_____

2. Denial _____

_____

_____

3. Projection _____

_____

_____

4. Rationalization _____

_____

_____

5. Regression _____

_____

_____

7. Examining Defenses People Use

Can you think of other kinds of defenses people use to protect themselves from past pains and current hurts?

1. _____   _____

_____

_____

2. _____   _____

_____

_____

3. _____   _____

_____

_____

4. _____   _____

_____

_____

8.   Developmental Differences between Men and Women

Using the concepts as presented by Kohlberg and Gilligan, discuss
your views on how men and women approach moral reasoning. What
differences and/or similarities do you see between how men and
women approach morality?

9.   Examining Differing Perspectives on Abnormal Behavior

Respond to the following statements concerning abnormal behavior.

1. Using a *situational* point of view, make an argument for abnormal
   behavior being a function of one's surroundings.

2. Using a personality development perspective, make an argument
   for abnormal behavior being a function of early child rearing.

3. Using the perspective of Laing and Szaz, make an argument that
   abnormal behavior is a normal reaction to stressful life events.

4. Using a genetic and biological orientation, make an argument for
   abnormal behavior being determined.

10.   Using the *DSM III–R*

Go to your college library reserve desk and obtain a copy of the *DSM
III–R*. Pick one diagnostic category and review the behavioral charac-
teristics of that disorder along with possible etiology of that disorder.
In class, discuss the varying diagnostic categories you found.

6

Systems: What Are They, and How Do We Work with Them?

General Systems Theory
Boundaries and Information Flow in Systems

Family Systems
The Development of the Healthy Family / Dysfunctional Families / Family Guidance, Family Counseling, and the Role of the Human Service Worker / Individual Counseling versus Family Counseling

Group Systems
A Brief History / Defining Support Groups, Guidance Groups, and Counseling and Therapy Groups / Group Membership Behavior / Group Leadership Styles / Stages of Group Development

Community Systems
Society and Subcultures / Social Service Systems: America's Response to Inequities / Understanding the Social Service System in Which You Work

Ethical and Professional Issues
The System and Confidentiality / Rules of Group Behavior / Training and Competence

The Developmentally Mature Human Service Worker: Using a Systems Approach in Understanding the Complexity of Interrelationships

Summary

Experiential Exercises

The concept of *system* thus treats people and events in terms of their interactions rather than their intrinsic characteristics. The most basic principle underlying the systems viewpoint has been understood for some time. An ancient astronomer once said, "Heaven is more than the stars alone. It is the stars and their movements." (Baruth & Huber, 1984, p. 19)

My sister is 5 years older than I, my brother 5 years younger. My father, who died when I was 26 years old, was a hard-working, kind, thoughtful man, somewhat on the quiet side and not particularly expressive of his feelings. My mom was (and still is) a nurturing, sometimes opinionated yet mostly supportive woman on whom we could always rely in time of need. Both my parents were college educated and first generation in this country.

Dinner was a very special time for my family. My mother (and sometimes my sister) would prepare dinner while the rest of us would watch television in the den. During dinner we would often have lively discussions about politics or other contemporary issues. As much as I loved these family interactions, I clearly remember being both overwhelmed by and particularly in awe of my sister's ability to argue her point of view. Because I was sickly as a child and overweight, my self-esteem was not very high. Although I loved the family interactions, I had a sense that I could not hold my own in the nightly discussions; I would often find myself going inward to my feelings rather than relying on my intellectual ability during these nightly discussions. I remember arguing over such issues as capital punishment and the war in Vietnam. My arguments often became very passionate because I had become comfortable in the feeling world and less comfortable presenting a factual argument. It seems as if we began to take on particular roles in the family—my father being the strong yet quiet debater; my sister, the verbally fluid family member; my mom, the mediator; me, the passionate member; and my brother, being the youngest and perhaps because the feeling and verbal roles were already taken, seemed on the quiet side. There was a kind of balance in the family. Things seemed a little off if we suddenly were out of our family roles. Perhaps it's not surprising that my sister became a lawyer; I, a mental-health professional; and my brother, an engineer—professions that match the personality characteristics of the roles we chose.

My first therapeutic experience was in a counseling group in college. It is not accidental that I was the advocate for "expression of feelings," for invariably the roles we took on as children in our families are repeated in these groups. A woman of that same group, who had always taken on what might be considered male qualities, wanted to experiment with her feminine side. Therefore, she decided to try to act more feminine in the group. A third member of the group was always considered the outcast in school. He quickly took on this role in the group, and the group leader helped him examine why this continually happened to him.

My first real job was at a street-front crisis and drop-in center. There we would often have homeless people seeking shelter. These people, most of whom had abusive or deprived childhoods, were often unkempt and uneducated, and many had emotional problems. Unfortunately, because of their inability to communicate effectively, which many times was a function of early roles played out in their families of origin, they would sabotage their attempts to receive aid from local social agencies. I remember when we hired Vanessa, a woman who had been on welfare herself, how effective she was in helping these individuals work with the local social service systems.

When I accepted my current job at Old Dominion University, I discovered that a colleague of mine, Garrett, had grown up in an Irish-American neighborhood a few miles from my predominantly Jewish neighborhood in Queens. I had not even known that his neighborhood existed. Despite the fact that we both were brought up close to each other, our neighborhoods were so insulated that there was little shared between these cultures. These closely knit neighborhoods had somewhat rigid boundaries that prevented a sharing of cultural wealth.

What do all of the above vignettes have in common? They all are expressions of the complex interactions in systems. From the family systems in which we grew up, to the groups in which we now interact, to the community and organizational systems in which we live and work, systems play an important role in our lives. In fact, in a recent survey of graduates of human service programs, a vast majority of respondents rated knowledge of organizations, families, and groups as particularly significant (Sweitzer & McKinney, 1991).

In this chapter, we will examine how human service workers can use knowledge of systems to enhance their work with clients. In addition, we will discuss ethical and professional issues related to working in systems. Finally, we will examine the importance of understanding the complex interactions of systems for the developmentally mature human service worker.

General Systems Theory

Although knowledge of the amoeba may seem like a far cry from our understanding of systems, in actuality there is much we can learn from this one-celled animal. The amoeba has semipermeable boundaries that allow it to take in nutrition from the environment. This delicate animal could not survive if its boundaries were too rigid or too permeable. Boundaries that are too rigid would prevent it from ingesting food, and boundaries that are too loose would not allow the amoeba to maintain and digest the food it has found. "Living systems are processes that maintain a persistent structure of relatively long periods despite rapid exchange of their component parts with the surrounding world . . ." (Skynner, 1976, pp. 3–4).

General systems theory was developed to explain the complex interactions of all types of systems including living systems, family systems, and community systems (Bertalanffy, 1934, 1968). Each system has a boundary that allows it to maintain its structure while the system interacts with other systems around it. Thus, the action of the amoeba, a small living system, affects the surrounding environment. Similarly, the action of a family unit will affect other families with which it interacts, and the action of a community group will affect other aspects of the community.

Components in a system tend to maintain their typical ways of functioning, whether those actions within the system are functional or dysfunctional. A much-used analogy is that of the thermostat in the house. When the temperature drops in the house, the thermostat, based on the temperature setting, switches on. If the thermostat is set for 70 degrees and the temperature drops below that, the heater turns on. However, if the thermostat is set for 40 degrees, the heater will not turn on until the temperature drops below 40 degrees. This tendency toward equilibrium is called **homeostasis**.

In families and in groups, members take on typical ways of behaving, regardless of whether these typical patterns are dysfunctional. Because families and groups become comfortable with their typical ways of behaving, members in these systems will exert covert or overt pressure to have atypical behaviors suppressed. For instance, it was unusual for any member of my family to express anger. When I was a teenager, the few times I got very angry I distinctly remember my mother saying "I don't understand why you're so angry; maybe we should take you to see a psychologist." My anger was atypical (as opposed to wrong), and the family system was attempting to deal with this unusual behavior of mine.

Boundaries and Information Flow in Systems

A healthy system has **semipermeable boundaries** that allow new information to enter the system and be processed and incorporated. When a system has **rigid boundaries**, information cannot flow easily into or out of the system, and the system has difficulty with the change process. Alternatively, a system that has **loose boundaries** allows information to flow too easily into and out of the system, resulting in the individual components of the system having difficulty maintaining a sense of identity.

Regardless of whether the system has semipermeable, rigid, or loose boundaries, the regulatory mechanism of the system maintains the homeostasis. Therefore, finding families and community groups (for example, religious organizations) with a fairly rigid set of rules that maintains their functioning in relatively healthy ways is not unusual. Alternatively, there are also families and community groups that allow for a wide range of behaviors within the system (for example, encounter groups). Although American culture allows for much variation in the permeability of various systems, systems that have very rigid or very loose boundaries have a tendency toward dysfunction. Sometimes these systems have disastrous results when breakdown occurs (see the story of Jim Jones).

Jim Jones and the Death of a Rigid System

In the 1950s and early 1960s, Jim Jones was a respected Methodist minister in Indiana. However, Jones soon became increasingly paranoid and grandiose, believing he was Jesus. He moved his family to Brazil and later relocated to California where approximately 100 of his church followers from Indiana joined him. In California he headed the People's Church, and he began to set more rigid rules for church membership. Slowly, he became more dictatorial and continued to show evidence of paranoid delusions. He insisted that church members prove their love for him, demanding sexual intercourse with female church members, having members sign over their possessions, sometimes having them give their children to him, and having members inform on those who broke his rules. In 1975 a reporter uncovered some of the tactics Jones was using and was about to write a revealing article about the church. Jones learned about this and, just prior to publication of the article, moved to Guyana, taking a few hundred of his followers with him. As concerns about some of the church practices reached the United States, California Congressman Leo Ryan and some of his aides went to Guyana to investigate the situation. Jones and his supporters killed the congressman and his aides. Jones then ordered his followers to commit suicide. Hundreds killed themselves. Those who did not were murdered.

Jones developed a church with a rigid set of rules. The publication of a revealing article as well as the congressman flying into Guyana were threats to the system. As in many rigid systems, attempts at change from the outside were seen as potentially lethal blows to the system. Jones dealt with the reporter's threat to the system by moving his congregation to Guyana. Then, rather than allow new information into the system, Jones killed off the system, first killing the congressman and then ordering church members to commit suicide. The members had become so mired in the rules of the system that nearly 900 of them committed suicide or were murdered. This is a tragic example of how dysfunctional a rigid system can be.

Family Systems

> Divorce has ripple effects that touch not just the family involved, but our entire society. As the writer Pat Conroy observed when his own marriage broke up, 'Each divorce is the death of a small civilization.' When one family divorces, that divorce affects relatives, friends, neighbors, employers, teachers, clergy, and scores of strangers. (Wallerstein & Blakeslee, 1989, p. xxi)

Today, nearly 50% of marriages end in divorce. So great is the impact of divorce on the family that Wallerstein and Blakeslee (1989) found that in a 5-year follow-up of children of divorce, a great majority of them were still negatively affected by the breakup of their parents' marriage. They also found that the effects of divorce can have a major impact on the children as they grow into adulthood. Families are systems, and each unique family system affects other systems around it. In this section, we will explore the family system, how it functions and dysfunctions, and the roles of human service workers in their encounters with families.

The Development of the Healthy Family

As in all systems, healthy family systems have semipermeable boundaries. A healthy family system allows information to flow in, evaluates the information, and through healthy communication channels, makes

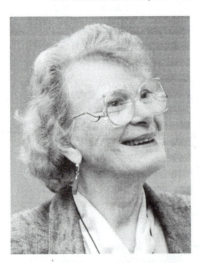

Virginia Satir, world-renowned family therapist (1916–1988), noted that the actions of one family member resonate throughout the family system.

changes as needed. A healthy family has parents or guardians who are the main rule makers (a healthy family system can also have a single parent or guardian). Although rules will change from family to family, healthy families have a clear sense of hierarchy. This means that the parents are the main rule makers and children, although possibly consulted in the rule making, are the recipients of those rules. Virginia Satir (1967) noted that when one member of the family feels pain, the whole family is affected. This is because the family is a system with a delicate homeostasis and the actions of one member resonate throughout the whole system.

Minuchin (1974) sees families as going through **situational crises** and **developmental cycles**. He states that families may face unexpected problems that are situationally specific *and* will encounter predict-

A Situational Family Crisis

When I was between the ages of 8 and 13, I had a heart disorder called pericarditis. This was a somewhat debilitating illness that enlarged my heart, caused me much chest pain, and left me periodically bedridden with a resulting mild depression. Although not considered extremely serious, this illness certainly affected my life in a major way. However, it also affected my parents' lives and the lives of my siblings.

Although my illness potentially could have been a threat to the homeostasis in the family, it became clear that the family was strong enough to deal effectively with this situation. Because my parents' marriage was solid, the added stress did not dramatically affect their relationship. In addition, they were able to maintain the functioning of the family in a relatively normal way. This normalization of family patterns during a period of stress speaks highly of the strength of the family.

able struggles as the family ages and goes through the life stages. For example, when a couple has their first child, the husband/wife dyad faces its first potential crisis. The husband and wife will face a disruption in their relationship because rules in their family change in order to deal with the new family member. As children age, families will continually face developmental crises (see Chapter 5) that necessitate changes in family rules. A healthy family has the mechanism to successfully pass through these developmental stages. Like Satir, Minuchin notes that when one member of the family is affected by a situational crisis or developmental milestone, the whole family is affected. If the family has healthy ways of communicating and if the family can support one another as individual members go through changes, then the family will survive in a healthy manner.

Dysfunctional Families

All husbands and wives bring to their marriage **unfinished business** from their pasts. Invariably, this unfinished business will affect their relationship. The more serious the issue, the more likely it will affect their marriage and, from a systems point of view, affect the family. A wife who was sexually molested as a child and has not worked through her pain will undoubtedly bring this unfinished business into the relationship. For instance, she might have developed mistrust of men and therefore unconsciously chosen a man who is distant (and safe). Perhaps he is a "workaholic." Alternatively, a man who has difficulty with intimacy might unconsciously pick a wife who allows him to be distant (and safe). As the relationship unravels, each spouse's issues get played out either on one another or on the child. The husband may become stressed out at work and take this out on his wife and/or children. The wife may crave more intimacy, become discontent with the marriage, and take this out on her husband and/or children. Is it surprising that there are so many affairs and divorces?

When spouses are discontented with each other and when they unconsciously take out their anger on a child rather than work it through with each other, that child is said to be a **scapegoat**. When a member of the family is scapegoated, he or she often becomes the **identified patient** in the family, or the member that is identified as the "one with the problem." In actuality, the whole family has the problem. When a

An Example of a Dysfunctional Family

When I was in private practice as a psychologist, a 12-year-old boy was referred to me by his school counselor because his grades had dropped considerably and he was acting out in school. I asked him and his parents to come in for family counseling. For the first 2 months, the parents insisted that everything was fine in their marriage. As I continued to explore the situation, I could not understand why this boy was doing so poorly in school and was demonstrating such a dramatic personality shift. Then, during one session, the father revealed to me that he was extremely depressed—in fact, suicidally depressed. His depression stemmed back to his childhood. Soon, the mother revealed that she was bulimic, and later I discovered she was having an affair. The secretness of the father's depression and the mother's bulimia and affair were symptoms of deep discontent in the marriage, and all stemmed back to issues in their childhoods.

Rather than dealing with these very painful issues with each other, the couple had taken out their discontent on their oldest child. They did this through the mother becoming overly protective, the father becoming overly distant, and, whenever they would get angry at each other, both focusing on their son's problems. When the school tried to involve them in assisting the boy, they sabotaged whatever they were asked to do, as if they had something at stake in keeping him the identified patient. In essence, as long as he was seen as the one "with the problem," they did not have to deal with their problems. As soon as they became aware of what they were doing, the mother became less protective, the father became closer with his son, and the couple stopped "scapegoating" their son and began to deal with their own issues. The son's acting-out behaviors immediately stopped, and his grades improved dramatically.

child acts out in the family, in school, or in the community, it is often the result of that child being the member carrying the pain for the family.

Family Guidance, Family Counseling, and the Role of the Human Service Worker

Therapists who do **family counseling** have in-depth knowledge of family systems and how to facilitate change in the family. Such counseling often involves the whole family being involved in intensive family sessions. Although human service workers do not have the training to do family counseling, knowledge of family systems can help them provide family guidance. Family guidance does not include intensive family counseling; however, human service workers may refer to family counselors, suggest workshops to attend, offer reading materials regarding how families interact, and give basic advice on family matters. It is important that the human service worker makes an assessment about the seriousness of the family dysfunction and acts accordingly.

Individual Counseling versus Family Counseling

When should a family member be referred to individual counseling as opposed to the whole family being referred for family counseling? Although some therapists might suggest it is always appropriate to refer the whole family for counseling rather than just one member (Napier & Whitaker, 1978; Satir, 1967), most therapists today agree that it is often a matter of making a decision based on an assessment of the situation. For instance, a child who comes from an extremely dysfunctional family may be better off seeing a therapist individually because working with the family may be an extremely long process whereas individual counseling may give some immediate relief to the child. Or it may be prudent to refer a spouse for individual counseling to work on his or her unfinished business because this will facilitate change in the whole family. Also, individual members in a family will often seek out individual counseling *while* the family undergoes family treatment. If you are unsure what might be the best referral for a client, seek advice from a more experienced human service professional.

Group Systems

Like members of families, group members will bring in their unfinished business, which may cause problems in the healthy functioning of the group. Groups tend to create their own homeostasis, and members may be scapegoated in this process. Therefore, when a group member is scapegoated, he or she is reflecting problems within the whole system. Although community and social groups have always existed, groups whose intent is to explore human interaction are relatively new.

A Brief History

Gladding notes that prior to 1900 the purpose of group treatment was to assist individuals in very "functional and pragmatic ways" (1991, p. 4). This often revolved around helping people with daily living skills and arose out of the social group work movement where individuals like Jane Addams organized group discussions that centered on such things as personal hygiene, nutrition, and self-determination (Pottick, 1988). Using groups as their vehicle, social reformers like Addams were particularly concerned with community organizing as an effort to assist the poor.

At the turn of the century, schools began to offer "Vocational and Moral Guidance" in group settings. These efforts were often "preachy" in their nature, and group members had little opportunity to discuss personal matters in reflective ways. However, with the spread of psychotherapeutic theory and with the beginnings of sociological concepts concerning group interactions, the first use of counseling and therapy groups that had more of an introspective nature arose in the 1920s and 1930s. (Gladding, 1991).

In the 1940s the modern group movement emerged. It was during this decade that Carl Rogers brought together therapists to discuss what problems they might encounter in working with returning war veterans. He soon found that within this group setting there was a deepening of expression of feeling and, in many instances, an uncovering of new awarenesses concerning themselves. Thus began the **encounter group** movement (Rogers, 1970). At about the same time, Kurt Lewin and other nationally known theorists developed the **National Training Laboratory** (NTL) to examine **group dynamics** or the ways in which groups tend to interact (Capuzzi & Gross, 1992; Shaffer & Galinsky, 1974). NTL still exists today and continues to train individuals in understanding the special dynamics of groups. Over the years, many different types of groups with unique characteristics have arisen. For instance, we have seen the proliferation of support groups, guidance groups, and counseling and therapy groups.

Defining Support Groups, Guidance Groups, and Counseling and Therapy Groups

Although systems dynamics occur in all groups, there are some differences in the functioning of support groups, guidance groups, and counseling and therapy groups (Trotzer, 1989). However, regardless of the type of group, all groups have rules regarding membership behavior, leadership style, technical issues (for example, when and where to meet, number of group members, length of meeting times), and ground rules (for example, limits of confidentiality, socializing outside of the group, nature and purpose of the group).

Support groups and personal growth groups. The growth of **support groups** in this country has been phenomenal over the past 20 years. From Alcoholics Anonymous (AA), to codependency groups, to eating disorder and diet groups, to men's and women's groups, to support groups for the chronically mentally ill, the kinds of support groups that have emerged seems endless. Their purpose is the education and affirmation of the group member. Usually, a leader focuses the discussion and helps define the rules of the group. Support groups are *not* indepth psychotherapy groups and therefore do not require a vast amount of self-disclosure. Instead, they usually encourage individuals to reveal only that amount that feels comfortable for the member. In fact, many of these groups might discourage intense self-disclosure because that would be more appropriate for individual or group counseling. Support groups are generally free or have a nominal fee and can be facilitated by a trained layperson or mental-health professional.

A Men's Support Group

For the past 1-1/2 years, I have been a participant in a men's support group. This group was started by 10 men who had an interest in discussing issues particularly relevant to our maleness. Although there has been no defined leader, we have all taken a leadership role at various times. When we first started meeting, we defined some of the rules of our group. We decided *not* to have designated topics to discuss (although generally, the discussions revolve around male issues—for example, relationships with women, how men express feelings, our relationships with our fathers). We decided to meet every Sunday for 2 hours and use our homes as a meeting place on a rotating basis. We also decided that we would not share details of our talks with others outside the group, although we felt it was all right to talk in generalities about what we discussed in our group. Our group has afforded each of us a place where we can feel supported, discuss issues about being male, and receive feedback about ourselves from other group members. Although, as in all groups, we have had our ups and downs, generally we all agree that the group has been a positive experience.

Personal growth groups are special kinds of support group. These groups arose in the 1970s and were known by a variety of names including sensitivity-training groups, encounter groups, and human relations groups (Yalom, 1985). Although the names might vary, they basically had the same goal: to offer support to the group members while encouraging expression of feeling and exploration of individual dynamics. Although there often is a designated leader, some personal growth groups can be leaderless, originated by a group of individuals who have a desire for self-reflection. One can find such groups in many settings including college counseling settings, private agencies, community centers, and even as required courses in undergraduate and graduate programs in the helping professions.

With support groups and personal growth groups, the number of group members, length of meeting times, and atmosphere of the group setting can vary considerably. Some groups might have 200 members, whereas others might be limited to just a few people. Some groups might meet in the basement of a church, whereas others might meet in the comforts of a therapist's office. Support groups might be ongoing, others may be time-limited, and some might demand confidentiality, whereas others will not.

Guidance groups. As opposed to support groups, **guidance groups** always have a designated, well-trained group leader and generally have as their purpose the education and support of the group member. Leaders will usually offer a *didactic* presentation, and although there is *not* much in-depth self-disclosure, there may be an opportunity for some sharing of personal information. With their purpose being more educational than psychotherapeutic, the end result of this group is to increase knowledge on the part of the member. Such groups may be ongoing or can occur on a one-time basis. Guidance groups can vary

An AIDS Guidance Group

Jonathan is a human service worker who works for the local AIDS awareness center. His main job is to go to local schools, businesses, and community centers, presenting workshops on how one contracts HIV, current diagnostic procedures for HIV, and treatment of AIDS. His 2-hour workshop is information-based, and he allows time for questions and self-disclosure when appropriate. When requested, he will extend his presentation for one to four additional meetings. He also provides referrals to AIDS support groups and to therapists who work with HIV-positive individuals, their families, and their friends.

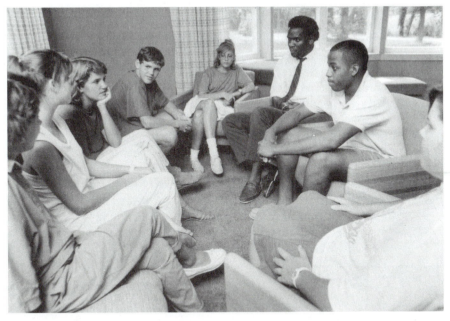

Groups can offer a safe environment in which one can share feelings and gain feedback about oneself.

in their length, and other technical issues can also vary depending on the focus of the group. Like support groups, guidance groups may be free of charge; however, some guidance groups involve a fee.

Counseling and therapy groups.   Like individual counseling and therapy, many people differentiate a **counseling group** from a **therapy group** by the depth of self-disclosure and the amount of personality reconstruction expected during the therapeutic process. However, counseling and therapy groups probably have more similarities than differences. For instance, both counseling and therapy groups have a designated highly trained leader. Generally, there are between 4 and 12 group members. Such groups usually meet for a minimum of eight sessions, and some may continue on an ongoing basis. Most counseling and therapy groups meet at least once a week for 1–3 hours, and confidentiality of the group is a must in that individual members are asked not to reveal information about other members outside the group. Although leadership styles may vary, members usually will have the opportunity to freely express their feelings and to eventually work on behavioral change. Many of the counseling and therapy approaches noted in Chapter 3 have been adapted for this group process.

William's Therapy Group

William has been struggling his whole life with mild depression. Upon getting married 2 years ago, he thought he would "feel better." However, after an initial period of "being pretty mellow," his depressive feelings again began to emerge. He entered individual counseling and began to work on some of his issues, discovering that he often had expectations that women in his life would bring him happiness. He found that he often relies on them for comfort and nurturing and becomes upset when they do not meet his needs. After some initial gain in self-awareness during individual counseling, his therapist suggested that he might want to enter a mixed (male and female) counseling group to experiment with new ways of relating to women. Although he has found this to be difficult, as he continues to build trust in the group, he is beginning to examine his behaviors more closely and explore new ways of relating.

Group Membership Behavior

We all have typical ways of behaving in life. These typical patterns are repeated in groups as they are in our daily interactions with friends and acquaintances. Therefore, groups are often called *minilabs* of our world, and they give us the opportunity to look at how we present ourselves to others. In addition, they allow us to obtain feedback about our typical ways of interacting. In counseling, therapy, and support groups, we will often be given the opportunity to examine these behaviors and work on changing those that we might identify as maladaptive. As members pass through the stages of group development, their typical patterns of behavior will emerge. Some group specialists have identified certain characteristics or roles taken on by members (Vander Kolk, 1990). For instance, some members may be dominators, mediators, manipulators, caretakers, nurturers, or facilitators, whereas other members may be withdrawn, hostile, or opinionated. These are just a few of the types of roles members may assume. Can you think of others?

Members may take on differing roles as the group process continues. The various stages of group development may affect individuals in differing ways. For example, whereas some members may be withdrawn near the beginning stages of group, others may become withdrawn at later stages.

Group Leadership Styles

Although leadership styles will vary depending on the leader's theoretical orientation (Gladding, 1991), all leaders need to be aware of basic group theory and process to facilitate groups appropriately (Brown, 1992). Therefore, knowledge of systems, familiarity with membership roles, awareness of group stages of development, and adeptness at basic as well as advanced counseling techniques are crucial. Good leaders are aware of the composition of their group and have adjusted their style to the needs of the group. A good leader will be strong without being authoritarian, knowledgeable about the rules and technical issues, yet flexible in the ways they are implemented. He or she can facilitate the interactions of the group members as they pass through the stages of group development. Such a leader feels comfortable working with a vast array of member behaviors and can set the stage for the group to unfold in a natural way.

Stages of Group Development

Over the years, many authors have identified typical stages of group development (Gladding, 1991; Tuckman & Jensen, 1977; Ward, 1982; Yalom, 1985). Although the terms for these stages vary from author to author, general characteristics of membership behavior are exhibited as group members pass through these stages.

The initial stage. This beginning stage of group behavior is often highlighted by anxiety and apprehension on the part of group members (and to a lesser degree, by the group leader). Members are learning about the rules and goals of their group and are wondering whether they can trust the other members. Because of this initial apprehension, members will often avoid talking about in-depth feelings, and discussions are relatively safe. Corey and Corey call this "self focus vs. other focus" (1987, p. 115). Therefore, members commonly talk about things not related to their lives.

During this initial stage, group members are often self-conscious, worried about how others might view them. The major task for the group leader is to define the ground rules and to build trust. In building trust, the ability to set limits, to use empathy, and to show unconditional positive regard is crucial. As members become comfortable with the ground rules and as they begin to feel comfortable with one another, they move on to the next stage of group development.

The transition stage. During the beginning phase of the transition stage, group members understand the goals and rules of the group but continue to maintain anxiety concerning the group process. This anxiety is sometimes manifested by hostility toward other members or the leader. Hostility during this stage can be viewed as a type of resistance that gives members a way to avoid dealing with their issues. The leader needs to be aware of any scapegoating that may occur as one manifestation of this hostility. Although empathy is still crucial, the leader must actively prevent a member from being scapegoated or attacked. Therefore, the leader will often take an active role in preventing coalitions from forming and in preventing verbal attacks on members.

As this stage continues, group members begin to settle in and can focus more on themselves. This is highlighted by a sense of self-acceptance of the member's life predicaments. Members now demonstrate the ability to take ownership of their feelings, to talk in the here and now, and to not blame others for their problems. This is an important step toward actually making change that occurs in the next stage. As members move into this part of the transition stage and begin to take more responsibility for their feelings and actions, the leader's role becomes much easier. No longer is it necessary for the leader to "protect" members, and during this part of the transition stage the leader can usually relax and let the group develop on its own.

The work stage.   As group members gain the capacity to take ownership for their feelings and life predicaments, a deepening of trust and a sense of cohesion emerge within the group. Members experience a sense of readiness to work on their identified problem areas. During this stage, the group has developed its own homeostasis. Now it is important that the group leader prohibit members from becoming too comfortable in their styles of relating because this can prevent change and growth. Members readily give feedback to other members, and as they identify problem areas, they begin to take an active role in the change process. It is at this point that members might attempt new ways of communicating, acting, or expressing feelings. The leader can best facilitate movement by asking questions, using problem-solving skills, giving advice, offering alternatives, encouraging feedback by members, and affirming members' attempts at change.

As members accomplish their goals, they begin to gain a sense of high self-esteem. This is a product of receiving positive feedback from other members as well as a personal sense of accomplishment for the work that they have done. As members meet their goals, they are near the completion of the group process.

The closure stage.   As group members reach their identified goals, there is an increased sense of accomplishment and the beginning awareness that the group process is near completion. During this stage, the leader will often summarize the learning that has taken place and begin to focus on the separation process. Because members typically have shared deep aspects of themselves, a sense of togetherness, cohesion, and warmth has developed. Therefore, saying good-bye can be a difficult process for many, and it is important that the leader facilitate this process in a direct yet gentle fashion. Often this is done by members sharing what they have learned about themselves and one another, through expression of feeling toward one another, and by defining future goals for themselves. This important final stage in the group process allows members to feel a sense of completion and wholeness about what they have experienced.

The leader might actively encourage members to express their feelings concerning the group process as well as their feelings about ending the group. Asking questions and encouraging members to express their feelings might accomplish this. Of course, using empathy to listen to members' feelings regarding the closure of the group is extremely important.

Conclusion.   Whereas all types of groups should pass through these stages to be effective, the depth of work and intensity of feeling expressed will vary depending on the nature of the group. For instance, guidance and support groups will work on more superficial levels as they pass through these stages, whereas counseling and therapy groups will deal with deeper levels of experience for the client; in these groups, the work accomplished will be at the level of personality reconstruction. Therefore, when conducting groups, expectations of group behavior should be partially based on the type of group being offered.

Community Systems

Society and Subcultures

Despite the fact that American society has passed sweeping economic development and civil rights laws, divisions based on culture and economics still exist. In any city, you will find sections that are mostly African-American, Asian-American, Irish-American, Italian-American, wealthy, poor, and so forth. The same rules that govern the functioning of biological, family, group, and social systems operate within these community systems. These rules remain intact because within each subsystem there is shared history and beliefs that create a unique homeostasis that by its nature discourages change (information from the larger system flowing into the smaller system) and because the larger system, society, has a stake in the maintenance of the smaller systems. A breakdown of these smaller community systems would resonate throughout society and create chaos. As most individuals are uncomfortable challenging the status quo (homeostasis), even if it is dysfunctional, the subsystems within society are maintained. This sometimes results in a lack of cross-cultural sharing and in disparities within society. Some argue that these smaller systems are being scapegoated by the larger system (Alinsky, 1971).

Despite many negative aspects attributed to a lack of breakdown of this class system, there are also some positive features. For instance, due to the continued integrity of these systems, the United States is one of the few countries in the world that can truly claim to have a society highlighted by cultural diversity and freedom of expression. Cultural integrity in the thousands of communities around this country allows individuals to experience a sense of belonging and identity within their subculture. It also allows for a wealth of cultural information to be shared with the larger society. We see this diversity in the language (because much of the language is spotted with words and phrases from other cultures), in the foods that are eaten, in the ways that people interact and, more subtly, think about the world.

Social Service Systems: America's Response to Inequities

One way that American culture has attempted to equalize the inequities found throughout society is to provide social service agencies that work with the poor, disabled, and deprived. Many of these agencies offer free or low-cost aid to individuals in need. In almost any community today, we find state and federally supported programs such as mental-health centers, shelters for the homeless, vocational rehabilitation, child protective services, Medicare and Medicaid programs, food stamp programs, Aid to Families with Dependent Children (AFDC), and so forth.

Understanding the Social Service System in Which You Work

In most social service agencies, we can find human service workers providing crucial services to those in need. Their ability to effectively serve client needs is central to American society's attempt to change the face of American culture (Bell, 1987; Richan, 1988). For the human service professionals to work effectively with clients within these agencies, they must clearly understand the rules, the hierarchy, and the information flow within the system. Hopefully, the system in which you may work will be healthy in that it has semipermeable boundaries, which allow for information to come into the system from other systems. This allows for flexibility and change.

Knowledge of hierarchies in systems is important when the human service worker needs consultation concerning a client. Not consulting with a supervisor can create animosity and can prevent additional feedback concerning client problems. This ultimately can be detrimental to the helping process. Sometimes, the system's rules may be contrary to your ethical guidelines. For instance, a system may have a rule that any use of illegal substances on the part of the client should be reported to the police. Because this rule is contrary to the ethical guidelines of confidentiality, the human service worker needs to make adjustments to work within the system under these rules while discussing this discrepancy with the supervisor and/or other administrative individuals.

Once you understand the system's rules, the hierarchy, and the information flow, you are ready to get to work. This usually involves a number of steps including diagnosing client problems, assessing client needs, setting client goals, making appropriate referrals, and following up.

Diagnosing client problems.   Whenever you first meet with a client, a thorough diagnosis of the problem is needed. With a good diagnostic interview, you may find that what the client presents as the problem is not the major source of stress. For instance, Dawn comes into a community health service complaining of heart palpitations and depression. Following a physical that reveals no medical problems, you interview Dawn and discover that she is a single parent with five children, who has not been able to secure employment. Additionally, she has had difficulty finding daycare for her two youngest children who are not of school age. You discover further that the added stress in her life has caused her to have a "short fuse" with her children. She recently has moved to the area and is not aware that she is entitled to receive AFDC. You assess that her unemployment and her financial concerns, coupled with her concerns for her children, are the cause of her great stress and account for her presenting complaints.

When diagnosing client problems, using the counseling skills identified in Chapter 4 is important. Therefore, empathy, effective questioning techniques and listening skills, encouragement, challenge with support, modeling, self-disclosure, and problem-solving skills are essential ingredients to diagnosing the client's problem.

Assessing client needs.   Assessing client needs is a natural outgrowth of the diagnostic interview. After you have determined what client problems are most pressing, making a hierarchy of client needs is important. This is often done informally; however, with some clients who have numerous concerns, writing a list of client needs in order of importance may be appropriate. In the case of Dawn, client needs might include reducing stress, defining career goals, and finding ways to deal effectively with her children.

Setting client goals. As the needs hierarchy is identified, you are ready to help the client set goals. This step should be a consultative process; that is, you and your client discuss what goals seem reasonable and reachable. Many human service workers will make a **contract,** either verbally or in writing, that describes client goals. This acts as a reinforcer and a reminder to clients about their stated goals. Goals can be redefined at any time, and clients sometimes do not attain their goals due to a misdiagnosis of the problem. For Dawn, her goals might include accomplishing a career assessment, finding appropriate outlets for her stress, and establishing daycare for her children.

Making appropriate referrals. A major part of setting goals for the client is making appropriate referrals. To make such referrals, human service workers must be familiar with local, state, and federal agencies. There are many agencies established to assist individuals with their concerns. For instance, one community services directory of the Tidewater, Virginia, area has over 600 listings of community agencies (McCarthy, 1991). With so many agencies to choose from, being familiar with your local community support system is extremely important. In making referrals for Dawn, you may include the state employment office, the local AFDC office, community and civic groups that might assist a family in need, and perhaps the local mental-health center.

Following up. The work of the human service worker is not finished when the client leaves the office. Follow-up to ensure that clients have accomplished their goals is important for a number of reasons. First, some clients may come across roadblocks and, for various reasons, may feel uncomfortable coming back for additional assistance. Second, follow-up can act as a means of encouraging clients to meet their goals. Finally, follow-up can help human service workers assess the quality of work they have done. Follow-up may be done by a phone call, a letter, or a more involved assessment (see Chapter 8 for more detail on assessment). With Dawn, accomplishing her goals would mean a decrease in stress and depression, more effective parenting, and employment. For you, the human service worker, her accomplishment would mean that the work done with Dawn was effective.

Ethical and Professional Issues

The System and Confidentiality

Human service workers have a responsibility to protect the confidentiality of the client, whether it be in individual, group, or family counseling. The proposed ethical guidelines of NOHSE/CSHSE state that "the client has a right to confidentiality except when such confidentiality would cause harm to the client or to others" (see Appendix A). However, the guidelines go on to state that confidentiality may be limited by agency guidelines or by local, state, and/or federal laws. Therefore, it is the responsibility of human service workers to be aware of any agency regulations and of laws that may affect their work with clients in respect to confidentiality.

When working with groups or families, human service workers can assure clients that they will not break confidentiality except in the above circumstances; however, human service workers cannot ensure that group or family members will uphold such standards. Therefore, when working with groups or families, stressing that confidentiality be maintained is important. When the human service worker becomes aware that a group or family member has broken confidentiality, appropriate action must be taken. Such action may be simply to discuss the breaking of confidentiality; however, with more extreme cases in a group, a specific member may be asked to leave the group. Any such action should be done after careful reflection and with sensitivity to the client and the group.

In social service systems, client confidentiality also must be maintained. This means that your work with clients should *not* be discussed with your colleagues unless it is for consultative or supervisory reasons. The proposed ethical guidelines of NOHSE/CSHSE state: "Although employers and supervisors have the right to all knowledge concerning client/human service worker interaction, they should attempt to respect the integrity of the confidential nature of the human services worker/client relationship." (See Appendix A.)

Finally, if human service workers are sharing information concerning their clients with other mental-health professionals, a signed release-of-information form should be obtained from the client prior to the sharing of such information. In addition, all client records should be secured so that only employers and supervisors have access to such records (see NOHSE/CSHSE proposed ethical guidelines, Appendix A).

Rules of Group Behavior

Depending on the type of group you are leading, rules may vary. Rules are often determined by the leader but can be altered after consultation with the group members. In determining the rules of the group, the following questions should be considered:

- What are the limits of confidentiality?
- Can members socialize outside the group?
- Can members date outside the group?

- What expectations do you have concerning attendance in group sessions?

- What expectations do you have concerning self-disclosure of members?

- What are the repercussions and limits of physical acting out during group sessions?

- Are there expectations concerning the types of things to be discussed during group sessions?

- What expectations do you have concerning members being punctual and staying for the whole group meeting?

- What expectations do you have concerning how members communicate during group sessions?

- What is your responsibility to a member and to the group should you suspect that a specific member might cause harm to himself, herself, or others?

- What other agency rules might determine specific conduct within the group?

Any group rules that are determined by the leader should be clearly defined to the group members. Members can then give their informed consent to these rules or decide that they do not want to participate under such conditions.

Training and Competence

The proposed ethical guidelines of NOHSE/CSHSE state that "human service workers should know the limit and scope of their professional knowledge and seek consultation, supervision, and/or referrals when appropriate" (see Appendix A). Therefore, when working with families or groups, human service workers need to know the limits of their professional competence.

Many human service workers have the training to lead guidance and support groups, but, generally, counseling and therapy groups should be left to more highly trained professionals. Similarly, human service workers are not trained to do family counseling and family therapy but may offer family guidance as an aspect of the human service worker's job function. In either case, when human service workers believe that their training is not at the level to work effectively with specific clients, they need to either refer those clients to other mental-health professionals and/or seek out supervision and consultation (Cogan, 1989).

Finally, all of our training does not take place in school. Depending on the circumstance, additional training can be gained through workshops or other continuing education activities. Ultimately, human service workers need to carefully review the helping relationships in which they are working and decide whether their training is adequate for each specific situation.

The Developmentally Mature Human Service Worker: Using a Systems Approach in Understanding the Complexity of Interrelationships

Developmentally mature human service workers do not view clients in isolation, unaffected by the systems in which they interact, but instead understand the complexity of the interactions in the clients' world. Mature human service workers understand that families, groups, and social systems have a large impact on the client. Therefore, they view depression, anxiety, economic deprivation, acting out behavior, and so forth as both symptoms of client problems and as issues related to the systems in which clients interact. Many times I have seen human service workers make statements such as "that client just has no motivation to change; he will do nothing for himself." If one were to take an individualistic view of this client, then such statements may seem to be true. However, human service workers who view clients as being affected by the systems around them understand the power that such systems may have on the behavior of clients. When working with clients, viewing them from both an individual and systems' perspective is important.

Summary

We examined the complex interactions of systems. General systems theory states that all systems have regulatory mechanisms that maintain their homeostasis. In addition, all systems have boundaries that are rigid, loose, or semipermeable. Members of systems will act covertly or overtly to maintain the homeostasis of the system. Healthy systems change by permitting information to flow into the system and allowing this information to be evaluated by the system.

One system, the family, is affected by situational factors and developmental milestones. Healthy families have semipermeable boundaries that allow for change, and such families can deal with stress if the hierarchical rules are clear. Although all spouses bring in their unfinished business to the family, healthy families can work through these issues, whereas dysfunctional families allow their issues to have a deleterious effect on them. This is often seen as scapegoating of one or more family members, often the children. With some background in understanding systems, human service workers can provide family guidance; family counseling and family therapy, however, are usually reserved for more highly trained therapists.

We also examined a second system, the group. As do all systems, groups develop a homeostasis with rules that govern their behavior. Often, a group leader's role is to gently challenge this homeostatic regulatory mechanism in order to induce change. Support groups, guidance groups, and counseling and therapy groups are three of the major types of groups that facilitate growth for clients. Groups can be viewed as minilabs of the world; that is, typical styles of behavior will be repeated during the group process.

Although all groups can be expected to pass through stages of development, the intensity of change during the process will be partially based on the type of group. Leadership styles will vary from professional to professional and will be based on the type of group being offered. In addition, membership roles in groups will vary, and leaders need to be aware of how to work effectively with different types of member roles. Membership roles will change as the group passes through the stages of group development.

The community system was the final type of system we examined. Systems theory can be applied to communities because they represent smaller systems within the larger system, society. There continue to be large racial and economic divisions in American society, and social service agencies represent one attempt to equalize some of the inequities. The human service workers' effective work with clients within these agencies is one means of ameliorating some of these problems. Effectively working with clients involves a number of steps, which include understanding the system in which you work, diagnosing client problems, assessing client needs, setting goals for your client, making appropriate referrals, and following up.

We also examined the ethical and professional issues of rules of group behavior, confidentiality, and training and competence as they relate to systems. Finally, it was noted that developmentally mature human service workers can use a systems approach in understanding the complexity of the interrelationships of clients' lives.

Experiential Exercises

1.   Reflecting on Your Family of Origin

After reflecting on your family of origin, write responses to the following questions.

1. What roles did your family members take on as your were growing up?

2. Do you think your family had rigid, loose, or semipermeable boundaries?

3. Were there predictable patterns of behavior that you could identify in the various members of your family?

4. What would happen if a member in your family acted differently than expected?

5. Was there a family member who was scapegoated and/or an identified patient?

6. How did your family handle conflict?

7. When your family experienced periods of stress, how was it handled?

8. What situational crises did you or members of your family experience? How was it handled?

9. What developmental cycles did you or members of your family experience? How was it handled?

2. Developing a Group Guidance Program

Develop an outline of a group guidance program on a topic of your choice. Discuss the following issues in the development of your program:

1. The title of the program

2. A brief outline of your program

3. Technical issues related to your program

   a. Number of sessions

   b. Number of clients

   c. Ground rules

   d. Type of meeting place

4. Expected responses of clients as they pass through the group stages of development

5. How you would handle closure of the program

6. Any follow-up you might do

3.   Developing a Support Group Program

Using the outline in Exercise 2, develop a support group program on a topic of your choice.

4.   Working with a Family in Need

Read the following description of a family that sought aid from your agency. Then respond to the questions that follow.

The family. David, Jan and their three children have just moved to the area. They made the move because David thought he would have an easier time finding a job. Having left family and friends, they no longer have the support that they had at their prior residence. They noted that, when they first moved, they were living out of their car and then at the "hotel from hell," but they recently moved into a low-income subsidized housing project.

David is an unemployed construction worker, and Jan works part-time at the local convenience store. David is age 28 and Jan is age 29. They have been married 10 years. Jan states that David "sometimes drinks too much"; David denies this. David states that Jan has "gotten too fat"; Jan admits having gained some weight but states that "David should love me anyway." During your meeting with them, you find that they often argue with each other about work, the children, and Jan's weight.

Mark, the oldest child, is 11 and has been autistic (out of touch with reality) from birth. Jan and David have received disability for him in the past and previously placed him in a residential treatment center. They are unsure about how to care for him now that they have moved. Jordan, who is 9 years old, has had a behavioral problem in school and has been involved in some vandalism in his neighborhood. Jan thinks he may be "drug running" for some of the older kids in the neighborhood. Jordan is entering the third grade (he was held back 1 year at his previous school). David and Jan are unclear on how to register Jordan in his new school. In fact, they're not sure where his new school is located. They describe their youngest child, Jessica, as "their gem." She is 6 years old and entering the first grade. They state that she is the only one who has not caused them problems.

As you work with this family, respond to the following questions:

1. Do you think this family's boundaries are rigid, loose, or semipermeable?

2. Do you think any member(s) of this family is (are) being scapegoated?

3. Is there an identified patient in this family?

4. What counseling skills would you need to work effectively with this family?

5. How would you diagnose the problem areas in this family?

6. What needs does this family have?

7. What goals would you help the family set for itself?

8. What referrals would be appropriate for this family?

9. What type of follow-up would you want to do?

5.   ## Working with an Individual in Need

The following description is of an individual who has sought aid from your agency. Read the description, and then respond to the questions that follow.

Alice. Alice is a 16-year-old single female who is 3 months pregnant. She seeks your advice concerning her pregnancy. She lives with her parents and her 15-year-old sister. She has not told her parents about the pregnancy and is concerned that they will find out before long. Her family has little money, and she is concerned about paying for the pregnancy and birth. Her parents do not have medical insurance.

Alice has come to your agency because she is depressed and feels at the "end of her rope." She is looking for help. When you meet with her, she sobs throughout the interview and at times seems to whine.

Alice's father Arnold, who is 36 years old, is a part-time truck driver. Alice states that he has rigid views and tends to be rather "authoritarian." She also thinks that he will "lose it" if he learns she is pregnant and will want to "take care of the situation" to make it go away. Although he has not abused her in the past 2 years, when she was younger he would often "take a belt to me." At times he drinks too much, and there seem to be conflicts between him and his wife. He was married at age 18.

Alice states that her mother "cares a lot about me"; however, she also notes that her mother would never go against her father's wishes. Alice's mother Linda, who is 35 years old, works part-time at a fast food restaurant and is very concerned about her daughter's well-being. Because she got married when she was pregnant with Alice, Alice thinks that her mother will probably understand her situation.

Joan is Alice's 15-year-old sister. Alice states that Joan is a good student but at time acts like a "wise-ass." She feels as if Joan has always received all the attention in the family; now that she is pregnant,

Alice is concerned that she will be even more of an outcast. Alice notes that Joan has many friends and is often out of the house doing things rather than staying home with her "drunk dad" and her mom.

As you work with Alice, respond to the following questions.

1. What counseling skills would you need to work effectively with Alice?

2. How would you diagnose Alice's problems?

3. What needs does Alice have?

4. What goals would you help Alice set for herself?

5. What referrals would be appropriate for Alice?

6. Would you consider a referral for family counseling or family guidance for Alice and her family?

7. Do you think this family's boundaries are rigid, loose, or semipermeable?

8. Do you think any member(s) of this family is (are) being scapegoated?

9. Is there an identified patient in this family?

10. Would you consider a referral to a group for Alice?

11. What type of group might you consider?

12. What type of follow-up would you want to do?

6.   Wearing Labels

Using the phrases listed below or having your instructor come up with new terms, do the following exercise in class. Have the instructor cut out each of the phrases listed below and tape them on each student's forehead (students should not know which phrase they have on their foreheads). Then find an open space and "mill around," responding to one another based on the phrase you have on your forehead. After a few minutes, sit in a large circle and, without removing the phrase, discuss your response to how people interacted with you.

Look at me intensely.

Walk away from me.

Tell me you like what I'm wearing

Look at my shoes.

Frown at me.

Act as if I don't exist.

Be loving toward me.

Yell at me when I speak.

Speak softly to me.

Be angry at me.

Look at my stomach.

Treat me humanely.

Act as if you like me even
  though you don't.

Touch me when you talk to me.

Act disgusted toward me.

Be nice to me.

Treat me like an object when you
  talk to me.

Be rude to me.

Talk to me but don't listen to me.

Disagree with anything I say.

Reflect back anything I say.

Discuss the following questions:

1. What's it like being labeled?

2. Do we all wear labels as we go through life? (Are there certain personality characteristics that we tend to exhibit?)

3. If we do exhibit certain personality characteristics, is it possible that we create other people's responses to us by the personality characteristics that we exhibit?

4. How can the group process help us understand the labels (personality characteristics) that we tend to exhibit?

7. A Detailed Examination of an Agency

To fully understand the nature of an agency system, a thorough review of its policies and practices is needed. Using the following guidelines, you and a partner pick a social service agency and interview someone who can respond to the items. Write down the individual's responses and compare agencies in class.

1. What is the name of agency?

2. What is the agency's address?

3. What is the number of total staff at the agency?

4. What is the number and type of administrative staff?

5. What are the approximate salaries of administrative staff?

6. What are the number of direct-service personnel (mental-health professionals who work with clients)?

7. What are the types of direct-service personnel (for example, mental-health aides, therapists, supervisors, program coordinators, group leaders, family counselors)?

8. What are the degrees held by direct-service personnel?

9. What are the approximate salaries of direct-service personnel?

10. What are the number and type of support staff (for example, secretaries, clerical staff)?

11. Is this a private or a public agency?

12. Where does the agency get its funding?

13. Does the agency have a policy and practices statement (a written statement that explains the functions of the agency and the roles of the staff)?

14. Who are the clients of this agency?

15. How does the agency obtain its clients?

16. What happens when a client initially contacts this agency?

17. Is there a process where client problems are diagnosed, client needs are assessed, goals are established, referrals are made, and follow-up is accomplished?

18. How do clients pay?

19. What type of counseling and/or assistance takes place at this agency? (for example, individual, group, family)?

20. How long are typical counseling/interviewing sessions?

21. What kind of paperwork is necessary for the direct-service personnel to fill out?

22. How many hours, days, weeks, months, or years would a typical client spend at this agency?

23. How are services for the typical client terminated?

24. How does the agency evaluate itself?

25. Does a staff development effort take place at the agency (for example, in-house workshops, guest speakers, monetary support for conferences)?

26. How does the agency deal with ethical concerns related to confidentiality and counselor training and competence?

27. Does the policy and practices statement of the agency match what is actually going on within the agency?

7

The Human Service Worker in a Pluralistic Society

You scorn us, you imitate us, you blame us, you indulge us, you throw up your hands, you tell us you have all the answers—now shut up and listen. (Lamar, 1992, p. 90)

Growing up in New York was a world unto its own—the ethnic foods, the multicultured music, the people; oh how I loved to watch the people. Walk down a Manhattan street and you could watch a sea of endless people, a sea that seemed to change color as it flowed by you. A sea whose shape transformed constantly, and if you flowed with it long enough, you could visit every part of the world. There is no question that New York gave me a multicultural perspective that many people don't have an opportunity to obtain. However, despite this exposure to a variety of cultures and ethnic groups, I really never got "below the surface." I could taste the foods, I could see the people, and I could listen to the music, but that experience alone was still from a detached perspective. Even though I might see the brightly colored clothes of the Nigerian, I still didn't know that person. Even though I could taste the sushi, I didn't understand the world of the Japanese. And even though I could listen to the Latino music, I didn't really understand the people.

When I lived in New Hampshire, I learned to adapt. No longer would I be this brash New Yorker. I mellowed. New Hampshire's population has a very large percentage of Catholics. My friend John, a priest at the Catholic college at which I worked, would often tell me that some of the nuns thought I was on the verge of a conversion. They saw me as searching. Maybe I was . . . a little, but not enough to convert to another religion. These nuns could not understand how a person with my values could not be more religious. They didn't really know me. Perhaps, if they had taken the time to find out who I was, they could understand me.

From New Hampshire I moved to Norfolk, Virginia—from an area that was mostly Catholic to a part of the country that had many fundamentalist Christians. I found that a small minority of these fundamentalist Christians would confront me on my religious orientation. For instance, one day I was eating lunch with a friend and a friend of hers. As my friend momentarily got up from the table, her friend slowly reached into her purse, pulled out some fliers, and placed them in front of me without saying a word. I looked down and was aghast to see that they were "Jews for Jesus" fliers. I said to her, "Are you trying to tell me something?" She responded that perhaps I would be interested in this. I felt intruded upon. I felt disrespected. Not unlike the nuns in New Hampshire, here was another person trying to place her values on me. If she had tried to talk with me, tried to understand me, tried to have a conversation regarding different approaches to religion, I would have talked with her.

This chapter is about differentness. It is about understanding people. It is about cultural and ethnic diversity. In this chapter, we will examine the cultural mosaic that makes up the United States. From the different cultural and ethnic groups, to the varying religious orientations, to understanding sexual orientation and gender sex-role issues, we will try to make sense out of the varying lifestyles that make up the United States.

Besides gaining knowledge about diversity in the United States, we will examine ways in which the human service worker can be effective with clients from diverse backgrounds. Finally, we will examine the professional issue of individual rights and personal dignity of our clients and how the developmentally mature cross-cultural helper can gain increased sensitivity toward working with diverse clients.

Some Definitions

In examining differences within American society, Baruth and Manning (1991) distinguish between culture, race, ethnicity, and social class and highlight how stereotyping, prejudice, racism, and discrimination can negatively affect our work with diverse clients. Understanding the differences between these and other terms can assist us in working with individuals from diverse populations.

Culture

Culture represents those common values, norms of behavior, symbols, language, and life patterns that people may share. All Americans have a similar cultural heritage because within the society there is a shared language, a common set of experiences, and patterns of behavior with which we are all familiar. Any American can travel throughout the United States and feel at least somewhat familiar with the community and the people. Within our broader culture, **subcultures** have distinguishing patterns of behaviors and values that in some ways may differ from the larger culture. Examples of some subcultures include gays and lesbians; various racial, ethnic, and religious groups; subcultures based on gender; subcultures based on the region of the country in which on lives (for example the South); and so forth (Porter & Samovar, 1985).

In attempting to delineate cultural identity, Whitfield, McGrath, and Coleman (1992) identify 11 elements that can be used in helping to understand specific cultural patterns. Each element can be defined for any culture and include how members in each culture tend to:

- Define their sense of self
- Communicate and use language
- Dress and value appearances
- Embrace certain values and mores
- Embrace specific beliefs and attitudes
- Use time and space
- Relate to family and significant others
- Eat and use food in their customs
- Play and make use of leisure time
- Work and apply themselves
- Learn and use knowledge

Race

Whereas the concept of culture has been based on such characteristics as shared personality traits, values, belief systems, and life patterns, **race** has traditionally been based on biological classification (Krogman, 1945). Therefore, people who are of the same racial group share a similar genetic heritage. This definition, however, becomes blurred when we realize the extent of intermarriages as well as the large differences in personality and physical characteristics of those who are of a similar racial heritage. It is for this reason that the concept of race is one that is not always as clear as we might believe.

Ethnicity

When a group of people share a common ancestry, which may include specific cultural and social patterns, they are members of an ethnic group (Davis, 1978; Rose, 1964). Ethnicity, as opposed to race, is not based on genetic heritage. **Ethnicity** is usually based on long-term patterns of behavior that have some historical significance and may include similar religious, ancestral, language, and/or cultural characteristics. Therefore, Jews, who share religious and perhaps similar ancestral characteristics, may be considered an ethnic group but may not share the same culture. Similarly, Asian people may be considered a race by some but may not share the same culture or the same ethnic background.

Social Class

One's **social class** may cut across a group's common ethnicity, cultural identification, or racial heritage. Therefore, even though individuals may share similar cultural, ethnic, or racial heritage, they may have little in common with one another due to differences in social class. For instance, an African American who is poor may find little in common with a wealthy African American. Hannon, Ritchie, and Rye (1992) state that social class is the "missing dimension" in understanding diversity.

Power Differentials

It is important to keep in mind that, in this fast-changing American culture, **power differentials** may represent greater disparities between people than the culture, ethnic group, race, or social class to which the individuals belong. Therefore, the Mexican American who holds an upper-management position in a business may be disliked because of the power he holds over his employees rather than his ethnic and cultural background. Or the Asian youth who is a gang leader may be disliked by the White gang member because of her position in the gang hierarchy.

Stereotyping, Prejudice, and Racism

Stereotyping people is often the leading cause of racism. In describing stereotyping, Brislin (1981) states that such views are often negative generalizations about a group that results in the people who are holding the **prejudices** blaming the out-group, not admitting uncomfortable feelings about themselves, and organizing and structuring their own world according to their rationale (cited in Lum, 1986). Some authors take the position that **racism** is a disease, noting that, like other mental disorders, racism is based on a distortion of reality (Skillings & Dobbins, 1991).

Discrimination

Whereas prejudice and stereotyping represent attitudes held by people, **discrimination** is an active behavior, such as gay bashing or unfair hiring practices, that negatively affect individuals within ethnic or cultural groups (Lum, 1986).

Table 7-1 Percentage of Discrimination and Prejudice Americans Think Various Groups Face Today

	Tremendous Amount	A Lot	Some	A Little	None	Not Sure
African Americans	16	50	22	8	3	2
Jews	4	22	39	22	11	2
Italians	1	7	29	32	27	4
Homosexuals	21	53	14	6	4	3
Catholics	1	8	24	29	36	2
Whites in general	2	11	25	26	35	1
Women	5	29	37	20	8	1
Asians	3	26	38	21	9	4
Hispanics	6	32	37	16	6	3

Does racism exist in the United States? A study by the Anti-Defamation League (ADL, 1992) found that, in surveying American households, many people believe that a wide variety of subcultures in this country experience prejudice and discrimination (see Table 7-1).

The Changing Face of the United States

In summarizing the changing face of the United States, Sue, Arredondo, and McDavis (1992) note that in the year 2000, one-third of the U.S. population will be ethnic minorities and that these groups will represent a majority by the year 2010. These changing demographics are a function of a number of factors including differential birth rates between culturally diverse populations and that the immigration rates are currently the largest in U.S. history. Compared with earlier immigrants who came mostly from Europe, current immigrants are now largely Asian (34%) and Latino (34%). These new immigrants are more likely to maintain their cultural heritage partly because they do not share the European heritage that was held by the majority of past immigrants.

Current ethnic and cultural changes in the United States are related to the changing face of religion across the country. As increased numbers of Asians, Latinos, and people from the Middle East arrive, we find more individuals with varied religious backgrounds. But even in the more traditional Protestant culture, diversity in the various Protestant religious groups has become prevalent as we now clearly distinguish between those who might be fundamentalist Christian, Methodist, Baptist, and so forth.

Besides the changing ethnic and cultural diversity, there are changes in sex-role identity. The "macho" male is no longer considered a model for maleness, and women no longer are expected to stay at home and rear the children. There is also increased awareness of the gay and lesbian subculture. Whereas in the past many homosexuals felt a need to hide their sexual orientation for fear of discrimination, today we find an increasing number of gays and lesbians "coming out." This is partly a function of the AIDS epidemic, but it is also a result of our changing values toward this subculture.

Finally, changes in federal, state, and local laws have given us an increased sensitivity to and awareness of special groups such as the disabled, older persons, the chronically ill, law violators, and so forth.

I have found that, when teaching human service workers, many students are unaware of the amount of diversity that exists in the United States. The United States is truly a multicultural society, a **cultural mosaic** that embraces a myriad of traditions, customs, and patterns of behavior that represent diverse ethnic heritages and cultural backgrounds. In an attempt to help us gain knowledge about some of the diversity that abounds in the United States, the following is a quick overview of many of the ethnic, religious, and cultural groups found across the United States.

A Brief History of Cultural and Ethnic Diversity in the United States*

People of Early North American Origin

The indigenous people of the United States are of three major groups: Native Americans, Aleuts, and Inuits. Native American (or Amerindians), were numerous when Columbus landed in America; however, due to disease brought by the Europeans and the wars they initiated, today there are only about 1.5 million Native Americans. Approximately one-half of all Native Americans live on reservations. Unemployment in reservations is high and general living conditions are not good. Today, Native Americans face myriad social problems, many of which can be traced back to the uprooting of their civilization (Heinrich, Corbine, & Thomas, 1990).

Approximately 10,000 years ago, people from Siberia crossed over the Bering Strait land bridge to what is now Alaska. Some of these people headed westward toward the Aleutian Islands and are now called Aleuts, whereas others headed north and east and are now

*Partially condensed from *We the People: An Atlas of America's Ethnic Diversity* (Allen & Turner, 1988).

called Inuits. Many Inuits were converted to Christianity by missionaries, and because of their close proximity to the former Soviet Union, many Aleuts became Russian Orthodox. Today, there are approximately 40,000 Inuits and 14,000 Aleuts.

People of Western European Origin

English, Scottish, and Welsh heritage (British heritage). With approximately 50 million Americans identifying themselves as having some English heritage, this group represents the largest number of Americans. In actuality, this figure is probably quite low because many people of English heritage have lost track of their roots. Because many individuals of English heritage immigrated during colonial times, much of American culture (for example, language, food, habits) can be traced to England. The term *WASP* (White-Anglo-Saxon-Protestant) has been associated with English heritage and is a somewhat derogatory expression, which has come to represent the influence of this British ancestry.

Like the English, the Scottish and Welsh immigration history dates back to the colonial period in the United States. Today, nearly 10 million Americans identify themselves as having Scottish ancestry, and 1.6 million have some Welsh ancestry.

Irish heritage. Irish Protestants of Scottish descent originally settled in this country in the early 1700s and by 1790 they represented nearly 10% of the population. In the 1840s, following the potato famine in Ireland, many Irish Catholics settled in this country, particularly in Boston and New York. Today, nearly 40 million Americans identify themselves as having some Irish ancestry.

German heritage. In 1790 10% of the population identified themselves as being of German heritage. In the 1800s there was a large number of German immigrants, although many of them tended to identify themselves with their religious affiliation or with the part of Germany from which they came. Although a large number of these immigrants were Roman Catholics, many were associated with Lutheran, Reformed, and Evangelical groups. Today, over 48 million Americans identify themselves as having some German heritage.

French, Dutch, Belgian, and Swiss heritage. More than 14 million Americans identify themselves as having some French heritage; 6.3 million, Dutch heritage; 1 million, of Swiss lineage; and a lesser number, of Belgian ancestry. Many of these individuals immigrated in the 1600s and 1700s.

Many Swiss immigrants identify themselves by their religious affiliations, which are predominantly Catholic, Mormon, Amish, Mennonite, Protestant, and nonaffiliated religious Swiss. Many of the Amish and Mennonites settled in America in the 1600s to escape persecution in Switzerland.

People of Northern European Origin

Approximately 9 million individuals identify themselves as having Scandinavian roots; that is, a heritage that can be traced to Norway, Denmark, or Sweden. Most of these individuals immigrated in the late 1800s and early 1900s and many immigrated to the Great Lakes region. This is also true of many of the close to 600,000 individuals of Finnish heritage. Many came from rural areas, became farmers, and converted to the Mormon religion.

People of Eastern European Origin

A number of ethnic groups are collectively called Slavs because they have languages that have similar linguistic properties. These include individuals of Austrian, Polish, Russian, Czech, Serbo, and Croatian heritage. Because people from Hungary, Romania, Albania, Latvia, Slovenia, the Ukraine, and Lithuania come from a similar area in Eastern Europe, many Americans have also identified people from these areas as Slavs. Jews, who lived in many of these Slavic countries, are a another ethnic group from Eastern Europe. Because many people from this part of the world identify with an ethnic group but live in a country other than their ethnic group, understanding their heritages becomes complicated. Today, more than 24 million Americans identify themselves as being of Eastern European origin, with a large percentage of these being Jewish (5.2 million), Polish (4.4 million) or Russian (2.8 million).

Many immigrants from Eastern Europe came to the United States at the turn of the century. As industrialization spread across the United States, many Eastern Europeans came to find economic prosperity, and others came to avoid military conscription. In addition, many Jews came to escape the pogroms—"campaigns of beating and killing and home burning" (Allen, & Turner, 1988, p. 81)—that began about 1881 in Russia, whereas others came because of restrictions on land ownership and because limitations were placed on which occupations they could pursue.

People of Southern European Origin

More than 14 million immigrants in the United States identify themselves as having roots from four areas in Southern Europe: Greece, Italy, the Basque Provinces (southern France and northern Spain), and Portugal, with the vast majority (more than 12 million) coming from

Italy. Many people of Southern European heritage came during the late 1800s and arrived for hope of a better life; some were attracted by the California gold rush.

People of Middle Eastern Origin

Immigrants from the Middle East can be classified as Armenian, Arab National, Assyrian, or of Israeli origin and make up less than 2 million Americans. Many of Mid-Eastern origin settled in the United States between 1890 and World War I, with a second wave of immigrants arriving as a result of the Immigration Act of 1965.

Those of Arab ancestry are mostly from Syria, Lebanon, or Egypt; number over 1.5 million Americans; and are mostly Christian, Muslim, or Druze. Assyrians, who are mostly from Iran, Iraq, and its surrounding areas make up a smaller number; Armenians, who mostly came from Turkey and to a lesser degree from areas near Turkey controlled

Cheryl Evans—An African American

Forty-six-year-old Cheryl Evans was born outside Boston in the oldest continuous African American community in the Northeast. From a very young age, she remembers being aware of her color because she was treated in a prejudicial manner and/or was made aware that she was "different" from others

Cheryl's family history is as diverse as most African Americans'. Some of this history includes a great-grandmother who was Native American, a great-grandmother who was born a slave, a great grandfather who was a "traveling preacher," a Lithuanian Jewish grandmother who was illiterate and immigrated to this country when she was 12 years old, a grandmother who was disabled at an early age from a stroke, an African American grandfather who worked for the railroad, and a grandfather who was an Ethiopian "Falasha"—a Jewish rabbi who immigrated to this country via Europe and Jamaica.

Because Cheryl's mother was a child of a mixed marriage, her mother and her mother's siblings were taken away from their natural parents and brought up in foster homes. Although Cheryl's parents were married in the Catholic church, she describes her mother as always being a "seeker"; therefore, Cheryl was exposed to a number of religions, including Jehovah's Witnesses, Islam, Mormonism, and Judaism.

Cheryl's parents, particularly her mother, strongly encouraged education, and Cheryl always found herself in the honors classes in school. Cheryl's mother stressed to her that others could take away by the former Soviet Union, make up approximately 200,000 citizens. Those whose ancestry is of modern-day Israel (since 1945) number about 50,000.

People of African Origin

With more than 26 million Americans being of African heritage, African Americans make up about 11% of the population. Of these, close to 90% are descendants from slaves. A small number of African Americans came from Cape Verde as whalers in the 18th and 19th centuries; more recently many of those of East and West African ancestry have come to the United States for educational opportunities.

Because many African Americans were brought to the United States as slaves, by 1790 19% of the population were of African heritage. Despite the fact that slave trading was made illegal in 1809, slave breeding and slave trading within the South (which was encouraged

her material things, but they could not take away her education. Being one of the few African Americans in her classes, she tended to feel highly visible and responsible for the whole race. By the age of 10, Cheryl became more aware of the civil rights movement; as she grew older, it was not uncommon to find her at a civil rights protest march or listening to Malcolm X or Martin Luther King, Jr. Cheryl speaks emotionally about the impact that Malcolm X, Martin Luther King, Jr., and other leaders of the times had on her.

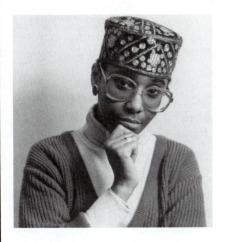

In her adult life, Cheryl has been a teacher of human development at a college, worked for a major radio station in Boston, helped run "Manpower" for the Dukakis governorship, recruited African American students for Rutgers University, administered a business for women, and ran for political office. In addition, Cheryl obtained her master's degree and is now working on her doctorate. With all of this, Cheryl has also found time for one of the major driving forces in her life—building bridges between diverse groups.

by Northern merchants) continued until the Civil War. With the end of these practices following the Civil War and due to the continued immigration of Whites, the percentage of African Americans in this country dropped to its current level.

As a function of agricultural development, most slaves lived in the South and were forcibly brought to farm the lands. In fact, in 1860, 90% of African Americans lived in the South. Conditions in the ships that brought the slaves were deplorable, and it is estimated that 6 to 10 million people died in passage. After the Civil War, many African Americans remained in the South, becoming sharecroppers or working for White farmers. Restrictive work laws and lack of education made it difficult for African Americans to leave the South. From the 1930s until the 1960s, because of changes in the economy and increasing violence, many African Americans moved from rural lands in the South to urban centers where there were hopes of better educational and career opportunities. However, more recently there has been a reversal of this trend, with better-educated African Americans moving to the South and obtaining higher-level jobs.

People of Central and South American and Caribbean Origin

People of Central and South American origin make up a large percentage of the American population. Most of these immigrants are Mexican (close to 9 million), Puerto Rican (over 2 million), Cuban (close to 1 million), or of "other" Spanish origin (over 3 million). A lesser number have come from such countries as Haiti, Guatemala, Panama, the Dominican Republic, Brazil, Jamaica, and the West Indian islands.

Many Mexican Americans (Chicanos) first immigrated to the United States in the middle 1800s, traveling north from Mexico to the Southwest and West, looking for gold in California, good grazing land for cattle, and economic prosperity. A second wave of Mexican immigrants arrived in the late 1800s and early 1900s, with many moving to California. Today, 52% of the Mexican American population live in California.

Most Puerto Ricans settled in the United States following their independence from Spain and after Puerto Rico became a U.S. territory. Many Puerto Ricans moved to New York City where there were hopes of a better life; more recently, there has been a large westward migration of Puerto Ricans in search of better employment opportunities.

Most Cubans immigrated in the late 1950s and early 1960s following Fidel Castro's overthrow of the Cuban dictatorship under Batista. They came out of fear of persecution and imprisonment and because of ideological differences with the Communist regime. The vast majority of Cubans settled in southern Florida, although there are sizable communities in New York, Chicago, and Los Angeles.

Dr. Martha Muguira—A Woman of Mexican Heritage

Dr. Martha Muguira was raised in Mexico City in a family that included her parents and three younger siblings. Marty, who is a naturalized citizen, considers herself Mexican, as opposed to Mexican American, because she was raised in Mexico.

Marty's paternal and maternal great-grandparents were of Spanish and Mexican-Indian descent. Marty notes that the population of Mexico is mostly Catholic and the rituals include many Indian customs that are not ordinarily found in the United States. She comments that, until recently, light-skinned Mexicans (usually Mexicans of Spanish heritage) were treated preferentially in the country. She mentions that Mexico has tended to be a male-oriented society with preferential treatment toward men, particularly concerning careers.

As a female, Marty remembers that she received mixed messages from her parents. On the one hand, they valued education, particularly bilingual education, and sent her to an American school in Mexico City. In fact, when Marty was 17 years old, she received a scholarship to live in North Carolina with a banker's family and go to a private school. On the other hand, even though Marty received this scholarship, her father encouraged her to stay in Mexico, pursue a more traditional education, and have a family. Despite these mixed messages, Marty went on to finish her doctorate, raise a family, and now works at a counseling center at a university in Virginia.

Although Marty states that she has not experienced overt discrimination, she notes that throughout her life people would have expectations of her because of her Mexican heritage. For instance, while living in North Carolina, she was asked to "fit in" better by wearing American- rather than Mexican-style clothes. Also, when she worked at a Veterans Administration hospital, she was "chosen" to run a special program for Spanish-speaking employees, mostly because she was Mexican.

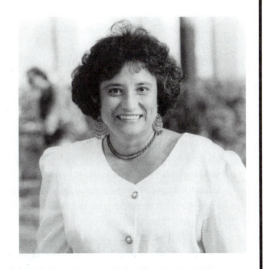

Dr. Muguira is proud of her Mexican heritage, values her bilingual education, and is another prime example of the diversity in the United States.

In the United States today, there are also a sizable number of Americans of Spanish descent who arrived here from Central and South America. Many of Spanish descent settled along the Rio Grande, and in the 1800s there was a migration of people of Spanish descent from the Rio Grande area to New Mexico, Arizona, and Colorado. From the 1960s until recently, due to political turmoil in their own country of origin, many people from Central America have migrated to the United States.

People of Asian and Pacific Islands Origin

People of Asian and Pacific island origin are a varied population, which includes fairly large numbers of Chinese (800,000), Japanese (700,000), Filipinos, (800,000), Koreans (350,00), Indians (350,000), Vietnamese (250,000), and native Hawaiians (160,000). Lesser populations of Laotian, Thai, Samoans, and Guamanians also immigrated to the United States. Since the changes in the immigration law in 1965, there has been more equity in who can immigrate to the United States. This has resulted in an increase in immigrants from Asia and the Pacific islands.

Chinese heritage.   Many Chinese immigrated to the United States in the mid-1800s during the Californian gold rush to escape poverty in China. However, Whites ousted many Chinese from the mines, and many ended up taking low-paying farm and blue-collar jobs. Because of prejudice and poor working conditions, many Chinese dispersed to midwestern and eastern cities. In addition, the development of "Chinatowns" represented a haven for many Chinese. Today, many have moved out of the Chinatowns, and these areas now generally house the poorer Chinese.

Japanese and Korean heritage.   In the late 1800s a large number of Japanese and Koreans also settled in California and, like the Chinese, took low-paying farm jobs. During World War II, many West Coast Japanese-Americans were forcibly removed from their homes and placed in internment camps. In 1943 some of the Japanese who were interned were able to leave the camps if they promised not to live on the West Coast. Many of these moved to the Midwest whereas others waited to the end of the war when they were allowed to resettle on the West Coast. Surviving Japanese-Americans who were placed in internment camps recently won a monetary settlement from the government for their hardship.

Filipino heritage.   After the U.S. takeover of the Philippine Islands in 1898, there was an influx of Filipinos to the United States. Many went to Hawaii and worked as sugar growers. In the 1920s and 1930s, many Filipinos moved to California and Alaska—some for low-paying jobs, others to pursue an education. In addition, until recently Filipinos could enlist in the armed services, and many have relocated to naval cities such as Norfolk, Virginia.

Korean and Vietnam heritage.   Following the Korean and Vietnam wars, large numbers of Koreans and Vietnamese immigrated to the United States. Many of the Korean immigrants were war brides, war orphans, and professionals, whereas many of the Vietnamese immigrants were refugees from the war in Vietnam and were brought to this country following the fall of South Vietnam to the Communists.

Indians and Pakistanis.   Prior to 1965, many Indians moved to California after having been recruited by Canadian railroad companies in British Columbia. After the changes in the immigration law in 1965, many highly educated Indians moved to metropolitan areas including New York, Chicago, and Washington, D.C. The majority of Indians in recent years have been Hindus, although some have been Muslims and Sikhs. Pakistanis, most of whom are Muslim, largely moved here since 1965 and, like the Indians, have generally been highly educated and have moved to metropolitan areas.

Religious Diversity in the United States

Knowledge of religious differences in the United States can make human service workers more sensitive to differences in personality styles of their clients. Assuming that we are a "Christian nation" and that we all share the same beliefs can hinder the helping relationship.

The religious makeup of the American people has shifted in dramatic ways over the past four decades—and there is every indication that those trends will continue in the future. In general, the nation has become less distinctly Protestant and more pluralistic in character (Gallup & Castelli, 1989).

As is its ethnic and cultural background, the United States is truly diverse when it comes to religious orientation. In the United States today, there are more than 80 religious groups that each have over 50,000 members. Of the 147 million Americans who report some affiliation with a religious group, 60% of them are Protestant. But even in this religious tradition, there is considerable variability in beliefs and traditions. Besides these diverse Protestant groups, a large number of Americans identify themselves as Roman Catholic (57 million), and lesser numbers are Muslim (around 6 million), Jewish

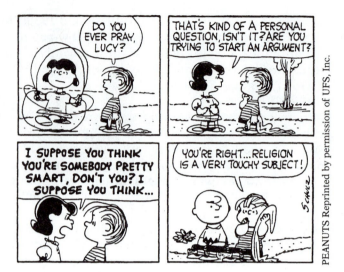

PEANUTS Reprinted by permission of UFS, Inc.

(close to 6 million), Eastern Orthodox (over 4 million), Old Catholic (close to 1 million), Buddhist (19,000), or other non-Christian religions (for example, Unitarian and Baha'i) (U.S. Department of Commerce, 1991; *World Almanac*, 1992). With 69% of Americans claiming membership in a church or synagogue and 87% stating that religion is fairly or very important in their lives (Gallup, 1991), it is clear that understanding the diversity of religious beliefs in the United States is extremely important.

Although most of us may not be familiar with the many Christian religious orientations in the United States, because Christianity is so prevalent in the culture, I have chosen not to review those religions. Instead we will spend a little time examining four religions of which you may have less knowledge. Keep in mind, however, that there are many Christian religious affiliations with which you may not be familiar. You are strongly encouraged to explore these religions in more detail as well as obtain more information about the religions that we now will discuss in brief, as well as about other religions you might encounter.

Judaism

Judaism is a monotheistic religion that began to coalesce around 1300 B.C.E. (before the common era). It is an evolving religious civilization whose purpose is to transform what is into what should be: peace and cooperation, the love and acceptance of others, and a progressive view

A Jewish-American Woman

Eleanor is a 70-year-old widowed Jewish woman. Both her parents immigrated to the United States from Eastern Europe and Russia when they were children. They came looking for a better life and to escape anti-Semitism in their countries of origin. Like many Jews who came to the United States around the turn of the century, they came with little and had to work hard to survive in their new homeland. Due to the turmoil when leaving their countries of origin, Eleanor notes, there is little history of her family genealogy.

Eleanor grew up in a mostly Jewish section of New York and states that this resulted in her maintaining her sense of Jewish heritage. For instance, even though she might have entertained the idea of marrying someone outside her faith, because her community was exclusively Jewish and because she would only meet Jewish men, this would have been unlikely. Although Eleanor was brought up speaking English, it was not uncommon for Yiddish to be spoken among her parents and grandparents. (Yiddish is a mixture of German and Baltic languages. Some common English words today are of Yiddish origin—for example, *kibitz, chutzpah, oy-vey.*)

Even though Eleanor does not view herself as being highly religious, she identifies herself strongly as a Jew, noting that for her, being Jewish today is mostly cultural and brings to her "a sense of belonging and an association with people who are more or less like me." Although Eleanor states that she has encountered little anti-Semitism in the United States, she feels this is partly a result of living mostly around other Jews. One example of anti-Semitism that she did encounter was when she applied for a bookkeeping position with the Navy during World War II. Having passed the interview, she was about to be hired when the officer asked her what her religious affiliation was. Upon telling him she was Jewish, he threw her application in the trash.

Eleanor is proud of her Jewish heritage and maintains a sense of her ethnicity through affiliation with friends, membership in a synagogue, and attendance at Jewish cultural events.

toward life. Judaism is based on the Hebrew Bible, which includes the five books attributed to Moses (called the Torah), the writings of the Prophets, and the writings of the ancient historians, kings, and wisdom teachers. Later writings called the Talmud, which are interpretations by teachers (rabbis) and judges of the early writings, are also used as a basis for knowledge and worship.

Adherence to Jewish laws varies from those who are very orthodox to those who are very liberal, although the majority of Jews in the United States are somewhere in between on this continuum. Some of the major holidays include Rosh Hashanah, the new year; Yom Kippur, the day of atonement for one's sins; Hanukkah, the festival of lights; and Passover, which celebrates the liberation of Jews from slavery in Egypt centuries ago and is symbolic of liberation in general. Finally, the Bar Mitzvah and the Bas Mitzvah, religious celebrations of male and female children, respectively, entering adulthood at age 13, are other major Jewish ceremonies to which many Jews adhere.

Buddhism

Founded around 525 B.C.E. in India by the Buddha, Gautama Siddhartha, Buddhism is based on the *Tripitaka*, teachings of the Buddha, and the *Sutras*, which are comments about Buddha's teachings. These texts are philosophical in nature and speak to the monastic life. Four truths of Buddhism include (1) the truth of suffering; (2) the cause of suffering, which is desire; (3) the cessation of suffering, which is the renunciation of desire; and (4) the way that leads to the cessation of suffering (Bach, 1959). Related to these truths are the Buddhist beliefs that reality is an illusion, that one lives and is reborn due to attachment to an illusory self, and that Nirvana is reached when, through meditation, you can transcend attachment to the illusory self. Actual practice of Buddhism varies greatly depending on the sect to which the person belongs.

Hinduism

Hinduism began to develop around 1500 B.C.E when Aryan invaders of India intermixed their religious practices and beliefs with the native Indians. The sacred texts include the Veda, Upanishads, Bhagavadgita, Mahabharata, and Ramayana. These texts are mythological and philosophical commentaries about life. Although the religion speaks to many gods, heroes, and saints, Hindus believe in one divine principle—that many gods are aspects of a single divine unity. Hindus believe that people are born and reborn based on their *samsara*, or separation from the divine and that one's *karma*, or total way of acting and being, can be improved through pure actions and meditation. Through these pure acts, one can eventually become closer to the divine. Hindus believe that reincarnation is the road to unity with the divine, and that it answers many perplexing questions such as why there are so many personalities in this world.

Islam

In the name of Allah, the Merciful, the Beneficent
Praise be to Allah, Lord of the worlds,
The Beneficent, the Merciful
Master of the day of Requital.
Thee do we serve and Thee do we beseech for help;
Guide us on the right path,
The path of those upon whom Thou hast bestowed favors,
Not those upon whom wrath is brought down,
Nor those who go astray.
(From the Koran, in Bach, 1959, p. 98)

This mostly nonauthoritarian and egalitarian religion was founded in 622 by Muhammad, the Prophet. Muslims believe that Allah (God) is the creator of the universe and is merciful, kind, and all powerful. Humans are seen as the highest creation of God and are capable of sin and of being misled by Satan. If a person repents, he or she can return to a state of sinlessness and go to paradise. Two of the major texts of Muslims are the Koran—which is said to be the true word of God, given by the angel Gabriel to Muhammad—and the Hadith. Muslims have five duties to which they should adhere: to profess their faith to Allah, to pray five times a day, to give regularly a portion of their material wealth to charity, to fast daily until sundown during the month of Ramadan, and to attempt to make at least one pilgrimage to Mecca.

Gender Differences in the United States

Differences in demographic characteristics between men and women are great. For example, women's labor-force growth rate has doubled that of men; today, more men take on child care as compared with the past (although women continue to do most of the child care); men own the vast majority of corporations in the United States; regardless of occupation, on average, women earn less than men; women have lower death rates than men; widowhood is much more likely for women as compared with men; although as many women start college as men, women are less likely to finish; elderly women are less likely to commit suicide than elderly men; and on and on . . . (Chandras, 1991; Taeuber, 1991).

Besides demographic variations, the evidence is great that personality differences exist between males and females. In fact, some writers have suggested that the "male reality" may be different from the "female reality" (Gilligan, 1982; Miller, 1976; Schaef, 1981). Whether these differences are a function of genetics and/or of social forces is still unclear; however, it is obvious that, generally, the way men and women approach life is different. For instance, evidence suggests that, generally, men are more restrictive in their ability to express emotion, are less communicative, have more difficulty with intimacy, and are more competitive than women, whereas women are usually more nurturing, more concerned about how their actions affect others, and have more difficulty expressing anger than men (Basse & Greenstreet, 1991; DeVoe, 1990; Rabinowitz, 1991).

It is clear that the sex-role identity of men and women in today's society is changing. As these changes become more prevalent, women and men are more likely to take on new personality styles. In fact, some research seems to indicate that individuals who take on multiple roles, including nontraditional sex-roles, may be more satisfied in life than are those who do not (Hammond & Fong, 1988).

A human service worker who does not acknowledge these changing demographics and their psychological impact on men and women cannot work effectively with clients of either gender. The importance of recognizing and being knowledgeable about the differences between men and women has become an essential ingredient to being an effective helper.

Differences in Sexual Orientation in the United States

In the famous Kinsey studies of the 1940s (Kinsey, 1948), when examining male sexual orientations, Kinsey found that 50% of males have had some sexual history with other males in their adult life, 13% had more homosexual than heterosexual experiences, 8% were exclusively homosexual for 3 years of their lives between the ages of 16 and 55, and 4% were exclusively homosexual throughout their lives. Kinsey also found that most individuals are not "purely" homosexual or heterosexual but rather fall on a continuum between homosexual and heterosexual. When asked in a recent Gallup Poll (Gallup, 1989) if homosexual relations between two consenting adults should or should not be legal, 47% said it should, and 36% said it should not (17% had no opinion). When asked if homosexuals should have equal rights relative to job opportunities, 71% of Americans said they should.

Although many have viewed homosexuality and bisexuality as an illness, a considerable amount of evidence disputes these facts (Dworkin & Gutierrez, 1989; Sang, 1989). This evidence has led the American Psychological Association and the American Psychiatric Association to view homosexuality as a sexual orientation, not an illness. Although it is still unclear how we obtain our sexual orientation, it appears now that sexual orientation is determined very early in life and may even be related to biological and genetic factors.

Like racism and prejudice, **homophobia** can be seen as an individual's distortion of reality because the homosexual unconsciously might represent a threat to the homophobic's understanding of sexuality. Homophobic attitudes have led to harassment and acting out toward gays and lesbians (Croteau & Morgan, 1989). Like cultural and ethnic identity, religious orientation, and gender differences, sexual orientation is another example of the diversity that exists in the United States. The human service worker needs to be sensitive and knowledgeable about all types of diversity.

Other Special Groups

Diversity includes more than cultural and ethnic background, religious preference, sexual orientation, and gender differences. There are many groups that have unique characteristics of which the human service worker should be aware. For instance, Schmolling, Youkeles, and Burger (1993) identify a number of target populations that have unique needs. These include America's poor, the unemployed, children in need, the elderly, people with disabilities, the mentally ill, substance abusers, law violators, the mentally retarded, the homeless, and AIDS patients (some of these groups are discussed in Chapter 10). This list is just a sprinkling of the various groups of which the human service worker should be aware. Although no professional can know the characteristics of all diverse groups, it is the responsibility of each professional to have resources available that can inform the helper about the best ways to work with these clients. This is accomplished through reading journals of professional associations, using library resources, having consultants available, and attending continuing education workshops.

The Helping Relationship and Cultural Diversity

Every person is like all persons, like some persons, and like no other person.*

Existentialists have noted that in trying to understand the individual we need to be aware of his or her uniqueness (*Eigenwelt*), the common experiences of a group or culture (*Mitwelt*), and our shared universal experiences (*Umwelt*) (Binswanger, 1962, 1963). Keeping this in mind, we need to ask ourselves, "How can the human service worker be

*Paraphrased from Kluckhorn & Murray, in Speight, Myers, Cox, & Highlen, 1991, p. 32.

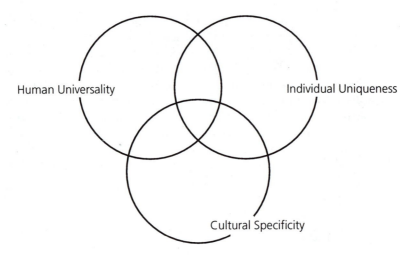

Human Universality

Individual Uniqueness

Cultural Specificity

Figure 7-1   Each sphere represents a unique aspect of the individual. Where the spheres overlap suggests that we can only
understand the totality of our clients' situation if we can understand the uniqueness of these three components.

SOURCE: From "A Redefinition of Multicultural Counseling," by S. L. Speight, J. Myers,
C. F. Fox, and P. S. Highlen, 1991, *Journal of Counseling and Development, 70*, 29–
36. Copyright 1991 American Counseling Association. Reprinted by permission.

effective with culturally different clients?" Using the above existential
framework, one model of working with all clients assumes that each
client has specific issues related to his or her culture, is unique unto
himself or herself, and shares universal issues common to all people
(Speight et al., 1991, p. 32)(see Figure 7-1).

Barriers to an Effective Multicultural Helping Relationship

In working with clients, Midgette and Meggert (1991) note a number
of barriers that hinder our effective work with clients of diverse backgrounds. We will discuss some of these in the following pages.

The melting pot myth.   For many years, there was a misnomer that
the United States was a melting pot of cultural diversity. This meant
that various values and customs of different cultures "melted" into the
larger culture. In actuality, most cultures want to maintain their
uniqueness and are resistant to giving up their special traditions. Assuming that clients should fit into and conform to majority cultural
values can turn off some clients. Probably, saying that the United
States is a cultural mosaic, a society that has a myriad of diverse val-

Counseling a Polish Mine Worker

As a therapist at a mental-health center, I had the opportunity to work with a Polish-American client who had recently retired from working most of his life in the coal mines in northeastern Pennsylvania. I quickly realized I knew little of his cultural heritage and little of what it was like to work in the mines. Because of this, I wondered how I would connect with this man who was depressed. My choices seemed clear: I could either ignore these cultural differences or find out more about his heritage and lifetime occupation. I therefore spent a number of sessions asking him what it was like working in the mines and growing up Polish-American. It was clear that this client wanted to share his background with me. I could see he was proud of his heritage and loved telling me about the mines. I could see that my ability to not feel defensive about my lack of knowledge and my desire to learn about his social and cultural heritage made him feel close to me. This created an atmosphere of trust, and I soon understood his depression, which was partly a result of his sense that he was no longer a productive member of his community.

Using the model presented in Figure 7-1, you can see that in working with this client I tried to understand his unique situation and tried to gain knowledge of the culture from which he came. My ability to gain an understanding of this client's uniqueness and cultural specificity made it easier for me to gain a deep understanding of some of the universal concerns with which he was dealing. These included his lack of meaning in life (which he had obtained partially through his work) as well as the sense of emptiness and loss he was currently experiencing.

ues and customs, more accurately represents the essence of diversity that we find today.

Incongruent expectations about counseling.   Throughout this text, we have talked about the importance of specific characteristics of the human service worker in creating a productive helping relationship. Along with these characteristics usually come certain expectations about how our clients should respond to our interventions. Some of these expectations might be that our clients should be self-disclosing and open-minded and be willing to take control of their lives. However, some cultures do not value self-disclosure and openness. Other cultures place value on the importance of authority figures making decisions for the individual. Human service workers need to be cognizant of and be able to adjust to these cultural differences.

Lack of understanding of social forces.   Some human service workers stress **intrapersonal** (internal) **factors** and ignore social and environmental factors that may be affecting a client from a minority culture. It is important to recognize that issues of racism, discrimination, and other social forces outside the individual may greatly affect the client's ability to make changes in his or her life.

Ethnocentric worldview.   Human service workers sometimes assume that their way of viewing the world is the same as their clients'. Although the importance of understanding a client's unique situation is always crucial to an effective helping relationship, this is particularly significant when working with minority clients whose worldview may be particularly foreign to our own.

Ignorance of self-racism and other's cultural identity.   Not being in touch with one's own prejudices and racist attitudes can negatively affect our work with clients. Understanding our own stereotypes and prejudices takes a particularly vigilant effort because our biases are often unconscious.

The Culturally Skilled Human Service Worker: Beliefs and Attitudes, Knowledge, and Skills

A number of authors have stated that to work effectively with clients, culturally skilled mental-health professionals must be aware of their attitudes and beliefs toward culturally diverse populations, have a knowledge base that supports their work with diverse clients, and have the necessary skills to apply to clients with diverse backgrounds (Pedersen, Draguns, Lonner, & Trimble, 1989; Sue, Arredondo, & McDavis, 1992; Sue et al., 1982).

Beliefs and attitudes.   Culturally skilled human service workers have an awareness of their own cultural backgrounds, biases, stereotypes, and values, and such helpers should have the ability to respect differences. Although culturally skilled human service workers may not hold the same belief system as their clients, they can accept differing worldviews as presented by the helpee. Being sensitive to differences and one's own cultural biases allows culturally skilled human service workers to refer a minority client to a human service worker of the client's own race or culture when a referral will benefit the helpee.

Knowledge.   Culturally skilled human service workers have an awareness of sociopolitical issues in the United States, have knowledge of the barriers that hinder culturally diverse clients from using social service agencies, and possess specific knowledge about clients' cultural or ethnic groups. Such skilled human service workers have or are willing to gain a knowledge of characteristics of specific cultural, racial, and ethnic groups (for example, personality styles, customs, traditions). At the same time, such human service workers do not assume that just because clients come from a specific cultural background, they necessarily have these characteristics. In other words, human service workers have knowledge of the group from which clients come, yet do not "jump to conclusions" about clients' ways of being.

Skills.   Human service workers who are effective with culturally diverse populations are able to apply generic interviewing and counseling skills with culturally diverse populations while being aware of and able to apply specialized interventions that might be effective with specific populations. Related to this, culturally sensitive human service workers understand the verbal and nonverbal language of clients and can communicate effectively with clients.

What happens when a helper does not have the knowledge, attitudes, and skills needed for an effective helping relationship? Robertiello and Schoenewolf (1987) note a number of mistakes that were made by helpers due to their own naiveté. In brief, a few examples include the following:

1. The liberal White therapist who refuses to deal with an African American client's mistrustful and suspicious dreams of him due to the helper's denial of the tension in the relationship.

2. The feminist helper who blindly encourages her client to leave her husband because he is a batterer. The client leaves her husband but ends up in another battering situation because the helper did not examine what part the woman was playing in picking abusive men.

3. The helper who reassures her client that the client's homosexual feelings do not mean she is a lesbian. The helper does this out of fear of dealing with the client's sexuality and instead tries to ignore the subject. The client may or may not be homosexual, but reassuring her that she is not does not allow the client to explore her sexuality.

4. The helper who refuses to hear his client's atheistic views because they are contrary to his religious beliefs. This had the effect of cutting off meaningful conversations in other areas because the client lost trust in the helper.

Blackbirds Sitting in a Tree

A White female elementary school teacher in the United States posed a math problem to her class one day. "Suppose there are four blackbirds sitting in a tree. You take a slingshot and shoot one of them. How many are left?" A White student answered quickly, "That's easy. One subtracted from four is three." An African immigrant youth then answered with equal confidence, "Zero." The teacher chuckled at the latter response and stated that the first student was right and that, perhaps, the second student should study more math. From that day forth, the African student seemed to withdraw from class activities and seldom spoke to other students or the teacher.

If the teacher had pursued the African student's reasons for arriving at the answer zero, she might have heard the following: "If you shoot one bird, the others will fly away." Nigerian educators often use this story to illustrate differences in worldviews between United States and African cultures. The Nigerians contend that the group is more important than the individual, that survival of all depends on interrelationships among the parts. . . . (Sue, 1992, pp. 7–8)

Some Practical Suggestions for a Helping Relationship with a Culturally Different Client

Some research has shown that clients of a different cultural background from the helper may experience the helping relationship more negatively than if the helper is of the same culture (Atkinson, 1985; Atkinson, Poston, Furlong, & Mercado, 1989). Because sensitivity to all cultures in the helping relationship is crucial (Pedersen, Draguns, Lonner, & Trimble, 1989; Sue, Arredondo, & McDavis, 1992; Sue et al., 1982), some helpful "tips" to working with culturally different clients may be important. In this context, Westwood and Ishiyama (1990) note a number of practical suggestions when working with culturally different clients, some of which may be particularly relevant to the human service worker (pp. 169–170):

- Encourage clients to speak their own language (words and phrases) to best illustrate how they are feeling at the moment.

- Because nonverbal expressions are often culturally based, check for accuracy of your interpretations when in doubt about clients' nonverbals.

- Make use of alternate modes of communication, other than a solely verbal exchange, to increase clients' comfort and involvement. Examples are acting, drawing, music, story telling, collage making, and so forth.

- Learn culturally meaningful expressions used by clients.

- Plan a show-and-tell session in which clients can bring items that might assist you in understanding their perspective (for example, book, photograph, article of significance, and so forth).

- Vary the helping environment to assist in communication and to break the monotony. Clients may prefer or enjoy having counseling sessions out of the office.

I'll add one suggestion of my own:

- Do not jump to conclusions about clients based on their outward appearance. Just because clients may look like they are members of a culture does not mean that they have been actively involved in that culture. The "effeminate" client may very well be straight, the "macho" male may be gay, the Asian-American client may know little about his or her heritage, and so forth.

Counseling the Culturally Different: An Ongoing Process

Despite the fact that throughout this text we have stressed specific methods of working effectively with clients, it should be stressed that counseling is not fixed, and, indeed, many international counseling theories may approach the helping relationship in ways foreign to the American helper (Locke, 1992). In fact, Usher notes that "it is widely acknowledged that current counseling theories are products of Western culture and, as such, are not universally applicable to cross-cultural counseling situations" (1989, p. 62). "Not ours, not theirs; no one way of counseling surpasses another in the international arena. As cultures differ, so must counseling" (Romano, 1992, p. 1).

In an effort to improve the ways in which the helper works with a variety of culturally different clients, Pedersen (1981, 1983) developed a training model in which a safe environment is created for the helper to learn about the culturally different client. In this **triad model**, the client, the counselor, an *anticounselor*, and a *procounselor* all meet together during an interview. The function of the anticounselor is to highlight the differences in values and expectations between the client and counselor, whereas the procounselor highlights similarities in values and expectations. In this model, the procounselor and anticounselor give continual and immediate feedback to the helper in an

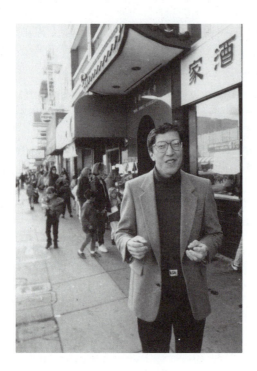

Dr. Derald Sue, one of the leaders in the field of multicultural counseling, has developed models for working with clients of diverse backgrounds and for incorporating cultural diversity in business, education, and mental-health organizations.

effort to increase the helper's ability to understand the client's perspective, recognize client resistance, recognize the helper's defensiveness, and learn how to recover from mistakes that the helper might make during the interview (Pedersen, 1985).

Sue and Sue (1990) note that working with culturally different clients should be viewed as a constantly changing process. In this context, they note that the helping relationship "is an *active process*, that is ongoing, and that it is a process that *never reaches an end point*. Implicit is the recognition of the complexity and diversity of the client and of client populations, and acknowledgment of our own personal limitations and the need to always improve" (p. 144).

Therefore, although it is important for us to be solidly based in our generic counseling skills when working with culturally different clients and aware of our own biases and stereotypes, we need to stay open to other ways of working with clients that may be more effective. Being open to new and different counseling techniques, which is supported by research, is the earmark of an effective cross-cultural counselor.

Ethical and Professional Issues

The Culturally Diverse Client's Right to Dignity, Respect, and Understanding

The culturally diverse client deserves a human service worker who has left his or her biases behind. Such a human service worker is knowledgeable about cultural and ethnic differences and is sensitive to the needs of the culturally different client. The importance of these attributes should not be underestimated. Examples of how mental-health professionals have negatively affected culturally different clients due to their own biases and prejudices abound in the literature (Cayleff, 1986). All clients deserve the respect and understanding of the professionals with whom they are working.

Our prejudices are often beyond our awareness. In other words, even though you may think you are not biased, unconscious prejudicial attitudes may seep out during interviews with clients. Because of this, ethical guidelines often speak to the importance of sensitivity to clients from diverse populations. For instance, the proposed ethical guidelines of NOHSE/CSHSE states the following:

Human service workers should be aware of multiculturalism in society and be responsive to the uniqueness of each citizen in regards to his or her cultural heritage and or personal belief system. . . .

Human service workers should advocate for the rights of all members of society, especially those who have been historically discriminated against. (See Appendix A)

Also, the Association for Multicultural Counseling and Development (AMCD), a division of ACA, has developed 31 multicultural counseling competencies that are viewed to be essential in the training of mental-health professionals. These competencies can be found in Appendix C, and you are encouraged to read them carefully.

The Developmentally Mature Human Service Worker: Open to the Continual Development of a Multicultural Perspective

Developmentally mature human service workers are able to work with clients of diverse backgrounds. They attempt not to be prejudiced or to hold stereotypic views and instead approach each client as a unique person. Such human service workers understand their limitations and are eager to learn about the culture or ethnic background of clients with whom they are working. This might be done by asking clients about their backgrounds but also by obtaining written materials about clients' cultural or ethnic backgrounds.

Along these lines, some advocates of a developmental multicultural perspective note that students proceed through predictable stages of development in gaining a multicultural perspective (D'Andrea & Daniels, 1991). These stages range from students who are in the affective/impulsive stage of racism, where they may respond impulsively and in a hostile fashion to individuals from diverse backgrounds, to the principled activist stage where students can understand and accept that culturally different people may hold varying values, beliefs, and may behave in ways different than the helper. In addition, students in this final stage actively work for systemic change in society.

Because helping students gain a multicultural perspective has become increasingly important, some authors have advocated weaving multicultural perspectives throughout human service programs (Garcia, Wright, & Corey, 1991), whereas others have spoken of the importance of having a separate course in multicultural awareness. Still others have suggested establishing peer-counseling programs for students of diverse backgrounds (Stokes et al., 1987).

Summary

We examined the increasing diversity found in our society and briefly looked at the differences in cultural and ethnic groups, religious beliefs, sex-role identity, and sexual orientations. We noted the diversity among other special groups and offered some explanations about how stereotypes and prejudices can lead to racism and discrimination. Such attitudes can often be unconscious and can deleteriously affect our work with clients.

We also examined barriers to an effective relationship with a culturally different client and offered examples of how culturally naive human service workers could negatively affect clients. In contrast, we examined the skills, attitudes, and knowledge base of the effective multicultural helper.

Being effective multicultural helpers is a developmental process in the sense that developmentally mature human service workers should be constantly striving to understand their own biases and vigilantly working toward improving their effectiveness with diverse populations. Finally, we stressed the importance of having knowledge, understanding, and respect for culturally diverse clients.

Experiential Exercises

1.   The Alligator River*

In class, do the following values clarification exercise, which is adapted from an exercise by Simon, Howe, and Kirschenbaum (1991).

First, read the following story.

Abigail is very much in love with Gregor who lives on the other side of the Alligator River. She wants to see Gregor but the bridge is out due to a recent flood. She would swim across the river, but she would get eaten by the alligators. Therefore, she goes to Sinbad, who is the only person with a boat on the river, and asks him to take her across.

Sinbad has always been in love with Abigail from a distance. He has a severe speech impediment, low self-esteem, and has rarely dated in his life. He makes a meager living taking people across the river. When Abigail asks him to take her across the river he states, "Abigail, I've always been in love with you, and I'll take you across the river if you'll make love with me." Abigail is initially disgusted, and she goes up to her friend Jaime and asks for advice. Jaime states, "This is your problem and you're going to need to work it out on your own." She ponders quite a while and then figures that she's slept with a lot of men, why not just do it, and then she'll be able to see Gregor. She agrees to make love with Sinbad (she insists that he use a condom).

Because Abigail has a very honest relationship with Gregor, she tells him the whole story. He becomes enraged and states, "Get out of my life, I never want to see you again." She becomes distraught, goes to her friend Slug, and tells him the whole story. He becomes infuriated with Gregor and punches him out.

Now, rate each of the five characters in the story on the following scale:

1. The person you liked most

2. The person you second best

3. The person you liked third best

4. The person you liked fourth best

5. The person you liked next to least

6. The person you liked least

---

*From the book, *Values Clarification: A Handbook of Practical Strategies for Teachers and Students*. Values Press, Sunderland, MA 01095, 1991, revised edition. For a list of other books on Values, phone Values Press, (413) 665-4800.

Have the instructor gather all the ratings and place them on a grid on the board with each name going across the top and ratings 1 through 6, on the side (*y*-axis). Count the number of 1s, 2s, and so forth for each person in the story and compare the distribution for each character.

Then, as a class, respond to the following questions:

1. What does the distribution tell you about how students in your class view individuals with differing values?

2. Did you assume that certain characters in the story were male and others female based on their names or roles?

3. If Abigail was a male, would you have rated the characters differently?

4. If Abigail was a male and Gregor a female, would you have rated the characters differently?

5. If the characters in the story were of differing ethnic, cultural, or religious backgrounds, would you have responded differently to them?

6. If you were in a helping relationship with any of the characters in the story, how would your positive and negative stereotypes affect your work with them?

2.   Examining Our Heritage

In class, form small groups of four or five. Then state your full name (if you're married and use your husband's last name, include your maiden name). Then discuss the origins of your name. Note such things as the origins of your last name, why you were given your first name, and any other information about your family history of which you may be aware. If you are not familiar with the history of your family name, ask a parent, guardian, or relative and see what they may know.

3.   Acknowledging Our Cultural/Ethnic/Religious Affiliation

In class, the instructor should ask each student to anonymously write on a piece of paper all ethnic, cultural, and religious groups to which each belongs (for example, Irish-American, Catholic, homosexual, individual with a disability). Then, have the instructor gather all papers and write on the board all the diverse groups found in your class.

4.   Finding Out about Other Cultural Groups
(Follow-Up to Exercise 3)

After the various ethnic, cultural, and religious groups are written on the board, each student should anonymously write any question he or she would like to ask about any of the diverse groups on the board. Have the instructor collect the questions, and as a class, all help answer the questions as best you can.

5. Interviewing a Person from Another Cultural Group

Using the following questions, interview a person from a different ethnic, cultural, or religious group. In class, share what you learned about that person.

1. What benefits does he or she attribute to being a member of that group?

2. What drawbacks does he or she attribute to being a member of that group?

3. What history does he or she know about his or her group?

4. What are the individual's feelings concerning stereotypes of the group?

5. What prejudice has he or she experienced?

6. How would he or she feel about seeing a helper of a differing ethnic, cultural, or religious background? Of the same background?

6. Experiencing Prejudice

Have the class divide up based on some physical attribute (for example, hair color, eye color, height). In addition, have the instructor randomly pick some of the groups to be below-average, average, and above-average intelligence. Within your group, come up with stereotypes of the other groups. During class, respond to one another based on your stereotypes and on the chosen intelligence level. At the end of class, process how the experience felt to one another.

7. Counseling Myths Questionnaire*

Read each of the following sentences and respond to each item accordingly. Each sentence should be rated twice according to the following scale:

SA	A	NO	D	SD
Strongly Agree	Agree	No opinion	Disagree	Strongly Disagree

*Adapted with permission from Dr. Richmond Calvin, Indiana University–South Bend.

First, indicate the extent to which you agree or disagree with *how it should be*; second, indicate the extent to which you agree or disagree with *how it is now*.

For instance, if you strongly agree with the sentence, you should circle as follows:

(SA) A NO D SD

If you have no opinion, you should circle as follows:

SA A (NO) D SD

How It Should Be   **How It Is Now**

SA A NO D SD   1. Certain clients should be avoided   SA A NO D SD
                   because of their past experiences.

SA A NO D SD   2. Cultural myths are unavoidable.   SA A NO D SD

SA A NO D SD   3. Cultural myths may become a   SA A NO D SD
                   cultural reality, even a norm, under
                   certain circumstances.

SA A NO D SD   4. Because clients are different, their   SA A NO D SD
                   behaviors are different.

SA A NO D SD   5. Helpers have fewer problems when   SA A NO D SD
                   they understand their clients'
                   backgrounds.

SA A NO D SD   6. Helpers should work only within   SA A NO D SD
                   their own cultural group.

SA A NO D SD   7. Most helpers believe that all   SA A NO D SD
                   culturally different persons have
                   problems if one member of that
                   group has demonstrated he or she
                   has a problem.

SA A NO D SD   8. Culturally different persons are   SA A NO D SD
                   usually sent to helpers from the
                   same cultural group as the client.

SA A NO D SD   9. Race and social class of both client   SA A NO D SD
                   and helper are significant factors in
                   the helping relationship.

SA A NO D SD 10. Cultural variations exist regarding   SA A NO D SD
                   verbal and nonverbal communication
                   across cultures.

How It Should Be   **How It Is Now**

SA A NO D SD 11. Everyone is culturally different;   SA A NO D SD
therefore, helpers need a model
that will serve all clients.

SA A NO D SD 12. All types of social services are   SA A NO D SD
available for all persons who
desire them.

SA A NO D SD 13. All cultures receive fair treatment   SA A NO D SD
in the helping relationship.

SA A NO D SD 14. Culturally different clients use   SA A NO D SD
profanity more often than
nonculturally different clients do.

SA A NO D SD 15. Nonculturally different clients are   SA A NO D SD
more likely to respond to helping
interventions than are culturally
different clients.

SA A NO D SD 16. Generally, clients from low-income   SA A NO D SD
poverty backgrounds cannot be
helped.

SA A NO D SD 17. Many culturally different persons   SA A NO D SD
have shown they do not trust
counselors.

SA A NO D SD 18. Family ties are extremely weak with   SA A NO D SD
many culturally different clients.

SA A NO D SD 19. Value systems for many culturally   SA A NO D SD
different clients are inferior.

SA A NO D SD 20. Poor minority clients do not trust   SA A NO D SD
nonminority middle-class helpers.

SA A NO D SD 21. Sociocultural history represents the   SA A NO D SD
most important ingredient in the
helping relationship.

SA A NO D SD 22. Culturally different clients do   SA A NO D SD
not possess qualities such as boldness,
initiative, and assertiveness.

SA A NO D SD 23. Many culturally different clients are   SA A NO D SD
not persistent, logical thinkers,
problem solvers, and adequate
decision makers.

How It Should Be		**How It Is Now**
SA A NO D SD	24. All helping relationships have a cross-cultural component.	SA A NO D SD
SA A NO D SD	25. Religious differences are *not* important in the helping relationship.	SA A NO D SD
SA A NO D SD	26. Age differences are *not* important in the helping relationship.	SA A NO D SD
SA A NO D SD	27. Gender differences are *not* important in the helping relationship.	SA A NO D SD
SA A NO D SD	28. Sexual-orientation differences are *not* important in the helping relationship.	SA A NO D SD

8

Research, Program Evaluation, and Testing

The inquiry of truth, which is the love-making, or wooing of it, the knowledge of truth, which is the presence of it, and the belief of truth, which is the enjoying of it, is the sovereign good of human nature. (Sir Francis Bacon)

While I was living in Cincinnati and working on my doctorate, I was walking down the street one day and a person came up to me and said, "Do you want to take a personality test?" I said, "Sure!" I was brought into a store-front office and spent about 30 minutes completing an inventory. When I finished, I was asked to wait a few minutes while they scored the instrument. Then, a person came into the room and said, "Well, you have a pretty good personality and you're fairly bright, but if you complete Ron Hubbard's course on Dianetics, you will have a better personality and be even brighter." Having taken some coursework in testing, I knew a number of things. First, I questioned whether the test truly measured personality and intelligence; second, I questioned the way in which the instrument was interpreted.

After finishing my doctorate and while teaching at a small New England college, I was supervising a graduate student's thesis. Her hypothesis was that there would be a relationship between the number of years of yoga meditation and self-actualizing values; that is, the more you meditated, the more self-actualized you would be. She went to an ashram (a yoga retreat center) and had a number of individuals fill out an instrument to measure how self-actualized they were; she then collected information from the individuals concerning how long they had been meditating. After collecting her data and performing a statistical analysis, she found no relationship. Because she herself had meditated for years, she strongly felt that she would find such a relationship. Upon finding no relationship, she said to me, "There must be something wrong with this instrument or this research because people who have meditated for years are clearly more self-actualized than those who have just started meditating." I suggested there was nothing wrong with the research or the instrument, but that perhaps she had a bias because of her own experiences with meditation. I explained that this does not mean that meditation does not affect people, but that in this one area, using this instrument, the evidence showed that no relationship existed. I told her that research is not how you *feel* something is but what you *find* something is. When she was able to see her own biases, she realized that perhaps I was right.

I once received a federal grant to train school counselors how to be aware of and intervene in cases of chemical abuse. To receive the grant, I had to explain the need for and purpose of the training, how the training was to take place, and how we would evaluate the effectiveness of the training. Explaining how I would determine the effectiveness of this training, through evaluation, was considered a crucial factor in deciding whether I would get this grant. In this case, evaluation was used as a check to ensure that what we were presenting to the counselors was effective. In addition, evaluation was also viewed as a measure of whether it would be worthwhile to do similar training in the future and to examine which areas to revise if future training were to occur.

Many human service workers have little knowledge of research, program evaluation, and testing, even though these three areas have permeated every part of our society and many aspects of our clients' lives. Mehrens (1992) notes, "There is much ignorance about very basic measurement, evaluation, and research topics among the practitioners . . . and among those who are ignorant, there is, on occasion, a fair amount of hostility toward some useful data" (p. 439). Research, program evaluation, and testing are important in helping us understand our clients and in determining whether what we are doing is of benefit to them. Although human service workers may not be directly involved in research, program evaluation, and testing, they will often come in contact with research concerning client outcomes, evaluation of social service programs, and tests that clients take. In this chapter, we will present an overview of these three areas.

Research

Conducting Research

Research answers the question "Are our hunches about the world correct, and how might what we are doing affect the future?" Best and Kahn (1986) define *research* as "the systematic and objective analysis and recording of controlled observations that may lead to the development of generalizations, principles, theories, resulting in prediction and ultimate control of events" (p. 18). In other words, researchers scientifically analyze information in order to make predictions about the future. Research can be anything from counting the number of times a child acts out during the day, to surveying opinions of human service workers, to performing a complex analysis of a specific counseling approach when working with clients. The next section provides a brief overview of a few of the major kinds of research.

The Hypothesis, the Research Question, and Literature Review

Kuhn (1962) said that all new knowledge is built on former knowledge and that, at times, shifts in our understanding of the world take place when former knowledge no longer explains current phenomena. In a sense, as Sir Francis Bacon said so eloquently, we are forever seeking the truth. In performing research, our first step in seeking current truth is to develop a **hypothesis** or **research question** to explore.

Such research questions are "testable propositions that are logically derived from theories" and prior research (Sommer & Sommer, 1991, p. 4). For us to come up with our hypothesis or question, we need to examine past research. This is done by doing a thorough **review of the literature**.

A review of the literature involves examining all major research done in the area we are exploring. This is accomplished by examining the literature, usually articles and books written on the topic in question. Most libraries today can provide us with a computerized literature review of the topic under question. Two such computer searches, ERIC and PSYCH LIT, provide abstracts of articles in the areas being examined. (Computer searches, such as ERIC and PSYCH LIT, are also valuable in helping the student identify sources for papers.) For instance, if I were interested in examining all the research that explored job satisfaction of human service workers, I might go to the computer and place in key descriptors; that is, major terms that the computer will search. In this case, such key descriptors might be *careers, occupations, human services, and social services*. The computer would print the abstracts of all articles that contained one or more of these descriptors. Then, I would most likely cross reference the descriptors *careers* and *occupations* with *human services* and *social services* as a method of retrieving only those articles that had research in these areas. After I read the abstracts, I would decide which articles I want to obtain, read them thoroughly, and develop a hypothesis or research question.

In the preceding example, one such research question might be "What are the major careers in the human service field?" A second question might be "How satisfied are human service workers in these careers?" Ultimately, I might want to set up a **research design** that examines this question.

Designing the Study

After deciding which research ideas to explore, carefully defining those variables that are being examined is important. A *variable* is "any characteristic or quality [for example, height, intelligence, self-esteem, job satisfaction] that differs in degree or kind and can be measured" (Sommer & Sommer, 1991, p. 83). In our example, the variables consist of satisfaction and careers in the human service profession.

Defining the Research Design

True experimental research.   Sometimes, as in **true experimental research**, you will be manipulating variables to see what effect they have on the outcome that you are examining. This type of research allows you to look at the causes of behavior. Usually, the variable that is being manipulated is called the **independent variable,** and the variable that you are measuring is called the **dependent variable**. For instance, if we could somehow randomly assign 1000 recent graduates from human service programs to different types of human service work (for example, mental health, social services, unemployment, rehabilitation), we could measure, at a later date, how satisfied these groups of individuals are and explore whether one group is more satisfied than another group. Clearly, this would be a difficult research study to undertake. Would you willingly participate in a study in which you were randomly assigned a specific type of job—one you perhaps did not want?

Quasi-experimental research.   Because experimental research involves random assignment and the manipulation of variables, it is often impractical or impossible to implement such research even though hypothetically it might be more sound. Therefore, **quasi-experimental**

A Failed Attempt at True Experimental Research

When I was living in New Hampshire, a colleague and I decided to do some research on the effects of aerobics on personality variables. After exploring the literature, we found some possible links between aerobics and the personality variables of self-actualization, depression, and anxiety. We approached our local YMCA, which was running a rather extensive aerobics program, and the staff agreed to let us talk with individuals who were about to start aerobics for the first time. They also agreed to let these people have 8 weeks of free membership at the Y if half of them (randomly chosen) would not start aerobics for 8 weeks. We found three instruments to measure our personality measures, with the intent of comparing, at the end of 8 weeks, the group that started aerobics with the group that waited. We excitedly met with approximately 50 new "aerobians." We told them our plans—they looked at us and said, "Are you kidding? We want to start now!"

Our good intentions obviously were not going to sway these individuals who were ready to start exercising. Unfortunately for us, we could not implement our study. Instead, we moved to a quasi-experimental study in which we compared individuals who had just finished 8 weeks of aerobics with those just starting. Because random assignment could not be used in this type of research study, it was not as solid a study as our original plan. I guess our desire to do research was not as powerful as the individuals' desire to exercise.

research, which allows us to examine variables of intact groups, is often employed. For instance, knowing that I could not randomly assign human service workers to differing groups, I decide to compare job satisfaction of human service workers who are employed at juvenile detention centers, in mental-health centers, and at unemployment offices. First, I would assign a satisfaction scale to each intact group. Second, I would examine statistical differences between the three groups. In other words, I would score the satisfaction scales and statistically analyze whether some groups are more satisfied than other groups. Because random assignment is not used in this case, any differences found cannot be attributed solely to the type of job (for example, perhaps people who are more satisfied pick certain jobs). Therefore, in this type of research, we cannot be assured that one variable causes another. However, this research can often give us a good sense of the relationship between variables.

Sociological research.   In sociological research, you are examining "the systematic gathering of information about people's beliefs, attitudes, values, and behavior" (Sommer & Sommer, 1991, p. 129).

Sociological research is generally divided into one of two categories. In **survey research**, a questionnaire is designed to gather specific information from a target population. For instance, we might send out a questionnaire to human service workers and ask them a series of questions regarding their job satisfaction. In this case, we could examine many variables like salary, number of years at the job, and educational level and perhaps ask them to rate their job satisfaction. We could then use charts and graphs to illustrate the differences between the various jobs on these variables.

To illustrate the type of information one can obtain from surveys, Neukrug, Healy, and Herlihy (1992) completed a survey of the types of ethical complaints lodged against licensed counselors. We surveyed licensing boards in each state that had counselor licensure. We found that more than 70,000 counselors are licensed in these states and that, since the inception of licensure, there have been over 1143 complaints (most states have obtained licensure within the past 5 years). We found that practicing without a license or other misrepresentation of qualifications was the most frequently lodged complaint (27%) and that having sex with a client (which is not only unethical, but illegal in many states) was the second most frequent complaint (20%). Other grievances, such as having a dual relationship with a client, lack of informed consent, and not properly forming a group, consisted of the rest of the complaints lodged.

Although survey research can be interesting, it cannot tell us the underlying reasons for our results. For instance, in our research on ethical complaints, we are not clear what percentage of complaints were actual ethical violations (as opposed to ethical complaints), and we can only make educated guesses about why we found misrepresentation and having sex with a client as the two most frequent types of complaints. Therefore, survey research can be limiting, although sometimes intriguing.

The second type of sociological research is called **participant observation** in which the researcher interacts with the group being observed. He or she may actually live with the group and take notes about their interactions (Burgess, 1984; Cole, 1975). Margaret Mead's famous research on aborigine youth in Samoa is an example of participant observation (Mead, 1961). Mead immersed herself with the people and their culture as she attempted to understand their lifestyle. This field research gives us a close-up view of the population we are studying. Although researchers involved in participant observation will attempt to be objective, such research may be subject to the biases of the researcher.

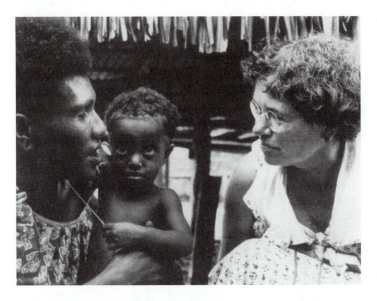

As a participant observer, Margaret Mead (1901–1978) gained a deep understanding of the culture she was observing by living with the people.

Examining the Results

Once you have completed your literature review, set up your design, and performed your study, you are ready to analyze your results. Many statistical analyses can be used in examining your research. Separate

Disruptive Observation of a Third-Grade Class

When I was working as an associate school psychologist in New Hampshire, I was asked to "debrief" a third-grade class that had just finished a trial period in which a young boy who was paraplegic and severely mentally retarded was mainstreamed into their classroom. During this trial period, a stream of observers from a local university came into the third-grade classroom to assess the students' progress. Because this was not participant observation, the observers sat in the back and took notes about the interactions between the students. This information was supposed to be used at a later date to decide whether it was beneficial for the student who was disabled to be in the classroom as well to decide whether having him in the classroom was disruptive for the third-graders.

When I met with the students, they clearly had adapted well to this young boy who was disabled. Although, because of his severe disabilities, they could not form any real relationship with him, his presence seemed in no way to detract from their studies or from their other relationships in the classroom. However, almost without exception, the students noted that what was annoying was the constant stream of observers interfering with their daily schedule. Perhaps if participant observation had been employed, where an observer interacted and was seen as part of the classroom, the students would have responded differently.

courses in both research and statistics, however, would be needed to comprehend the complexity of analyses that can be performed in good research. Briefly, when examining differences between groups or the relationship between groups, a number of analyses can be performed. Terms that you might see in the literature that examine group differences and relationships between groups include *t-tests, analysis of variance (ANOVA),* and *correlations* (usually found in true research and quasi-experimental research). To decide if there is statistical significance between groups, you will see a *probability level* set. Such levels tell you the probability that the results you have found could be found by chance alone. For instance, much research will set its probability at the .05 level. This means that there is less than a 5 out of 100 chance that the results you find happened by chance. Or, put another way, your results are probably due to the factors you are examining. In the literature, this is reported as $p < .05$ (p = probability, < = less than).

In the reporting of survey or sociological research, *descriptive statistics* are usually used. Descriptive statistics include measures of central tendency (mean, median, and mode), measures of variability (for example, range, standard deviation), percentages, and frequencies (see the section on measures of central tendency and measures of variability, page 229). These statistics are often presented in charts, graphs, and tables. This allows you to examine the overall results of the data you have collected. Table 8-1, based on a survey by Randolph and Lassiter (1985), is an example of a table using descriptive statistics with percentages.

Table 8-1 Mean Percentage of Time an Intern Spends at Various Functions According to Degree Level

Role/Function	Bachelor's	Master's/Post-master's	Doctoral
Casework/case management	32.9	20.9	13.7
Counseling and psychotherapy	25.5	37.9	39.5
Consultation and education	6.2	7.2	9.5
Testing/assessment	6.1	8.3	10.3
Research and evaluation	3.6	3.3	6.5
Supervision	7.9	9.7	10.6
Seminars	3.5	3.5	5.8
Vocational assessment/placement	5.3	4.4	.7
Other	9.0	3.2	3.7

SOURCE: Randolph and Lassiter (1985, p. 9).

Discussing the Results

Probably the most important aspect of research is the conclusions drawn from the study. These conclusions, based on the results, give the researcher an opportunity to discuss possible reasons that such results were found. Although discussions allow for some leeway, the researcher should not take giant leaps in an effort to present "the truth." For instance, in Table 8-1, one can easily see that doctoral student interns spend considerably less time doing case management activities as compared with master's- and bachelor's-level interns. However, any discussion about why this might be the case should be worded carefully because the research only presents the data and does not explore the reasons behind them.

Using Research in Human Service Work

Knowledge of basic research techniques is valuable for human service workers. First such knowledge enables human service workers to understand professional journal articles and to make conclusions concerning what might be the most effective interventions for their clients.

Second, research can validate what we are doing; at other times, it might suggest new ways of approaching client change (Lambert, Ogles, & Masters, 1992). Third, research might suggest new avenues to explore and is often the basis for future research. Finally, use of basic research techniques can be valuable for program evaluation.

Program Evaluation

Although many research concepts are used in evaluation, the purpose of program evaluation tends to be different (Burck & Petersen, 1975). Whereas research tends to examine new paradigms to expand understanding and knowledge, program evaluation has to do with "the extent to which a program has achieved its stated goals and objectives" and "the conditions under which a program is most efficient" (Engelkes & Vandergoot, 1982, p. 314). For instance, suppose I implement a new program that examines the effects of self-esteem training on job attainment. If I offer the program and have no method of researching its effectiveness, I will not know if the program is worth our time and effort. Therefore, I would want to find some mechanism of evaluating the program *while* it is occurring, as well as *after* it is completed. The two major types of evaluation that help us do this are process and outcome evaluation.

Process Evaluation

When presenting a program, workshop, or conference, assessing effectiveness through an ongoing evaluation process is important. **Process evaluation** involves the assessment of a program *during* its implementation in order to gain feedback about its effectiveness and to allow for change in the program as needed.

There are a number of ways to perform process evaluation. Probably the most basic way is to ask for verbal feedback from your audience. In this case, presenters need to be open to feedback, especially any negative criticism, and be willing to change their programs midway. A little less threatening, and sometimes more revealing, is to have participants write down reactions to the program while it is occurring. Doing this anonymously allows participants to express their feelings openly, without fear of repercussions. Along these same lines, participants can be asked to complete rating forms during the program in order to obtain ongoing feedback. The advantage of rating forms is that you can easily collate the data and get a sense of how the whole group feels about aspects of the program. The disadvantage is that rating forms do not allow for feedback outside the questions being asked. Of course, rating forms could be created that include room for written feedback.

Outcome Evaluation

Outcome evaluation involves assessment of the total training program *after* it is finished. Like process evaluation, outcome evaluation may involve asking for verbal feedback, written feedback, and responses to rating scales. However, some programs may also require a more systematic evaluation process that involves the use of research techniques. For instance, you might want to examine the effectiveness of two differing programs on attainment of effective parenting skills. You might randomly assign 20 parents to one group and 20 to a second group, run your training programs, and measure the effectiveness of the two programs. You can then contrast the effect of one program with the other, trying to determine if one type of training is more effective than another.

In some cases, you might expect training programs to have some far-reaching effects. For instance, I received a grant to train helpers in a local school system to identify, assess, and intervene with students at risk for drug and alcohol abuse. Some of the long-term outcome measures that we hoped to see from this training included the reduction in alcohol and drug use by students, a decrease in the dropout rate (chemical abuse has been shown to be related to dropout rate), and an increase in the age of first use of drugs or alcohol. To obtain information like this would be a major undertaking and would involve a large-scale assessment of students. Though not an easy project, these behaviors are measurable and could be an indication that our program was effective.

The Human Service Worker and Program Evaluation

At some point in your career as a human service worker, you will be asked to run a program for your clients. It may be a self-esteem program, a job-awareness program, a parenting program, or simply a program that explains the services of your agency to your clients. Whatever program you run, you will want to receive feedback about its effectiveness. To improve the program while it is occurring *or* to improve it for the next time that it might be given, process and outcome evaluation measures should be undertaken: "Without ongoing evaluation, it is difficult to know whether you are helping. If change seems to be occurring, you may not know what actually *is* helping the consumer" (Halley, Kopp, & Austin, 1992, p. 420).

Program evaluation also has an important place in examining the effectiveness of job-related behaviors at your agency. A responsible agency is willing to look at the effectiveness of its employees and its programs. Such evaluation can greatly assist in understanding what works and what needs to be changed.

In these times of fiscal crisis, the issue of **accountability** of programs and agencies has become extremely important. No longer can

Outcome Evaluation of a Drug and Alcohol Training Program

The following is an outcome evaluation measure that was used during a drug and alcohol awareness workshop (Project TRUST) for mental-health professionals in a school system in Virginia. The numbers on the right under "Mean" represent the average score, on each item, for all participants. The presenters were generally rated very high, as was the workshop itself. Based on this information, in which areas would you want to see improvement in the future?

Workshop Evaluation ($N = 52$)

Describe your reaction to each of the following statements in terms of this scale.

1. Never	3. Sometimes	5. Always
2. Seldom	4. Usually	6. Not applicable

Workshop presenters	Mean
1. Were well prepared.	4.7
2. Delivered material in a clear, organized manner.	4.7
3. Stimulated intellectual curiosity.	3.9
4. Showed respect for questions and opinions of participants.	4.6
5. Allowed for relevant discussion when appropriate.	4.7
6. Were concerned that participants understood them.	4.6
7. Were accessible for individual and group concerns.	4.6

Workshop TRUST	
8. Offered information applicable to one's field.	4.0
9. Was presented in a comfortable, conducive environment.	4.4
10. Provided a beneficial, educational experience.	4.1

programs and agencies deliver services without some account that what they are doing is working. The use of evaluation techniques is an important step in the accountability process and assures the public and funding agencies that you are performing essential and effective services for your clients (Ohlsen, 1983).

Testing

Norm-Referenced Tests and Criterion-Referenced Tests

Generally, tests are either norm-referenced or criterion-referenced. **Norm-referenced tests** are those instruments in which the examinee can compare his or her score with a peer or **norm group**. This means that an individual's score can be compared with conglomerate group scores of his or her peers. Many tests that are sold by national publishing companies are norm-referenced.

Criterion-referenced tests are those tests in which the examinee has specific goals to meet based on his or her rate of learning. This allows the individual to move at his or her own pace in accomplishing those goals. Criterion-referenced testing is used with the learning disabled because they may need additional time to meet learning goals as compared with other students in their grade level.

Standardized Tests and Informal Tests

Standardized tests are assessment instruments that are given in a standard fashion; that is, each test administration, regardless of where and when it is given, is given by the examiner in the exact same fashion. **Informal tests** are assessment instruments that are not necessarily compared with a norm group, and the way they are administered may vary during each test-taking situation. Teacher-made tests and rating scales are two examples of informal types of tests. Teacher-made tests measure what students have learned in the classroom. Because they are based on the teacher's sense of what students have learned, they are somewhat subjective. Rating scales are often used for evaluation purposes or for a quick overview of an individual's personality style.

Tests can be standardized and norm-referenced, standardized and criterion-referenced, informal and norm-referenced, or informal and criterion-referenced. Sometimes, criterion-referenced tests may also be norm-referenced. Some examples follow:

- A standardized, norm-referenced test might be an individual intelligence test in which the test is given the exact same way across the country and the individual's score is then compared with national scores of his or her peer group.

- A standardized, criterion-referenced test might be an individual achievement test given to a student who is learning disabled. The test is given the same way across the country, but the student will take only those parts of the test in which he or she has reached individualized learning goals.

- An informal, norm-referenced test might be a rating scale devised by a researcher to measure the amount of cynicism among a national group of human service workers and educators. The test could be sent to all members of NOHSE, and a score received by one human service worker can then be compared with the larger population of human service workers.

- An informal, criterion-referenced test might be a teacher-made test that has targeted learning goals for students.

- A criterion-referenced test that is also norm-referenced might be an individual diagnostic test that assesses for a possible learning disability in math. Being criterion-referenced, it has individualized learning goals. However, because it is also norm-referenced, it allows the examiner the opportunity to compare the individual to a norm group.

Types of Tests

Tests in the cognitive realm: ability testing.   Tests in the cognitive domain are generally called **ability tests**. These tests measure an individual's cognitive capabilities. Two major categories of ability tests include **achievement tests**, tests that measure what you have learned, usually in school; and **aptitude tests**, tests that measure what you are capable of learning.

Three major types of achievement tests include survey battery tests, diagnostic tests, and readiness tests. **Survey battery tests** measure general achievement and are usually given in large-group settings in schools. You are probably familiar with this type of test through your own education. The Iowa Test of Basic Skills (ITBS) and the Stanford Achievement Test are two examples of survey battery tests. The uses of survey battery tests are many and include the assessment of a student's ability level, the determination of teaching effectiveness, and the examination of the general level of ability throughout a school system.

Diagnostic tests delve more deeply into suspected problem areas and are often given one-on-one by an experienced examiner, usually a school psychologist or learning disabilities specialist. Following the results of a diagnostic test and in consultation with parents and teachers, it may be decided that a student has a learning disability; that is, in one or more specified areas, it is suspected that the student's ability is much lower than his or her average ability in other areas.

Readiness tests assess an individual's ability to advance to the next educational level. One major use of readiness tests is to determine if a child is developmentally ready to enter first grade. Because children at kindergarten age develop at different rates, some children

Public Law 94-142

In 1975 the **Education for All Handicapped Children Act** [Public Law 94-142 (PL94-142)] was passed (*Federal Register,* 1977). This landmark legislation ensured the right to an education within the *least restrictive environment* for any individual between the ages of 3 and 21 who had a disability. The importance of this law for individuals with a disability, particularly a learning disability, was enormous. To implement this law, diagnostic testing has become one of the main ways of determining who might have a disability. Subsequent laws have enhanced this landmark legislation (Gable & Hendrickson, 1990).

need additional time in school before they are ready to enter first grade. Readiness at this age does *not* imply innate ability but simply reflects differing stages of development at an early age in life. For instance, a very bright child may be developmentally too immature to enter first grade.

Four major kinds of aptitude tests include individual intelligence tests, cognitive ability tests, special aptitude tests, and multiple aptitude tests. **Individual intelligence tests**, such as the Stanford-Binet, are individually given to measure general intellectual ability and are usually administered by highly trained examiners, most often psychologists. These tests have a broad range of use; they help identify individuals who have learning disabilities, developmental disabilities, or are gifted and help us understand the total personality style of an individual. Usually, when a comprehensive assessment of an individual is requested, an individual intelligence test is included.

Cognitive ability tests are paper-and-pencil tests used to measure general intellectual ability. These tests, which are often given in groups, assess an individual's ability to do well in school. Therefore, they are sometimes used for placement in school, as part of determining learning disabilities and giftedness, and as predictors of ability for college (for example, Scholastic Aptitude Test, or SAT), graduate school (for example, Graduate Record Exam, or GRE), and so forth.

Special aptitude tests measure a specific, clearly defined segment of ability (for example, spatial ability, eye/hand coordination, mechanical ability). Special aptitude tests are sometimes used as part of the criteria for job placement and acceptance into specialty schools (for example, the use of a eye/hand coordination test to determine ability for operating complex machinery in a factory). **Multiple aptitude tests** measure a number of clearly defined segments of ability and often help an individual understand his or her broad range of abilities and how those abilities might be associated with occupational choice. The Armed Services Vocational Aptitude Battery (ASVAB), which is given by the military (often for free in the schools), and the General Aptitude Test Battery (GATB), which is given by an employment security office, are two examples of multiple aptitude tests.

Although both achievement tests and aptitude tests may be standardized, informal, norm-referenced, or criterion-referenced, most testing of this kind tends to be norm-referenced and standardized. A standardized test ensures that the comparisons with the norm group are of high quality and the use of norm groups allows for comparisons with large groups of examinees.

Tests in the affective realm: personality testing.   Three types of personality assessment most frequently used today are objective tests, projective tests, and interest inventories. **Objective tests** are often multiple choice or true/false paper-and-pencil measures that allow us to compare the individual's personality with his or her norm group. Therefore, individuals can compare personality traits such as depression, anxiety, interests, and introversion to individuals who exhibit such behavior or to the "normal" population. Objective tests are given in groups or on an individual basis. Some of these tests, like the Minnesota Multiphasic Personality Inventory-II (MMPI-II) can measure psychopathology, whereas others, like the Myers-Briggs, measure common personality characteristics. The use of objective tests are many and include helping make a clinical diagnosis, helping an individual understand his or her personality style, and determining emotional stability for certain types of jobs (for example, working in a nuclear missile silo).

Projective tests allow an individual to make an unstructured response to a stimuli. For instance, the Rorschach, a major projective test, consists of showing ten inkblots to an individual and asking the individual to state what he or she sees in the blots. Other types of projective tests include sentence completion, where the end of a sentence is omitted and the client completes it with the first thing that comes to mind; drawings, where the client is asked to make a specific drawing (for example, a drawing of the client's family all doing something together); and tests in which the individual is asked to develop stories from pictures that are presented. In all of the above, based on the client's responses, a highly trained clinician makes judgments about the client's personality style.

Interest inventories measure an individual's likes and dislikes as well as his or her personality orientation toward the world of work. These paper-and-pencil assessment instruments are most frequently used to help individuals discover those occupations and careers to which they would most likely have a good fit. The Strong Vocational Interest Inventory and the Self-Directed Search (SDS) are two of the more common interest inventories used today.

The Nature of Tests

Relativity of scores.   John receives a score of 47 on a test. How did he do? Jill receives a 95 on a different test. How did she do? If John's test score was 47 out of 50, he probably did pretty well. But, if 1000 people take the test and all but John receive a score of 50 out of 50, we might view his test score a little differently.

What about Jill's score? Is a score of 95 good? If the best possible score is 100, perhaps it is a good score. But what if the best possible score is 200, or 550, or 992? If 1000 people take the test and Jill's score is the highest, we might say that she did well, at least compared with this group. But if her score is at the lower end of the group of scores, then comparatively she did not do well. To make things even more complicated, what if a high score represents more of an undesirable trait (for example, cynicism or depression)? Then clearly, the higher Jill scores compared to her peer or norm group, the worse she has done comparatively. What's important here is the concept that in much of testing—particularly norm-referenced, standardized testing—scores are relative and an individual's raw score makes sense only in its relative position to his or her group.

Measures of central tendency and measures of variability.   When examining an individual's test scores to his or her norm group, understanding measures of central tendency and measures of variability of the test becomes very important. Measures of **central tendency** include the **mean**, the average of all the scores; the **median**, the middle score—that score representing the point where 50% of the examinees score above and 50% fall below; and the **mode**, the most frequent score. Two important measures of **variability** include the **range**, which represents the spread of scores from the highest to the lowest score; and the **standard deviation**, which represents how much, on average, scores vary from the mean. For instance, one test has a mean of 52, a standard deviation of 5. This means that most of the scores (about 68%) range between 47 and 57 ($\pm$ 1 standard deviation). Another group of scores also has a mean of 52 but a standard deviation of 20. This means that most scores (again, about 68%) on this test range between 32 and 72 (52 $\pm$ 20 points). Clearly, even though the two tests have the same mean, the range of scores around the mean vary considerably. An individual's score of 40 would be in the average range on the second test but well below average on the first test. If you know the central tendency and the measures of variability of the group of scores, you can compare your scores to these measures.

Reliability, validity, and practicality.   Before any test is given, it should be reliable, valid, and practical for the situation in which it is being used. A reliable test is consistent—that is, if individuals take the test a second time, and we have ensured that no learning has taken place between the first and second testings, then their test scores should remain about the same. A valid test accurately measures what it is supposed to measure. A test's validity is a function of how it is created. To create a valid test, one should do a thorough analysis of the literature concerning the test content, consult with experts about the test content, and compare the test with other tests of a similar nature. Using statistical analysis, test publishers will often report a number of different types of reliability and validity. To obtain a full understanding of these concepts, you would need to take a course in tests and measurement.

Practicality speaks to the issue of whether the test being given makes practical sense for the situation. For instance, although one might argue that individual intelligence tests should be given to many students, cost and time factors would make this a near impossibility.

Who Can Administer Tests?

The American Psychological Association (APA) defines three levels of test complexity that are associated with who can administer tests:

Level A tests are those that can be administered, scored, and interpreted by responsible nonpsychologists who have carefully read the test manual and are familiar with the overall purpose of testing. Educational achievement tests fall into this category. . . .

Level B tests require technical knowledge of test construction and use and appropriate advanced coursework in psychology and related courses (e.g., statistics, individual differences, and counseling). . . .

Level C tests require an advanced degree in psychology or licensure as a psychologist *and* advanced training/supervised experience in the particular test. . . . (APA, 1954, pp. 146–148)

Generally, the associate's- or bachelor's-level human service worker who has some coursework in tests and measurement can give a level A and, under some circumstances, a level B test. Level C tests require at least a master's degree along with advanced training in the test in question.

Using Tests with Minorities

Because tests have been shown at times to have bias against minorities and to be less predictive for some minority groups (Thorndike, Cunningham, Thorndike, & Hagen, 1991), the issue of whether to use tests with some groups has been hotly debated. No doubt, a well-made test can afford much information to an individual. However, not all well-made tests are accurate in their predictions for all people. The reasons for this are complex, and volumes have been written on this issue, but Walsh and Betz state it succinctly when they note that ". . . tests must be used in ways that, as far as possible, take advantage of the tremendous *utility* of test and other assessment data, while also facilitating optimal understanding and nurturance of a wide range of individual and cultural differences" (1985, p. 393).

Using Tests with Clients of the Human Service Worker

With literally thousands of tests in use today, the responsible use of assessment instruments can be a great adjunct to our work with clients: "Psychological tests and inventories, derived from and refined by scientific research, contribute to responsible practice by providing an empirical basis . . . for assessment and intervention" (Claiborn, 1991, p. 456).

Although the human service worker may not have the advanced training needed to administer many tests, it is not uncommon for a client to have taken some assessment instruments as a means of providing adequate goal setting. For example, tests are commonly used in many settings: the unemployment office where vocational assessments help clients find jobs, the community-based mental-health center where assessment is useful for diagnosis and treatment, or schools where assessment helps identify children with special needs as well as a measure of students' progress. No question, tests have become an integral part of our lives.

Even though human service workers will probably not be administering and interpreting most tests, consultation with examiners is a crucial step in working with our clients. Usually, examiners will provide a written test report that summarizes their results, and human service workers should be able to use these results in working with their clients. Therefore, basic knowledge of how tests are used is essential to our work with clients.

Ethical and Professional Issues

Informed Consent

Informed consent involves the client's right to know the purpose and nature of all aspects of client involvement with the helper. In reference to research and testing, clients have the right to know the general purposes of the research in which they are involved as well as how any tests they are taking are going to be used. Except in special cases (for example, court referrals for testing), clients also have the right to refuse to take part in any testing and research. Corey, Corey, and

Callanan (1993) note that when a client is not fully informed, the helper is open to liability concerns. Most ethical guidelines speak directly to the issue of informed consent. For instance, the proposed NOHSE/CSHSE ethical guidelines state that the "human service workers have the responsibility to inform clients of the purpose, goals, and nature of the helping relationship prior to its onset" (see Appendix A).

Today, an increasing number of authors are recommending that clients sign informed-consent forms indicating that they are fully aware of any therapeutic, testing, or research procedures in which they are participating (Bray, Shepherd, & Hays, 1985; Handelsman, Kemper, Kesson-Craig, McLain, & Johnsrud, 1986). As testing and research become more prevalent, and within this increasingly liability-conscious society, the issue of informed consent has become paramount (Bennett, Bryant, VandenBos, & Greenwood, 1990).

Use of Human Subjects

Stanley Milgram's "shocking" research on obedience (1965, 1974) dramatically affected the way future research would be done in the United States. Recruiting subjects through a local newspaper ad, he told them that they would be participating in research on the effects of punishment in learning. Assigning them to the role of teacher, he told the subjects that they would be administering an electrical shock to a learner every time the person did not complete a task properly. In actuality, the equipment was not hooked up, and the learner was an actor who would respond every time a "shock" was administered. As the experiment continued, the teacher was told to increase the voltage, and the learner, who initially was making mild grunting sounds following the shock, began to respond more strongly, eventually screaming. Despite the fact that many of the teachers protested what they were doing, with prodding by the experimenter, 65% of the subjects ended up administering 450 pseudo-volts to the learner, potentially enough to harm or kill a person had it been electricity. Although an interesting study, Milgram's research was much criticized for its potential psychological harm to the participants.

As a result of this study, as well as other research that had the potential to cause psychological or even physical harm to subjects, many restraints have been placed on the type of research in which people can participate. In fact, research like Milgram's could not legally be done today. Restraints on research that might cause physical or psychological harm are guided by ethical standards and, in many states, by legislation. Clearly, our sensitivity to research participants is much greater than it used to be.

Proper Interpretation and Use of Test Data

Human service workers are not experts in test administration and test interpretation. Therefore, they must rely on those who are. However, effective human service workers can use the results of test data in their work with clients. Therefore, they should carefully read the results of test reports and consult with experts in the field in order to understand how such data can best serve their clients. As noted earlier in this chapter, proper use of test data involves sensitivity to clients, knowledge of informed consent, and awareness of the cultural biases that are inherent in some tests.

The Developmentally Mature Human Service Worker: Understanding the Changing Face of Research, Program Evaluation, and Testing

The main purpose of research, program evaluation, and testing is to benefit our clients. Research helps us understand those interventions that are most effective with our clients, program evaluation helps us understand whether the programs we are offering benefit our clients, and tests try to give us insight into our clients. Research, as Kuhn (1962) notes, is an ever-evolving process that continually adds new knowledge to the field. Tests are always improving, giving us better insights into the clients with whom we work. Because the evaluation process relies heavily on research and testing, it too is an evolving process. Developmentally mature human service workers do not view research, testing, and evaluation as a stagnant process. Mature human service workers understand that new ideas, new tests, and new programs will be devised, and they are flexible enough to adopt those concepts that will best benefit their clients.

Summary

We examined the nature and purpose of research, program evaluation, and the use of tests in the work of the human service worker. Research adds knowledge to our field and therefore helps us make wise decisions concerning treatment plans for our clients. Differing types of research, such as experimental, quasi-experimental, and sociological studies, provide us varying ways to examine situations that may affect our clients.

Regardless of the type of research you are doing, certain steps in implementing research must be followed. They include reviewing the literature, developing a hypothesis or research question, designing the study, finding ways to analyze the data, and discussing the results.

Program evaluation ensures that the services we are offering our clients are of high quality. Basic research designs are sometimes helpful in evaluating our programs. Other times, we employ process or outcome evaluation techniques to examine the efficacy of our programs. In either case, evaluation ensures that we are ever vigilante in our efforts to improve services.

We noted the differences between norm-referenced and criterion-referenced tests, as well as standardized and informal assessments. In addition, we defined the varying types of ability tests and personality tests and discussed the qualities of validity, reliability, and practicality, three attributes that should be examined in determining whether a test should be used. Although human service workers do not generally have enough training to give many tests, they will be constantly exposed to test reports and test data. Therefore, the importance of close consultation with supervisors and experts in test administration is important.

Whether doing research or testing, the importance of fully informing our clients of the purpose and nature of their involvement is crucial. Clients have a right to informed consent concerning all aspects of their treatment. Finally, whether human service workers are involved in research, testing, or the evaluation process, it is important that these processes are seen as evolving; that is, as more knowledge is gained through research and evaluation and as tests are improved, developmentally mature human service workers are willing to examine and adapt these new concepts and materials in ways that will benefit their clients.

Experiential Exercises

1.   Critiquing a Journal Article

Obtain a research article from a human service journal, and using the following criteria, critique the article.

1. State and describe the type of research being employed (true experimental, quasi-experimental, sociological research—survey or participant observation).

2. On what basis is this experimental or sociological research?

3. Was the hypothesis or research question based on an adequate literature review?

4. What results were found?

5. What are the implications of the results for the human service worker?

6. What future research might arise out of this research?

7. Generally, what did you think of the article?

2.   Designing a Research Study

Have the instructor divide the class into four groups. Each group is to design a research study concerning the effectiveness of human service workers with their clients. One group is to design a true experimental study; the second group, a quasi-experimental study; the third group, a survey study; and the fourth group, a participant observation study. In designing your study, make sure you address the following issues:

1. Literature review

2. Hypothesis or research question

3. Research design

4. Results

5. Discussion

3.   Developing Evaluation Instruments

In small groups or as a class, develop a process and an outcome evaluation form for your class.

4.   Evaluating an Evaluation Form—Part 1

Most colleges and universities have some form of course evaluation that is completed at the end of the semester. Obtain a copy of the evaluation form that is used at your college and discuss any positive and negative aspects of that form.

5.   Evaluating an Evaluation Form—Part 2

Visit a local social service agency and see whether the agency has any evaluation forms that are used to assess client satisfaction, the effectiveness of programs, and/or the overall effectiveness of the agency. Share these forms in class.

6.   Sharing Experiences with Testing

In class, discuss any positive or negative experiences you have had relative to taking a test.

7. Advantages and Disadvantages to Testing

In small groups, discuss the following issues, pick a spokesperson, and report back to the class. Have the instructor write on the board the advantages and disadvantages that are noted by the groups.

1. The advantages and disadvantages of the SAT's

2. The advantages and disadvantages of individual intelligence testing

3. The advantages and disadvantages of personality assessment

8. Using Tests with Clients

Refer to the differing types of tests listed in the chapter and discuss the possible use of educational and psychological assessment for each of the following scenarios:

1. Johnny is a 12-year-old child in seventh grade. His grades have always been average, but recently his math scores have dropped considerably. In addition, he tells you that he found out not long ago that his parents are getting divorced.

2. William is 35 years old and recently separated. A few months following the separation, his wife accused him of molesting their 4-year-old child. He vehemently denies this accusation and states that she is "just saying those things in order to gain custody."

3. Judy is applying for a high-security job with the CIA. Following a background check, as a matter of course, they give her a number of assessment instruments.

4. Juanita is in lower management at a major computer firm. Her supervisor is thinking of recommending her for a promotion. Her new job would involve making quick decisions, and it requires a stable personality.

5. Jason is considering changing careers. He is not sure what career options are open for him and is unclear about what he likes to do. He is also unclear about what he is good at.

9. Ethical Vignettes

Discuss the ethics of the following scenarios:

1. Recently, there has been some research on the effectiveness of various drugs to combat the human immunodeficiency virus (HIV). To test if there is any effect, a drug company obtains permission to randomly assign individuals who have tested HIV-positive to two

groups. One group will get a new drug, and the second group will get a placebo (a sugar pill). Individuals do not know to which group they belong.

2. Based on the available research, a human service worker, who works at a 30-day rehabilitation center for chemically dependent individuals, founds a program on confrontation and humiliation. Although individuals can theoretically leave at any time, in this program, those who do not admit to their addictions and who do not begin to make major changes in their lives are heavily confronted by the whole group, are forced to shave their heads, and during "social time" are made to sit in their rooms and think about their lives.

3. To become more familiar with a local community religious group, a human service worker decides to become a participant observer and spends a week with the community at their retreat center. Part of their ritual is to smoke marijuana during their meditation times. Following the week at the center, he reports them to the local law enforcement agency for the illegal use of drugs.

4. During the taking of some routine tests for promotion, it is discovered that, based on the results of the tests, there is a high probability that one of the employees is abusing drugs and is a pathological liar. The firm decides not to promote him and instead fires him.

5. After receiving negative feedback concerning a workshop on communicating with teenagers, a human service worker decides "they really didn't want to learn how to communicate with their kids. I simply won't do workshops on this topic for 'those people' any more."

The Human Service Worker and the World of Work

When I was a young child, my father, a building contractor, took me around to various construction sites, and I would watch buildings slowly get built. As a teenager, during the summers, I would help a carpenter or general laborer at the sites. I remember getting picked up at five o'clock in the morning being crammed half-asleep, in the cab of a well-seasoned truck, to be taken on a bumpy ride to work. I would think to myself, "Is this what I want to do for the rest of my life?" Luckily, because I did well in school, I knew I'd be going on to college—but to do what?

Majoring in biology and thinking I was not bright enough to get into medical school, I chose dentistry as my eventual career path. My mind was made up, but something did not feel right. Although a part of me said "Go to professional school in a medical-related field," another distant voice said "This is not for you; you have other things to do in your life, other things that involve helping people." These divergent feelings were certainly an outgrowth of many things, including my family values and my placement in my family, my interests, my own emerging values, and my abilities. Although it was a tough decision, I eventually chose to listen to my distant voice, and I switched majors to psychology. Eventually, mostly through selected trial and occasional error, I ended up in the field of counseling. No doubt my life would have been made much easier if someone with training had assessed my likes and dislikes, my values, and my abilities; had helped me understand my personality style as it relates to the world of work; and helped me match these qualities with possible careers.

As I have proceeded on my career journey through life, I have continued to be faced with a number of choices. Should I go on for a graduate degree? Should I go toward clinical work or toward academia? Should I switch occupations totally? Again, my choices often seemed to be a product of trial and error. I would try something out to see if I liked it, if I was good at it, and would then make a decision about my future career direction. However, as I gained more awareness into myself and began to understand the career development process, I saw that I could choose my direction based on knowledge of my self along with knowledge about the world of work. No longer would my career decision making be an accident. I began to choose my future!

Despite the fact that I have been pretty satisfied at my work, there were times when my life did not feel complete. Therefore, other activities began to fill in some of the spaces. In my mid-20s I began to jog. As the years continued, running and aerobics became a focal point in my life. They offered an outlet for my stress, a place to meet other people, and an activity that took me away from my work. Recently, a foot injury has prevented me from working out at the level of activity I was used to. Now I am looking for other things to fill up the space that use to be taken up by exercise.

I have found my story, with its twists and turns, to be common. Many times when I've asked human service majors why they've chosen their major, I get ambiguous responses. Sometimes they'll say things such as "I like to work with people" or "I want to help people." Although these responses certainly may be one important component of choosing a career in the human service field, it is rare that I find individuals understanding how the dynamics of their family, their interests, their abilities, and their temperaments have affected the career choices they have made. The result is that, sometimes, a person chooses this field when another choice may be a better fit. As it is with human service workers, it is with people in general.

In this chapter, we will examine how individuals make career choices, what the future job outlook is for the human services, and how we can best facilitate our own and our clients' career choices.

Some Definitions

Although there are common meanings for many of the terms used in career development, our everyday definitions are not always the same as those we find in the literature. The following represents the definitions found in the career development literature, definitions we will use in this chapter.

> *Career.* "The course of events which constitutes a life; the sequence of occupations and other life roles which combine to express one's commitment to work in his or her total pattern of self-development; the series of remunerated and nonremunerated positions occupied by a person from adolescence through retirement, of which occupation is only one" (Super, 1976, p. 4).

> *Career development.* "The total constellation of psychological, sociological, educational, physical, economic, and chance factors that combine to shape the career of any given individual over the life span" (Sears, 1982, p. 139).

> *Job.* "A group of similar positions in a single plant, business establishment, educational institution, or other organization" (Shartle, 1959, cited in Isaacson & Brown, 1993, p. 13).

> *Occupation.* "A group of similar jobs found in different industries or organizations. Occupations exist in the economy and have existed in history, even when no man, woman, or child is engaged in them. Occupations, trades, and professions exist independently of any person. Careers, on the other hand, only exist when people are pursuing them" (Super, 1976, p. 4).

> *Career path.* "A term typically used in business and industry to describe a series of positions available in some occupational or spe-

cialized work area ordinarily connoting possibilities for advancement" (Herr & Cramer, 1988, p. 18).

Leisure. "Time free from required effort for the free use of abilities and pursuits of interests" (Super, 1976, p. 4).

Avocation. "An activity pursued systematically and consecutively for its own sake with an objective other than monetary gain, although it may incidentally result in gain" (Super, 1976, p. 4).

Career awareness. "The inventory of knowledge, values, preferences, and self-concepts that an individual draws on in the course of making career-related choices" (Wise, Charner, & Randour, 1978; cited in Herr & Cramer, 1988, p. 18).

A Little Bit of History

The Industrial Revolution brought about many demographic changes throughout the United States. Almost overnight, thousands of people moved from rural areas to the cities, numerous immigrants settled mostly in urban areas, and with this, a great number of children enrolled in city schools. Shifts in the types of available jobs were also evident, as was the need to assist these new city dwellers and students in their vocational development. In addition, social reform, as was evidenced by the settlement houses and charity organization societies, reflected the new focus on helping individuals determine their futures. All these changes led to the beginnings of the vocational guidance movement, which represented one of the first attempts to help individuals make vocational decisions.

One of the first persons credited with a systematic approach to vocational guidance was Frank Parsons. Parsons suggested that vocational guidance involve a three-step process: knowing oneself, knowing job characteristics, and making a match between the two through "true reasoning" (Parsons, 1909). Although undergoing some changes over the years, this **trait-and-factor approach to career guidance** has continued to be prominent in assisting individuals in the career-counseling process. Today, the trait-and-factor approach states that (Brown, 1984, p. 12):

- Each individual has a unique set of traits that can be measured reliably and validly.

- Occupations require that workers possess certain traits for success, although a worker with a rather wide range of characteristics can be successful in a given job.

- The choice of an occupation is a rather straightforward process, and matching is possible.

- The closer the match between personal characteristics and job requirements, the greater the likelihood for success.

In 1913 the increased emphasis on vocational guidance led to the founding of the National Vocational Guidance Association (NVGA). This association was a forerunner of the American Counseling Association (ACA). In the 1920s and 1930s vocational guidance was offered mainly in the schools and by the U.S. Department of Labor, and the testing movement began. The merging of vocational guidance with testing was a natural consequence because assessment offered a relatively quick and reliable means of determining individual traits. At around the same time, the U.S. Department of Labor published the first edition of the *Dictionary of Occupational Titles*, which represented one of the first attempts at organizing career information. Now individuals could assess their traits and match these traits to existing jobs.

In the 1950s a shift from vocational guidance to career development began. No longer was there an emphasis simply on making a job choice; instead, emphasis was placed on one's lifelong career patterns. In addition, with this new definition, postvocational patterns related to retiring were now included in the definition of career guidance. Donald Super, with his developmental approach to career guidance, was one of the leaders in changing the focus from vocational guidance to developmental career counseling.

With the emergence of the humanistic approach to counseling and government initiatives such as the **National Defense Education Act** of 1958, which stressed career guidance in the schools, new comprehensive models of career guidance were developed in the 1960s and 1970s. These models viewed career guidance in the broadest sense and included focusing on lifelong patterns of career development, helping individuals make choices that reflected their self-concept, defining career guidance as not only occupational choices but also as leisure and avocational options, and allowing for flexibility and change in one's lifelong career process (Herr & Cramer, 1988). In addition, these models emphasized the individual, not the counselor, as the career decision maker.

In the 1980s and 1990s, viewing career development as a life-span process has been increasingly emphasized; within this framework, career development models have been expanded to assist individuals in their lifelong pursuits. In addition, the computer age has brought about a wealth of accessible information that allows for quick exploration of the world of work. The evolution of career development models in conjunction with this new technology makes career exploration an exciting and in-depth process.

The Importance of Career Development

Many authors have highlighted the importance of career education and career counseling in facilitating one's career development. Work serves a number of economic, social, and psychological needs for the individual (Herr & Cramer, 1988) (see Table 9-1). In fact, lack of adequate career planning has been associated in numerous studies with job dissatisfaction, whereas a good match between one's personality and chosen occupation has been shown to lead to job satisfaction (Assouline & Meir, 1987; Spokane, 1985). In a similar vein, Isaacson (1986) notes that "unemployment, underemployment, or misemployment carry psychological costs borne by the individual in dissatisfaction, alienation, and lack of self-esteem, and by society as it is affected by those characteristics" (p. 32). These factors highlight the importance of adequate career counseling for the clients of the human service worker.

Despite the importance of work in our lives, our career development happens all too often by trial and error or hit or miss. Therefore, in the remainder of this chapter, we will examine some of the more prevalent theories that help us understand the career development process. In addition, we will explore sources of information that help us make informed choices. You will have the opportunity to examine the kinds of choices you have made in your life path and learn how you

Table 9-1 The Different Purposes of Work

Economic	Social	Psychological
Gratification of wants or needs	A place to meet people	Self-esteem
	Potential friendships	Identity
Acquisition of physical assets	Human relationships	A sense of order
Security against future contingencies	Social status for the worker and his or her family	Dependability, reliability
Liquid assets to be used for investment or deferred gratifications	A feeling of being valued by others for what one can produce	A feeling of mastery or competence
Purchase of goods and services	A sense of being needed by others to get the job done or to achieve mutual goals	Self-efficacy
Evidence of success		Commitment, personal evaluation
Assets to purchase leisure or free time	Responsibility	

SOURCE: From *Career Guidance and Counseling Through the Life Span: Systematic Approaches,* 3rd ed., by Edwin L. Herr and Stanley H. Cramer, p. 46. Copyright © 1989 by Edwin L. Herr and Stanley H. Cramer. Reprinted by permission of HarperCollins Publishers.

can apply some of these concepts to the clients with whom you work. Finally, we will examine how human service workers can optimize career choices for their clients and how developmentally mature human service workers view the career development process from a life-span perspective.

Models of Career Development

When I ask students how they chose their college major, I often get a response such as "Well, it was something I thought I'd like to do." Similarly, when I ask an individual how he or she ended up in a job, I find responses such as "The job was available" or "I always wanted to be a. . . ." Also, it is not unusual for a returning student to say to me, "I always knew I was in the wrong field; I don't know why I did that for so many years." These responses show me how little reflection and self-assessment have taken place when many people make one of the most significant decisions in their lives. If individuals had a broader understanding of their likes and dislikes, abilities, and personality characteristics, the reasons why they make these important choices would be clearer. In fact, greater awareness of individual traits, along with an understanding of the career development process, would probably lead many individuals in different directions from those in which they settled—directions that would yield greater career and life satisfaction.

Since the beginning of the vocational guidance movement, and particularly in the past 20 years, a number of career development models have been devised that have a common focus of helping the individuals understand their career choices. However, despite this common theme, people approach the career-counseling process in distinct ways. For instance, **self-efficacy theory** states that the types of choices we make in our lives are based on our beliefs about whether or not we can do certain behaviors (Bandura, 1977; Krumboltz, Mitchell, & Jones, 1976; McAuliffe, 1992). **Decision-making theory** views the individual's decision-making process as crucial in successfully making career choices (Tiedeman & O'Hara, 1963). On the other hand, **situational theory** states that often the choices we make are out of our control (for example, unavailability of jobs due to a recession) (Warnath, 1975).

Probably the two models that have been most prevalent in the field are the **developmental** and **personality approaches to career development.**

The Developmental Perspective

Like the developmental perspectives studied in Chapter 5, career development, from a life-span viewpoint, involves a series of stages through which individuals pass. Two of the major developmental theo-

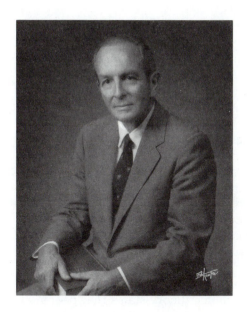

Donald Super, with his developmental approach to career guidance, was one of the leaders in changing the focus from vocational guidance to developmental career counseling.

ries are those of Eli Ginzberg (1972) and Donald Super (1984). Super, in particular, has extensively researched his career development theory, and this will be presented in brief form.

Super views career development as a lifelong process in which we attempt to make choices based on our view of self. He states that individuals differ in their abilities, interests, and personalities and that, despite these differences, there are a number of occupations in which each person can fit. He further notes that as we pass through the life stages, our perceptions of self may change and we may therefore shift our orientation toward the world of work.

Super views career development as a five-stage process. The **growth stage** (ages birth–14 years) involves the development of career self-concept through identification with others and beginning awareness of interests and abilities related to the world of work. Included in this stage is the very young child's beginning awareness of the world of work and the middle school youth who compares his or her abilities and interests with those of peers. In the **exploration stage** (ages 14–24 years), we begin to test out our occupational fantasies tentatively through work, school, and leisure activities. At the later part of this stage, the individual begins to crystallize his or her vocational preferences by choosing an occupation or further professional training. The **establishment stage** (ages 24–44 years) involves stabilizing our career choices and advancing in our chosen fields, and the **maintenance stage** (ages 44–64 years) encompasses the preservation of our current status in the choices we have made and avoidance of stagnation. In the **decline stage** (ages 64 to death), we begin to disengage from our chosen fields and focus more on retirement and leisure and avocational activities. Super has recently added a minicycle in which he suggests that we can cycle through the five stages at any point in our career.

Personality-Based Theories of Career Development

In 1956 Ann Roe developed a rather elaborate theory that based career choice partially on the kinds of early parenting received. This psycho-dynamic-oriented theory states that how our needs were satisfied as children lead us toward one of eight occupational groups, which include the following orientations: service, business, organization, technology, outdoor, science, general culture, and arts and entertainment. Despite the fact that her theory has not been supported by research, it was one of the first attempts to link early history with eventual career choices.

Although John Holland did not directly address how our personalities were formed, his vocational choice theory states that people express their personality through the types of career choices that they make. Holland proposes that there are six personality types, which he calls *realistic, investigative, artistic, social, enterprising,* and *conventional.* By taking an assessment instrument such as the Strong Interest Inventory (Strong, Hansen, & Campbell, 1985) or the Self-Directed Search (Holland, 1985), an individual can determine which type of work best fits his or her personality orientation. This is done by taking the top three personality codes in order and then matching one's personality orientation (code) to the jobs that best express those personality traits. Then an individual can generate a list of jobs to which he or she might be best suited.

Holland states that, regardless of ability, we can fit into a number of work environments based on our personality. For example, although I may not have the ability to be a physician, I still might enjoy working in the medical field. Much research has found that the better the fit between an individual's personality type and his or her chosen field, the more likely that person would be satisfied in his or her career (Assouline & Meir, 1987; Jagger, Neukrug, & McAuliffe, 1992). Although it is not as valid as taking one of the instruments listed above, Activity 9-1 will give you a sense of your personality code.

Now that you have examined your personality type, let's look at some of the work environments that fit various personality types. For example, some work environments for the various personality types include a filling station, a machine shop, a farm, a construction site, and a barber shop for the realistic type; a research laboratory, a diagnostic case conference, a library, and work groups of scientists, mathematicians, or research engineers for the investigative type; a play

Activity 9-1   Finding Your Holland Code

The exercise below can help you determine your personality orientation toward the world of work. Imagine that you are on a space ship traveling to another solar system. When you arrive at this solar system, you discover six planets, each of which is occupied by people who share one of the six qualities listed below. Which planet would you land on first? Then, if you left that planet, which would you go to next? And so forth.

Planet R: People who are practical, robust, have good physical skills, like the outdoors, and who avoid social situations intellectual pursuits, and artistic endeavors.

Planet I: People who like to investigate, think abstractly, do problem solving, but who avoid social situations and tend to be introverted.

Planet C: People who are concrete, like to work with data, and prefer routine problem solving. They prefer clerical tasks and tend to be neat, follow instructions, and look for social approval.

Planet A: People who express themselves through art, are creative and imaginative, like unstructured activities, and tend to be sensitive, introspective, and independent.

Planet E: People who are persuasive, self-confident, like to lead, and see themselves as stable, sociable, adventurous, and bold.

Planet S: People who are concerned for others, nurturing, introspective, responsible, like social situations, and are verbally skilled.

Starting with the upper left group of people and going clockwise, each planet represents one of the following Holland codes: realistic, investigative, artistic, social, enterprising, and conventional. In the order that you picked them, and taking the letter of the planet for each of the first three groups that you picked, what is your code? For instance, I picked the social group first, the artistic group second, and the enterprising group third. Therefore, my code would be SAE.

rehearsal, a concert hall, a dance studio, a study, a library, and an art or music studio for the artistic type; a school classroom, counseling offices, mental hospitals, religious settings, educational offices, and recreational centers for the social type; a car lot, a real estate office, a political rally, and an advertising agency for the enterprising type; and a bank, an accounting firm, a post office, a file room, and a business office for the conventional type (Isaacson, 1986).

To obtain a more comprehensive examination of the work environments, Holland and his colleagues have written a book called the *Dictionary of Holland Occupational Codes* (Gottfredson, Holland, & Ogawa, 1982). This books lists, by Holland code, approximately 12,000 jobs. After an individual discovers his or her top three codes, then by going through the book, he or she can make a list of possible jobs that are of interest. This is where the work begins. After making a list of potential jobs, the person needs to obtain information about them, which can be accomplished in a number of ways. First, the individual can use many sources to obtain information about specific jobs (see informational systems discussed later). Second, once the list has been narrowed, the person can go on informational interviews to hear first-hand about those jobs.

Integrating Models of Career Development

When working with clients, most career development experts use an integrative approach to career counseling. Let's use, as an example, a 17-year-old who is in the exploration stage of her career. You decide that it would be appropriate to give career-interest inventories and aptitude tests to understand the occupations in which her personality might best fit. Upon giving the Self-Directed Search and the Strong Interest Inventory, you discover that your client has high realistic, investigative, and enterprising codes. One possible occupation would be engineering. You offer varying choices to the student, including engineering, at which point she says, "Oh, I always thought about doing that, but I know I couldn't make the grades in college." Because this student has done well in high school and scored high on her aptitude test in the areas associated with engineering, there seems to be no objective evidence that this is true. Instead, it appears that this student's beliefs about herself are deterring her from at least one possible career. Therefore, working on examining and possibly changing her beliefs (self-efficacy theory) could help her find a satisfactory career, possibly in engineering.

After an involved career assessment, our client decides to enter college and major in engineering. However, just prior to graduating

Courage in Changing Career Paths

Fifty-six-year-old Roger is employed as an undergraduate academic advisor at a large public university. However, his route to this occupation was by no means direct. When Roger first started college, he had an interest in becoming a minister; however, because he was "totally turned off by religious courses," he gave up that idea. Although he considered veterinary medicine, he decided not to pursue this interest because he would have to transfer schools; he instead majored in math education and joined ROTC for the financial aid afforded through the GI bill. Although Roger wanted to enter pilot training, he was told that he would have to commit to the air force for 5 years, a commitment he did not wish to make. Therefore, he took a job in meteorology, which required only a 3-year commitment. Roger so enjoyed meteorology that he began to think that a career in the air force, being a meteorologist, might not be so bad. He became enthused about the field, received his master's degree, and traveled the world. Continually promoted, Roger practiced meteorology in the air force for 18 years.

Wanting a change, Roger then took a job as head of ROTC at a large Midwestern university and later worked at officer assignment in personnel. Then after 24 years in the air force, promotion to colonel, and having seen some friends become bitter and others start drinking too much, Roger began to feel that the air force was "not fun any more." So, he changed occupations in midstream.

Roger retired from the air force but not from work. He pursued a master's degree in business administration (M.B.A.) and subsequently took a position at the financial aid office at the university where he now works. However, feeling a lack of "fit," he stopped pursuing his M.B.A. and eventually took his current position in freshman advising. Finding he really enjoyed academic advising and wanting skills to match what he was doing, he started his master's degree in counseling. He is now considering obtaining a job as a school counselor, a career he had pondered when he was a freshman in college. Roger is a prime example of a person who has reached the midcareer stage of his life and has chosen change over maintenance or stagnation. He states that for the first time in his life his career choices are conscious and notes that until recently he more or less "went with the current," but now sees he can choose his future. His situation also shows the influence that situational factors can play in influencing one's career path (for example, joining ROTC for financial aid). Finally, Roger's career path shows us the importance of fit and of enjoying our life's work.

high school, her mother suddenly becomes chronically ill (situational factor), funds for college become depleted, and this young woman has to decide between going to college and taking out massive loans or delaying college and helping care for her ailing mother. At this point, the helper, having a good decision-making model, can assist this young woman in this very difficult decision.

This example shows the importance of understanding and being able to implement developmental and personality theories, being able to apply self-efficacy theory, recognizing the importance of situational factors, and using decision-making theory when struggling with major choices in life.

The Use of Informational Systems in Career Development

An extensive amount of information on all aspects of occupational information is available in the field of career development. In the career-counseling process, using some of these resources as a method of understanding the nature of different jobs, as well as examining long-range job forecasts, is usually important. In this section, we will examine some of the more prevalent informational resources available to helpers and their clients.

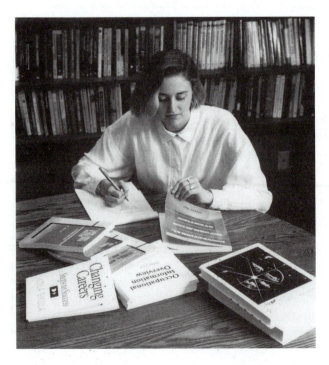

Sources of occupational information can greatly aid an individual's understanding of his or her career choices.

Dictionary of Occupational Titles

The ***Dictionary of Occupational Titles*** (*DOT*), which is published by the U.S. Department of Labor (1991), is a comprehensive classification system for occupations. The *DOT* provides a short description for each of approximately 20,000 occupations and offers a nine-code classification system for each job. The first three numbers of the classification system place jobs in general occupational groups, and the second series of three numbers present the complexity of worker traits related to the use of data on the job, the type of interactions with people at work, and the use of different types of things on the job (for example, equipment, food). Each of the three numbers ranges from 0 to 9, with the level of complexity decreasing as you approach 9. The last three digits distinguish jobs that have the same first six digits. For instance, psychiatric social worker and school social worker have the same first six digits but are distinguished by the last three digits.

An Example from the *DOT*: Social-Services Aide (DOT Number 195.367–034)

Assists professional staff of public social service agency, performing any combination of following tasks: interviews individuals and family members to compile information on social, educational, criminal, institutional, or drug history. Visits individuals in homes or attends group meetings to provide information on agency services, requirements, and procedures. Provides rudimentary counseling to agency clients. Oversees day-to-day group activities of residents in institution. Meets with youth groups to acquaint them with consequences of delinquent acts. Refers individuals to various public or private agencies for assistance. May care for children in client's home during client's appointments. May accompany handicapped individuals to appointments. (U.S. Department of Labor, 1991, p. 163)

Occupational Outlook Handbook

The ***Occupational Outlook Handbook*** (*OOH*) (U.S. Department of Labor, 1992–1993) includes information on the future outlook of selected occupations, the nature of the work of those occupations, the type of training that is needed for the job, and wage and employment conditions. Although the handbook examines only approximately 300 jobs and is not always perfect in its predictions, it is a good source of information concerning general categories of work.

Interest and Aptitude Testing in Career Counseling

Over the years a number of assessment instruments have been developed to assist in the career exploration process of individuals. Probably the most important of these have been the interest inventories. Inventories like the Strong Interest Inventory (Strong, Hansen, & Campbell, 1985), the Career Decision-Making System (CDM) (Harrington & O'Shea, 1988), and the Career Assessment Inventory (CAI) (Johansson, 1982) generally compare an individual's interests in such areas as school subjects, types of people, types of occupations, amusements, and/or personal characteristics to people in varying occupations. Therefore, one can obtain a sense of whether a client might share similar interests with people in those occupations. Other interest inventories like the Self-Directed Search (Holland, 1985) and the Strong Interest Inventory (again) examine an individual's personality orientation toward the world of work and usually provide occupations in which the client might find a good fit.

Aptitude testing has also been a valuable aid in the career assessment process. These tests allow an individual to examine whether occupational preferences match the individual's ability. For instance, an individual who has interest in becoming a researcher but has little math ability may have a difficult time achieving his or her occupational goals. Some of the aptitude tests that include this type of career assessment program include the Differential Aptitude Test (DAT) (Psychological Corporation, 1977), and the General Aptitude Test Battery (GATB), which is published by the U.S. Department of Labor, Employment and Training Administration.

Computer-Generated Assessments

The expansion in the use of personal computers has made career information systems available to a vast array of individuals. Computers offer an easy and quick method of assessing large amounts of career information. Numerous computer programs allow us to assess such traits as abilities, interests, values, and skills and match them to occupational or educational preferences. In addition, career information systems allow us to examine the types of information we might find in such sources as the *DOT* and the *OOH*. For instance, computer systems such as Guidance Information System (GIS) (Riverside Publishing Company, 1992) and System for Interactive Guidance and Information (SIGI) (Educational Testing Services, 1993) allow the individual to examine his or her values, interests, skills; have information concerning occupations, college, and trade schools; and give information on such things as financial aid. Many of these programs can be found in schools, colleges, business and industry, public employment and labor-related agencies, and private career-counseling agencies. No doubt, the use of computers in the career development process is here to stay.

Other Sources of Occupational Information

The amount of occupational information that is available is enormous, and much of it is free. Isaacson (1986), in his book on career counseling and career information, devotes six chapters to various types of career materials that are available. For instance, he notes that printed materials can be obtained from a number of government agencies, commercial publishers, professional associations, educational institutions, and periodicals. In addition, he notes that many colleges and trade schools have career centers available for student use, and sometimes for the general public. One excellent paperback that can assist you or a client in the career exploration process and gives a rather comprehensive list of available career resources is *What Color Is Your Parachute?* (Bolles, 1993).

Choosing a Career in the Human Service Profession

Am I in the Right Field?

How do you know if the human service field is a good choice for you? After reading this text, you should have a sense if you are the type of person who has or wishes to strive for the personality characteristics considered important in human service work (for example, empathy, caring, being nondogmatic, living life as a process). However, you may still be wondering, "Is this something I really want to do?" The job characteristics of the human service worker (discussed in the next section) might help you decide if you wish to enter the field; however, you might also want to examine your abilities and interests to see if there is a fit between your personality type and the work environment of the human service field. You did this to a small degree in Activity 9-1. However, if you want a more comprehensive understanding of your personality style, see if the career services center at your college or university can help you understand your career aspirations. Roger, in our example earlier, did not have the opportunity to have a comprehensive career assessment for himself. Perhaps such an assessment might have assisted him in his career search through life. In addition to self-knowledge, such assessments can be a valuable exercise in helping you understand how to work with clients who are wondering about their career direction.

Job Titles and Job Characteristics for the Human Service Worker

The types of jobs in which you might find the human service worker vary and are associated with a number of job titles including social service technician, case management aide, social work assistant, residential counselor, alcohol or drug abuse counselor, mental-health technician, child abuse worker, community outreach worker, and gerontology aide (see *DOT* for specific job descriptions) (U.S. Department of Labor, 1991). Collison and Garfield (1990) list a number of occupations within a variety of human service fields, including school settings, postsecondary school settings, college settings, business and industry, private practice, public and private agencies, federal and state agencies, health care facilities, residential treatment centers, and agencies that work with special populations. Their book, *Careers in Counseling and Human Development*, gives a quick overview of human service occupations and can probably be found in your local library.

Like job titles, the functions and roles of the human service worker vary. Some human service workers help clients obtain various types of social services. Others might provide valuable supportive services in crisis centers, community centers, shelters, group homes, and halfway houses. Others might assist clients in daily living skills at day-treatment programs, at vocational rehabilitation centers, or in group residential settings. Still others might provide individual counseling, group guidance, and family guidance. Most human service workers will be responsible for maintaining client psychosocial records.

Qualifications, Training, and Earnings

Although some employers might hire human service workers with a high school degree, human service workers generally have an associate's or bachelor's degree in human services, social work, counseling, sociology, psychology, rehabilitation, or special education. Some kind of on-the-job experience and/or internship is often required for employment, along with a caring and patient attitude and desire to help others. Advancement in the field usually requires the minimum of a bachelor's degree, with more agencies wanting a master's degree in a human service field (for example, counseling, social work, psychology, human services). In 1990 the starting salary of human service workers ranged between $12,000 and $20,000, with experienced workers making between $15,000 and $25,000 (U.S. Department of Labor, 1992–1993). Those who obtain a master's degree and an administrative position can earn well above $25,000.

Job Forecasts

The *OOH* has some optimistic job forecasts for individuals in the human service profession. It notes that the estimated number of human service workers in 1990 was 145,000 and that there will be 103,000 more human service workers between 1990 and 2005 (a 71% increase): "Employment is expected to grow much faster than average for all occupations [in the human service field] through the year 2005. Opportunities for qualified applicants are expected to be excellent, not only because of projected rapid growth in the occupation, but because of substantial replacement needs" (U. S. Department of Labor, 1992–1993, p. 119).

If this is a field to which you are committed, jobs seem plentiful, at least for the near future. The down side is that jobs in the human service field often have high burnout and low pay. Consider what you can do to prevent burnout, and if more money is important to you, give thought to what you can do to advance yourself into higher paying jobs in the human service profession.

Finding a Job

Networking

You have taken some interest inventories, examined your aptitudes, reflected on your life, examined the job characteristics and job forecasts, and have decided that the human service field is where you want to be. You have finished your training and now are ready to find a job. What do you do? If you want to get a head start on the process, join the professional associations before finishing your training. Joining the local, state, and national associations is one of the best ways to get networked. When people know you, you get jobs.

Getting Networked, Getting Involved, and Getting a Job

Randy is a former student of mine who was enthused about the human service field. He joined his professional associations, worked on research with me, and participated in professional activities whenever possible. Because Randy was so involved, he had the opportunity to present a workshop at a state professional association conference. His enthusiasm showed during the workshop. At the end of the workshop, one woman who attended the presentation was so impressed with him that she offered a job—right there. Thus, we see the importance of getting involved and being enthused.

Developing a Résumé

Besides getting networked, there are a number of other things one can do to find a job. First, have a good résumé. Make it readable, attractive, and to the point. Do not worry about how long it is. It should be as long as is necessary to show your important qualifications. Do not put anything on the résumé that might prevent you from getting an interview (for example, marital status or a goal statement that is too focused), and make sure it is grammatically correct and neat. For a more detailed look at résumés, get a good book on résumé writing (for example, see Donaho & Meyer, 1976, and Biegeleisen, 1976).

Devising a Portfolio

Besides having a good résumé, other materials can strengthen the chances that you will get the job you want. For instance, French (1993) suggests developing a portfolio that "can furnish the prospective employer with proof of [the student's] knowledge and skills that correspond with the requirements of the job. . . ." (p.1). Such things as transcripts, reports that you have written, written statements presenting your philosophy of working with individuals, outlines of workshops you might have presented, and so forth can add depth to your presentation to a potential employer.

Looking Good

Finally, look good and present yourself well. I have often seen potentially good employees or students applying to a job or graduate school present themselves poorly. I am not talking about getting dressed in a business suit. I mean dressing appropriately—dressing in a manner that will not offend your potential employer. Keep in mind that it is generally better to be overdressed than underdressed. Also, know what you are going to say if you are meeting someone. Of course you cannot predict all the questions that may be asked of you, but you probably can have a pretty good sense. Therefore, practice responses. Practice with yourself, and practice with your friends. Feel confident that you know what to say.

Now that you have your résumé and a portfolio, you are networked, and you look good and sound good, what do you do? Chances are you have identified a few different types of jobs in the human service field. Find some people who have these jobs and go on some informational interviews. These interviews will allow you to get a closer look at exactly what people do in these jobs and will help you make a decision regarding whether you would really want to pursue a particular position. Although you should not expect this, sometimes through informational interviews you can learn of specific job openings.

If you have done the above and are still looking, you can use a number of methods to obtain a job. For instance, apply directly to an employer. Jobs often become available, and if your call and résumé get to the right person at the right time, you may be hired. Some other methods include responding to or placing an ad in a newspaper or professional journal, going to a private or state employment agency, and utilizing your college or university placement office.

Helping Clients Choose a Career

If you have had enough training and background, you can help your clients make comprehensive career analyses. Such training involves some in-depth knowledge of career development theory, a basic course in assessment, and application of counseling skills. Applying these skills and giving clients access to career information resources can greatly help clients understand their career development process. However, even if you have not had such training, you can help clients understand that career development is a lifelong process, that one's career choices can always change, that satisfactory career choices are closely linked to personality fit with the occupation chosen, and that many career resources are available. Having a list of career counselors who can work with your clients is always essential.

Finally, if you have helped your clients define some career options and they are now looking for jobs, the process that your clients go through differs little from what you would go through if you were looking for a job in the human service field. Clients should become knowledgeable about their fields and the specific jobs for which they are applying, have a good résumé, present themselves well, and use all the possible means you would use to obtain an interview.

Ethical and Professional Issues

Optimizing Career Options—Being All That You Can Be

Over the years, I have heard many discouraging stories related to the career development process. For instance, a successful college student told me that her high school guidance counselor said she would never succeed in college and that she should find a job in a technical occupation. A 55-year-old man told me, upon losing his management job, that he was convinced he did not have the skills to make a career shift.

A number of female students in the helping professions have not pursued graduate school, particularly doctoral programs, because of fears of math. What do these scenarios have in common? They all speak to the limited focus that many of us have on our abilities or the abilities of others.

One should never tell another that he or she cannot succeed in a field. Although it is reasonable to tell a client specific qualifications for a field and to explore whether the client *currently* has those qualifications, it is condescending to assume that another person cannot succeed in a certain occupation. As mental-health professionals, we should try to optimize the choices that individuals have. Although a person may not currently have the ability, if he or she is motivated, we need to encourage the client to reach for his or her potential. As good helpers, the best we can do is to point out an individual's strengths and weaknesses, listen carefully, and help the client decide what options seem best.

We do a service for clients when we allow them to explore many options that might be of interest to them, and we let them make informed choices, based on their knowledge of the fields. We would be violating our ethical code of being competent helpers if our biases and actions limited our clients' choices.

The Developmentally Mature Human Service Worker: Viewing Career Choice as a Life-Span Process

Developmentally mature human service workers see the career development process from a life-span perspective. They view this process as a flowing river that twists and turns, with parts that seem shallow, dangerous and scary and parts that are deep, still, and stable. Developmentally mature human service workers see this river as starting to flow in young childhood when youngsters wonder about the world of work; picking up speed in adolescence when teenagers begin to explore their interests, values, and abilities; moving more rapidly and dangerously in young adulthood when individuals tentatively choose careers; becoming deep but maybe twisting and turning in mid-adulthood when middle-aged workers feel established in their careers or individuals decide to take a fresh look at career choices; and finally slowing down in later life when individuals move out of work and into leisure activities or shift the type or amount of work they are doing. Developmentally mature human service workers are willing to flow, for a short while, along this river with their clients; perhaps, if helpers are good navigators, they can help guide the client down the river along the most direct and stable route.

Summary

We examined the career development process and looked at the important position that career plays in our lives. From giving us the ability to purchase things, to feeling good about ourselves, to building friendships, to being part of what forms our identity, career is a vital part of our lives.

We explored the beginnings of the career-counseling and career education movements, noting the importance of Frank Parsons and his trait-and-factor theory and the later developmental models of Donald Super and the personality theories of Ann Roe and John Holland. We discussed how the career development process is viewed from a developmental perspective and why understanding one's abilities, values, and interests is so important in decisions relating to occupational choice. We also talked about the importance of becoming familiar with some of the interest and ability tests available, knowing about some of the many informational systems such as the *Dictionary of Occupational Titles* and the *Occupational Outlook Handbook*, and being aware and perhaps using some of the recent, comprehensive computer-generated career assessments.

We also took a specific look at the job characteristics, job forecasts, and qualifications and earnings of jobs in the human service field. We noted that human service workers who are actively looking for jobs are well networked, know how to write a résumé, can present themselves well, and are knowledgeable of the ways to find job vacancies. We pointed out that the process of finding jobs for human service workers is similar to the process for clients.

Finally, we noted that professionally astute human service workers optimize and expand job options for their clients. These human service workers do not assume clients *cannot* be successful in certain fields. Instead, effective human service workers point out the qualifications required for various occupations; note the skills, values, and interests of the client; and help clients make wise choices for their future. Along these lines, developmentally mature human service workers can optimize client choices throughout the life span, whether it be helping the 5-year-old in his first awareness of the world of work or in assisting the 85-year-old in deciding what activities would give her the most pleasure in this part of her life.

Experiential Exercises

1.   Developmental Career Strategies

Divide the class into small groups, assigning each group to one of Super's five developmental stages. Each group should develop ways to assist individuals in their career development on the basis of developmental stages.

2.   Finding Out about an Occupation

Interview an individual in a occupation about which you would like more information. Ask the following questions as well as any others you might find interesting:

1. Do you view your current job as part of your career or as a transitory job?

2. How long have you held this job?

3. If you view this job as part of your career, when did you first start to think about doing what you are doing?

4. What early family factors affected your eventual career choices?

5. What situational factors affected your career choices?

6. What interests, abilities, and values do you hold that seem to fit with your career choice?

3.   Exploring the *DOT* and *OOH*

Gather the information that follows and discuss the varying information you received in small groups in your class.

1. From the *DOT*, choose one occupation to examine. Copy the general description of the job, along with information about the level of skills needed for people, data, and things (the middle three digits of the nine-digit code).

2. From the *OOH*, choose one occupation to examine. Copy the job's *DOT* nine-digit code, information about job characteristics, job forecast, and earning power. Then examine the job characteristics in the *DOT*.

4.   Finding Potential Jobs

Do one or more of the following activities and make a ten-item (or more) list of potential occupations that you might like.

1. Take an interest inventory and have it interpreted.

2. Look through the newspaper want ads and write down all jobs that seem interesting to you.

3. Do Activity 9-1 and make a list of all jobs that seem interesting to you. If you can obtain a copy of the *Dictionary of Holland Occupa-*

tional Codes (check your library or career services office), expand your list of potential jobs by looking up your three-letter code in the book.

4. Spend some time looking through the *DOT* to identify possible jobs you might like.

5. Include in your list *any* jobs about which you have fantasized, regardless of whether you think you could do that job.

5. Narrowing Your List of Potential Occupations

Take the top 10 or 20 jobs you listed in Exercise 4 and rank-order your list; that is, make a list, starting with the job you like best and ending with the job you like least.

6. Identifying Skills Needed for Your List of Occupations

From the list in Exercise 5, starting with your top-ranked occupation, write down the jobs on the left side of the page and identify the skills needed for those jobs in the space provided (use the *DOT* or *OOH* if needed). Then ask yourself if you currently have the skills needed for the job and if not, what you can do to obtain the skills. See the example that follows:

Job	Skills Needed	Do I Have the Skills?	How Can I Obtain Skills?
Social services aide	Interviewing	Yes	
	Empathy	Partly	Practice sessions, role-play
	Record keeping	No	Take course, obtain information from agencies
	Supervising clients	No	Internship
	Counseling	Partly	Role-play, internship,
	Consulting	No	Course, internship, speak to consultants about what they do

7. Assessing Your Developmental Stage

The following is a developmental checklist that is based on Super's developmental stages and was developed by Harris-Bowlsby, Spivack, and Lisansky (1986, pp. 17–18). In this checklist, Super's exploration stage is broken down into crystallization, specification, and implementation tasks. Go through the checklist and identify those areas in which you have not completed a task leading to eventual career choice.

	Not Yet Completed	Already Completed

Crystallization Tasks

Realizing that I need to crystallize my alternatives

Knowing how to organize occupations and programs of study in a meaningful way.

Knowing what interests me.

Knowing what my abilities/skills are.

Knowing what my values are.

Knowing how to use information about myself to focus my exploration of occupations and educational programs.

Applying the steps of a planful decision-making process to my vocational and educational choices.

Knowing which life roles I want to play.

Identifying several occupations for detailed exploration.

Identifying several educational programs for detailed exploration.

Specification Tasks

Selecting criteria that will assist in narrowing my occupational alternatives.

Gathering detailed information about high-priority occupations and educational programs.

Using information and criteria to make a tentative selection of occupational and educational programs.

Declaring a major or choosing a program of study.

Drafting plans to "reality test" three or more occupations.

	Not Yet Completed	Already Completed

Implementation Tasks

Drafting a plan for the implementation of possible educational or occupational choices.

Learning and using job interviewing skills.

Learning and using networking skills (to identify available jobs).

Finding a full-time job in the chosen occupation.

10

A Look to the Future: Trends in the Function and Roles of the Human Service Worker

A student asked a question in class that I thought I had answered a number of times. She asked it on a day that I had a cold and was not feeling well. I remember responding somewhat belligerently, saying something like "I've answered this question four times before!" After class I saw that she looked angry so I asked her what was going on. She stated, "I thought you were condescending toward me, and it makes me feel like not asking any more questions." I realized she was right, and I also knew that sometimes I get like that. I try my best to be accepting of students, but I know that sometimes I just "lose it." This has been a constant struggle for me—to try to hear each question and comment for what it is and not to lose my patience. This student reminded me again that I still have issues to work on. Change for me is not easy, and when I think of my clients attempting to make change and having difficulty, I try to remember that in certain areas of my life I, too, have difficulty.

I remember listening to a news report about President Clinton's first years as governor of Arkansas. When he was first elected, he apparently was overzealous about a number of issues and ended up alienating many people. He lost his next election. Trying to understand his loss, he spent much time listening to people and eventually realized that he had to work with people to make change. Change would take time. He couldn't just come in and get his own agenda passed. After this painful lesson, he was reelected and became a successful and popular governor.

I sometimes joke with my colleagues about the trends in the titles of conferences that have been held within recent years. Every conference seems to have a theme like "Human Services in the 21st Century and Beyond," "Transformation of the Counseling Profession," "Looking into the '90s," and "Change, Metamorphosis, and Trends for the Future." No question, change is on people's minds. Some workshops at these conferences are exciting because they present new, on-the-cutting-edge information about innovative ways to work with clients and systems. However, I find that more often than not, the changes aren't implemented or, at the very least, are implemented very slowly.

The tendency to maintain the status quo is great, whether it be within ourselves, our family and social systems, or organizations. Change keeps us alive. It allows the new information to be assimilated or accommodated by the existing system, but it is often an arduous process. In this chapter, we will explore the change process and examine what changes and adaptations seem imminent in the future of the human service profession. Some of these changes will assuredly take place, and others may fall by the wayside. Because we are looking toward the future and are considering adapting new methods of working with clients as well as innovative ways of working with social systems, we are a profession that is alive, willing to examine ourselves, and willing to move forward. We are not satisfied with staying with the status quo and are willing to walk down the sometimes rocky path of change.

We will examine some of the changes that say we are a profession that is willing to grow. We will explore current trends in working with some special populations including HIV-positive individuals; the hungry, homeless, and poor; older people; the chronically mentally ill; people with disabilities; and chemically dependent individuals. We will discuss the recent movement toward managed health care in the United States, the new emphasis on developmental trends in working with clients, the increased emphasis on consumerism and advocacy, the growing importance of multicultural awareness in the human service field, and the ever-increasing focus on credentialing in the mental health field. Finally, we will examine the effects that stress and burnout have on us and our work with clients, the importance of staying alive in this high-stress career, and the place of continuing education as one way of keeping us abreast of changes that are taking place.

Recent Trends in Working with Clients

Increased Focus on Special Populations

Human service workers have traditionally responded to the needs of special populations within this society. As societal trends have changed, so have the special populations with whom the human service professional has worked. Today, a number of special populations demand increased attention, and the human service worker will likely be at the forefront of this challenging work.

Working with HIV-positive individuals. In 1993 approximately 1 million people in the United States were infected with the human immunodeficiency virus (HIV), which causes AIDS. Since AIDS was first identified, 242,146 Americans have developed the disease, and 81,774 have died from it. Despite a massive education campaign, with 46,423 individuals having developed AIDS from October 1991 through September 1992, the disease is by no means tapering off (personal communication, Centers for Disease Control AIDS hotline, December 1992). With some insurance companies dropping health coverage for individuals who become chronically ill, the health care system in the United States does not seem prepared to deal with the AIDS epidemic. The cost to the health care system in responding to this epidemic is staggering.

The human service field's response to the epidemic has been varied and includes support group and counseling group programs for HIV-positive individuals and their families, needle-exchange programs, programs for children who have AIDS, prevention and education programs in the schools, condom-distribution programs, and hotlines to

The U.S. Supreme Court Says No Guaranteed Health Care Coverage for Insured Individuals with AIDS

The U.S. Supreme Court has denied an appeal that would have prevented insurance companies from dropping health insurance coverage for individuals with AIDS. This decision probably will be applied to all individuals who have catastrophic illnesses and means that all individuals cannot be assured that their health insurance coverage would continue following the onset of a serious illness. This generally applies to individuals who have independent health insurance (including small-group plan coverage), and the obvious result of this decision is that many individuals who have serious illnesses may find themselves without medical coverage.

respond to questions about AIDS (Kain, 1989). Workshops and articles about the AIDS virus and how to counsel individuals who have tested HIV-positive are now commonplace at conferences and in the professional journals. No doubt, unless a cure to this disease is found, which in the near future seems unlikely, AIDS will continue to have a major impact on the health care system in the United States.

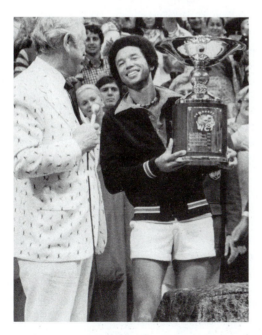 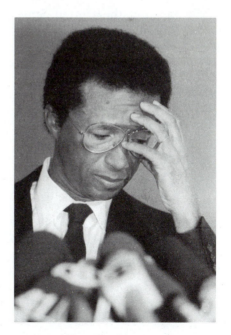

Arthur Ashe in the prime of his career (left) and, years later, announcing to the public that he had AIDS (right).

In the 1990s, the human service worker will be an important component in the education and prevention of this disease, the deliverer of counseling services for those who are already infected, and the supervisors of those many volunteers who are giving of their time and humanity to assist in the caretaking of those infected, their families, and their friends (Viney, Allwood, Stillson, & Walmsley, 1992; Williams & Stafford, 1991). Because sexual activity with an HIV-positive individual is potentially life-threatening, human service workers who are counseling HIV-positive clients may very well be challenged with ethical dilemmas concerning confidentiality toward their client versus the duty to warn those who may be infected by the deadly virus (Cohen, 1990). In the future, the responsibilities of the human service professional who works with AIDS-related issues will be great. The human service worker must be knowledgeable about the disease, about treatments for the disease, and about counseling techniques to use with HIV-positive individuals and their families and friends.

The hungry, homeless, and poor. As many as 3 million Americans may be homeless. While the number of homeless has grown considerably in the past 10–15 years, resources to serve these individuals have remained minimal. Many attribute this to a deteriorating economic situation, an economic situation that has especially affected the poor since the early 1980s. An astounding 178,828 emergency shelters now exist around the United States for homeless people (U.S. Department of Commerce, 1992a). Although homelessness has always existed throughout history, the homeless person is no longer the stereotypic hobo. The homeless today include children who have run away from home, intact single-parent families, intact families who have no place to live, poor single men and women, those who have minimum-paying jobs but cannot afford shelter, and the deinstitutionalized mentally ill. In addition, compared with those of the past, the homeless of today are more likely not to have shelter, are younger, are less apt to find employment, and are heavily overrepresented by minorities (Axelson & Dail, 1988; Rossi, 1990).

In the past, if individuals were poor, they were not necessarily at much greater risk of being homeless; however, being poor in the United States today is often one step away from not having a roof over one's head. The number of poor Americans was close to 36 million in 1991 (14.2% of the country). More than 14 million (40.2%) of these were children, and a staggering 22% of all children in the United States lived in poverty. More than 4 million of the poor were elderly. Only 40% of the poor over the age of 15 worked full time, year round, and as one might expect, a large percentage of the poor (18.6%) reported having no medical insurance. Poverty seems to be associated with race

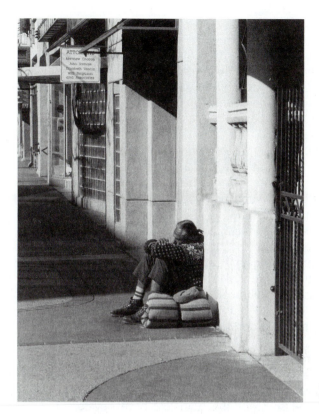

Many of the homeless in America have little hope for the future.

because 32.7% of African Americans, 28.7% of Hispanics, 13.8% of Asians or Pacific Islanders, and 17.6% of "other races" were below the poverty level. Poverty is also more prevalent in cities and in the South. Finally, poverty seems to be related to educational level because the more educated had lower poverty rates than those less educated (U.S. Department of Commerce, 1992b).

The negative results of homelessness and poverty are great. The homeless and the poor are at much greater risk of developing AIDS, tuberculosis, and other diseases. Homeless and poor children are much more likely to have retarded language and social skills, be abused, and have delayed motor development. The psychological and emotional response to homelessness and poverty can also be great and can result in despair, depression, and a sense of hopelessness (Blasi, 1990). Although the **McKinney Act** of 1987 provides job training, literacy programs, child care, and transportation funds and subsidizes counseling for the poor and homeless, the outlook for this section of society seems bleak (Waxman & Reyes, 1988).

An Interview with Al

Al is a 41-year-old homeless man in Norfolk, Virginia. Although raised in New York City, he and his family of origin now live in Norfolk. Having some college credits and growing up with modest means, he notes that "my Dad grew up in the Depression. I never thought that I would be in this situation." He goes on to state that being homeless can suddenly happen to anybody. Until recently, Al was staying with his parents, adopted sister, and her three children. However, after his father had a mild stroke, he felt that he was a burden on his family, so he took to the streets. He states that he believes things have become much worse in the past 10 years and notes that he made more money as a teenager than he does now.

Although Al is homeless, he usually has a roof over his head at night. Generally, he stays at one of the local church shelters or at the Union Mission. Every morning Al goes to a temporary job-placement service with the hope of finding work. Al states that obtaining food is usually not a problem because local religious groups and shelters provide some food daily. Al has a 23-year-old daughter and 4-year-old twin boys. He says, "It hurts that I don't have a job—hurts that I can't support them."

Al's sense of the homeless is that about one-third would work if employment was available, that some of the homeless are those who have been institutionalized for mental illness and are probably incapable of working, and that some of the homeless have developed "attitudes" from years of hopelessness. He says the street term for such people is "ate up." Being on the streets, according to Al, has a domino effect. A homeless person has few resources—no nice clothes, no place to keep personal things and records, and little hope. The result: Pulling oneself out of the situation is difficult. Al, however, seems to keep a positive attitude and states that "sometimes I slip into a blue funk, but I don't lose hope." He says that keeping a positive attitude is like a "mental volley."

As for hope for the future, Al says that it is important to have long-range goals and to hope that the next year will be better. He feels strongly that the Republican administrations of the past developed short-term programs and that more emphasis needs to be put on developing long-term programs aimed at assisting those in need to get out of their rut. Although homeless, with little to his name, Al is clearly a man with hope and vision.

Because of the economic recession of the early 1990s, an easing of conditions for the poor and homeless seems unlikely in the near future. Continuing high employment rates make this situation even more dismal because unemployment will lead to even more individuals becoming poor. Human service workers will increasingly see themselves working with the poor, underprivileged, and disadvantaged in a variety of settings, including homeless shelters, publicly funded mental-health centers, state social services, unemployment offices, and other agencies that will attend to this population.

Older people.   In 1900, 3% of the population of the United States was over 65 old. In 1960, this figure rose to 9.2%, and in 1989, 14.4% of the population was over age 65 (U.S. Department of Commerce, 1991). It is estimated that by the year 2030 fully 21% of the population will be over 65 years old (Special Committee on Aging, 1983).

Partly as a result of the changing demographics in the United States, there has been an increased focus on treatment and care programs for the elderly: day-treatment programs for the elderly at community mental-health centers, long-term care facilities such as nursing homes, home settings that are specifically geared toward older persons, senior centers that offer a variety of services for older people, and programs for the elderly offered through religious organizations and social services agencies (Myers & Salmon, 1984).

Although the population of the United States is aging and training in gerontological counseling is needed more than ever, such training is limited (Ganikos, 1979).

In conclusion, it seems clear that the climbing number of elderly alone will create the need for more counseling services. But beyond this quantitative

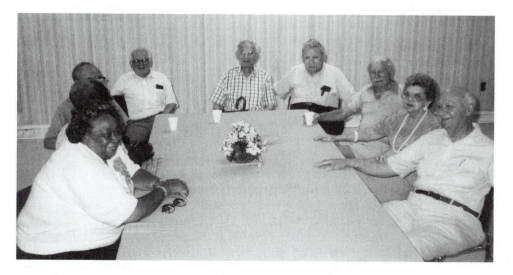

Seniors at a community center discuss some of the problems they face in older age.

aspect, burgeoning research will alter the standards upward for the quality of these services. As a result, the necessity for improved training for future practitioner has never been greater. (Cohen, 1984, p. 99)

An increasing number of graduate programs now emphasize the counseling of older persons (Myers, 1983; Myers, Loesch, & Sweeney, 1991), and more undergraduate human service majors and human service graduates are finding internships and employment in settings that focus on aging and gerontological issues (McGrath, 1991–1992). However, few undergraduate human service programs seem to offer specific coursework that focuses on gerontological counseling (Cogan & Wood, 1987; Petrie, 1989; Sweitzer & McKinney, 1991). With an increasingly larger number of elderly people in the United States, along with more programs to service this population, even larger numbers of human service workers will be employed in community centers for the elderly and in gerontological centers. As this field becomes more recognized, coursework in this content area hopefully will be added.

Needs of Older Americans

In an effort to understand some of the needs of older Americans, I visited a local community center that had organized senior services. These included meals at reduced prices, educational activities such as guest speakers on a variety of topics, and social activities such as movies and trips to local theater productions. At the center, I had lunch with Irving, Lasard, Izzi, Jeanette, Max, Joe, and some other senior citizens; their average age was about 80 years old. We had an informal discussion about a number of issues facing older Americans. Although there was some debate concerning the amount of federal subsidies that should be given to seniors, some of their major issues seemed clear. For instance, all felt that seniors are entitled to safe and secure housing, good medical care, transportation, healthy meals, and federal assistance in the delivery and implementation of these programs. Most of the group felt that they had spent a lifetime in hard work and now deserved something in return.

Finally, although the issue is not something that could be handled through legislation, it was clear that many of these seniors were dealing with losses in their lives—of spouses, friends, and relatives. This psychological component was clearly not being attended to by any of the existing available services.

The chronically mentally ill.   In 1988 the number of average daily in-patients in a psychiatric hospital was 227,900 (U.S. Department of Commerce, 1991). This compares to 560,00 inpatients in 1955 (Schmolling, Youkeles, & Burger, 1993). Although fewer individuals are now hospitalized for psychiatric problems on a daily basis, the number of psychiatric facilities that offer mental-health services is staggering: 138 Veterans Administration (VA) psychiatric hospitals, 286 state and county facilities, 757 free-standing psychiatric outpatient facilities, 886 private facilities, and 1486 other types of psychiatric facilities, for a total of 4941 mental-health facilities (U.S. Department of Commerce, 1991). As is evidenced by this large number of psychiatric facilities around the country, the reduction in the number of inpatients is not a result of a more mentally healthy population. Since the 1950s, a number of dramatic events have greatly reduced the number of individuals needing psychiatric inpatient care but have increased the number of individuals needing ongoing outpatient support.

First, the development of new psychotropic medications such as antipsychotics (for example, Haldol, Thorazine), antidepressants (for example, Prozac, Zoloft, Elavil), and antianxiety agents (for example, Valium, Tranxene) has made the management of severe emotional conditions possible outside the inpatient setting.

Second, the passage of the **Community Mental Health Centers Act** of 1963 funded the establishment of nationwide mental-health centers that provide short-term inpatient care, outpatient care, partial hospitalization, emergency services, and consultation and education services. This made it possible for those with severe emotional problems (as well as for those with adjustment problems to life) to obtain free or low-cost mental-health services. Approximately 600 community-based mental-health centers could trace their origins to this act (Schmolling, Youkeles, & Burger, 1993).

Third, the proliferation of social service programs, introduced through the Great Society Initiatives of the Johnson presidency, created a myriad of other types of social service agencies.

Finally, in 1975 the U.S. Supreme Court decision *O'Connor* v. *Donaldson* stated that a person who is not dangerous to self or others could not be confined in a psychiatric hospital against his or her will. This case and others were instrumental in the eventual **deinstitutionalization** of mental hospitals (Swenson, 1993).

These events have greatly shaped the delivery of mental-health services in the country. Those with severe emotional problems can no longer be confined against their will unless dangerousness can be shown, and the mentally ill are now able to receive a wide range of services through the massive "safety net" that now exists in the United States.

O'Connor v. Donaldson:
The Deinstitutionalization of Mental Hospitals

In 1975 the U.S. Supreme Court decided a case that would dramatically affect the status of mental hospitals in the United States. Kenneth Donaldson, who had been committed to a state mental hospital in Florida and confined against his will for 15 years, sued the hospital superintendent, Dr. J. B. O'Connor, and his staff for intentionally and maliciously depriving him of his constitutional right to liberty. Donaldson, who had been hospitalized against his will for "paranoid schizophrenia," said that he was not mentally ill, and that even if he was, the hospital had not provided him adequate treatment.

Over the 15 years of confinement, Donaldson, who was not in danger of harming himself or others, had frequently asked for his release; relatives had stated they would attend to him if he was released. Despite this, the hospital refused to release Donaldson, stating that he was still mentally ill. The U.S. Supreme Court unanimously upheld lower-court decisions stating that the hospital could not hold him against his will if he was not in danger of harming himself or others. This decision led to the large-scale release of hundreds of thousands of individuals across the country who had been confined in mental hospitals against their will and who were not a danger to self or others.

Although most of these events are seen as positive, there has also been a down side to these changes. For instance, the deinstitutionalization of the chronically mentally ill has resulted in a large number of individuals who are not hospitalized yet cannot adequately take care of themselves. Some of these find themselves in day-treatment programs or group homes; however, a substantial number can be found on the streets, and as many as 50% of all homeless people may have severe psychiatric problems. Also, for some of the chronically mental ill, psychiatric admissions have become a revolving door; the mentally ill decompensate after leaving the hospital, are rehospitalized and stabilized on medication, leave the hospital again, stop taking their medication and stop receiving services, and again need hospitalization. Some people even question whether deinstitutionalization has worked, noting the preceding problems, and, with fewer patients to serve, an expected drop in savings has not occurred (Johnson, 1990).

Undoubtedly, the human service worker will be intimately involved in the future of social services for the chronically mentally ill. This will take place in many settings including community-based mental-health centers, social services, programs for the homeless, group homes, and so forth. As advances in medications continue to be made and as long as the chronically mentally ill continue not to be hospitalized, management and care of these individuals will be an important aspect to many who work in the human services.

People with disabilities.   The estimated number of individuals with disabilities in the United States is staggering. It is thought that approximately 43 million Americans have a disability, of which 30 million are adults and 13 million are children. Of those who have been identified as having a disability, only one out of six are born with the disability (U.S. Department of Commerce, 1991). Some of the most common forms of disabling conditions include mental retardation, learning disabilities, emotional problems, and speech impairments; other disabling conditions include hearing impairment, visual impairment, orthopedic impairment, and multiple disabilities.

Two federal laws have greatly affected the ability of the disabled to receive services. The passing of the **Education for All Handicapped Children Act** of 1975 (PL94-142), ensures the right to an education within the *least restrictive environment* for all children who are identified as having a disability that interferes with learning. This law also mandates that the states are responsible for the funding of services for children with a disability. The **Rehabilitation Act** of 1973 ensures access to vocational rehabilitation services for adults if they meet three conditions: having a severe physical or mental disability, having a disability that interferes with their ability to obtain or maintain a job, and assessing that employment with their disability is feasible. Both

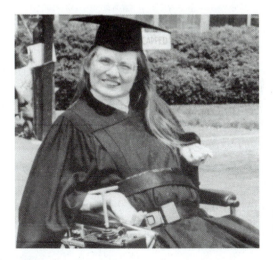

Despite being born with cerebral palsy and later having an accident that resulted in quadriplegia, Lisa Lyons obtained her master's degree in counseling.

PL94-142 and the Rehabilitation Act ensured client participation in individualized treatment planning or individualized educational planning (IEP's).

The **Americans with Disabilities Act** of 1992 updated these laws and ensures that qualified individuals with disabilities cannot be discriminated against in job application procedures, hiring, firing, advancement, compensation, fringe benefits, job training, and other terms, conditions, and privileges (Americans with Disabilities Act, 1992). More specifically, an employer must make reasonable accommodations to a qualified individual with a disability by (Americans with Disabilities Act, 1992, p. 1):

- Making existing facilities used by employees readily accessible to and useable by persons with disabilities . . .

- Job restructuring, modifying work schedules, reassignment to a vacant position . . .

- Acquiring or modifying equipment or devices, adjusting or modifying examinations, training materials, or policies, and providing qualified readers or interpreters.

This law specifies the responsibility of employers to employees with disabilities and applies to any employer with 25 or more employees. As of July 1994, the law includes any employers with 15 to 24 employees (U.S. Department of Justice, 1992).

Because federal laws have increasingly supported the rights to services for individuals with disabilities, the human service worker has taken an increasingly active role in the treatment and rehabilitation of the individual who has a disability. Lombana (1989) suggests that, along with this expanding role, we will see other changes associated with working with individuals who have disabilities. Some of these include the following:

- Reduction of the use of *terminology* in describing individuals with disabilities and an increased emphasis on the fact that we all have limitations

- Increased emphasis on individual treatment planning and education planning

- Increased use of assessment in determining which skills clients can use on the job

- Increased preservice and inservice training to help human service workers understand how to modify the client's environment in order to best meet the client's needs

- Increased emphasis on a team approach to working with those who have disabilities, especially in the schools.

As new medical procedures make it possible for individuals to live with disabling and chronic health conditions, we may even see an increase in the number of individuals with disabilities. This will result in additional needed services for these individuals, services in which we may find the human service worker taking an increasingly more active role. Finally, let us remember that we are all only temporarily able-bodied.

Individuals at risk for chemical dependence.   Although there has been some reduction in the use of certain illegal substances since 1979, the use and abuse of illicit drugs in the United States remains very high. For instance, a national drug abuse survey (U.S. Department of Health and Human Services, 1991) shows the following:

- Of youth between the ages of 12 and 17, 14.8% used an illegal drug within the past year, and 6.8% used an illegal drug within the past month.

- Of Americans over the age of 12, 6.2% use illicit drugs, with higher-use rates found for the unemployed, for individuals who live in the West, and for African Americans.

- Of Americans over the age of 12, 1.6 million use cocaine.

- Of Americans over the age of 12, 138 million drink alcohol, with 19 million of these drinking daily or almost daily.

- Of Americans aged 12 and older, 75.4 million have tried marijuana, cocaine, or other illicit drugs.

- 2.9 million Americans have tried heroin, and 700,000 have used it in the past year.

- An estimated 1 million Americans have used anabolic steroids.

- Of women in childbearing years, 7.7% have used an illicit drug within the past month.

Drug and alcohol abuse not only is widespread within the inner cities but also can be found within middle-class America. Such abuse not only affects the users but also has great impact on family members and society. Chemical dependence appears to be both a cause and an effect of many of the problems facing the United States, including increased crime, problems on the job, and the changing morals in society. Alcohol abuse alone appears to affect a vast majority of Americans, with estimates as high as 34 million Americans being identified as children of alcoholics (COAs) (Black, 1979). Woititz (1983) identifies 13 characteristics of adult children of alcoholics (ACOAs) and shows how serious the effects of alcohol abuse can be (p. 4):

1. ACOAs guess at what normal behavior is.
2. ACOAs have difficulty following a project through from beginning to end.
3. ACOAs lie when it would be just as easy to tell the truth.
4. ACOAs judge themselves without mercy.
5. ACOAs have difficulty having fun.
6. ACOAs take themselves very seriously.
7. ACOAs have difficulty with intimate relationships.
8. ACOAs overreact to changes over which they have no control.
9. ACOAs constantly seek approval and affirmation.
10. ACOAs usually feel they are different from other persons.
11. ACOAs are super responsible or super irresponsible.
12. ACOAs are extremely loyal, even in the face of evidence that loyalty is undeserved.
13. ACOAs are impulsive.

Similarly, many of these characteristics can be applied to children of drug-addicted individuals. Although there has been some minimal reduction in drug and alcohol abuse throughout the country, vast numbers of individuals are still being affected by the results of drug and alcohol abuse. The human service worker is going to continue to be an important link for providing the necessary services for these people.

Primary Prevention

Throughout the history of the mental health professions, there has been an enduring tension between those public policies and institutional goals which argue for serving all persons and those policies and goals which single out only some persons, typically those most distressed, as deserving treatment. Such has been the seeming dichotomy between *prevention* of mental illness and other emotional problems of living and the *treatment* of such maladies. (Baker & Shaw, 1987, p. 8)

In the last 10–20 years, there has been a major shift in the focus of working with clients. Whereas in the past mental-health professionals generally responded to crises in clients' lives or worked with individuals who were chronically ill, many professionals now provide consultation and education to prevent mental-health problems.

This change is partly a response to the fact that stress, burnout, and cynicism as well as other preventable problems like drug abuse have been cited as a leading cause of many psychological and medical problems (Smith & Pope, 1990). In fact, 60%–70% of Americans take a prescribed medication every day; about 10% suffer from high blood pressure; millions suffer from cardiovascular, pulmonary disease, and cancer; up to 80% of visits to physicians are stress-related; alcohol abuse affects at least one in ten families; various types of abuse affect a majority of American families; and only 6% of all Americans are totally healthy. Although genetic factors are related to many of these health problems, a large percentage of them could be treatable and even preventable.

With today's increased emphasis on primary prevention, many agencies and schools offer workshops on such topics as AIDS education, stress management, assertiveness training, anger management, motivation, birth control education, drug and alcohol awareness, and wellness. This focus has become so prevalent that many major federal and private funding organizations now offer grants in primary prevention. For instance, in 1991 the Carnegie Corporation funded $600,000 in grants for "the education and healthy development of young people" (Foundation Grants Alert, 1992), and the U.S. Department of Education now funds millions of dollars worth of training for drug abuse awareness and intervention in the schools.

This change in focus has greatly affected the roles and functions of the human service worker. Human service workers are more often assuming a consultation and education role by offering primary-prevention workshops and other activities for clients and the community at large. This changing focus will no doubt continue throughout the 1990s and beyond.

The Use of Technology in Human Service Work

In 1988 more than 9.5 million personal computers (PCs) were sold, and 45 million were in use in the United States (U.S. Department of Commerce, 1990). This is truly an amazing figure if one considers that the first IBM PC was sold in the early 1980s. Computers are showing up everywhere, from home to business to school. Computer literacy is often a requirement for obtaining a job.

Evidence suggests that the mental-health professions are adopting computer usage in a variety of ways (Lee & Pulvino, 1988). For instance, human service professionals use computers for case management, clinical assessment and diagnosis, testing of clients, documentation of client records, and billing. Computers have also been used to train helpers in the learning of counseling skills (Hammer & Hile, 1985; Libby & Walz, 1988; Neukrug, 1991; Nurius, 1990; Nurius & Hudson, 1989a). Computer use has become so important to the human services that the journal *Computers in the Human Services* was developed specifically to look at computer usage in the profession.

Computers, and other technology like interactive videos, are also used to help clients learn new skills such as parenting skills, assertiveness training, and vocational skills for specific jobs. As technological advances become more commonplace in the human service field, human service programs will need to integrate into their curriculum the understanding and use of advanced technology.

Managed Health Care

Within the past 20 years the cost of mental-health services has skyrocketed. For instance, 7–15% of health care costs of business and industry are now devoted to mental-health services. Very large increases have also occurred in the cost of mental-health care for the dependents of employees (Montgomery, 1988; Prospero, 1987). In addition, these costs seem to be rising at higher rates than are other medical benefits (Ludwigsen & Enright, 1988).

In the past, when individuals sought mental-health services, they almost always sought private counseling from private-practice practitioners or from mental-health agencies, and, usually, an employee health care package would include a certain amount of coverage toward individual, group, and/or family counseling. However, due to the steadily rising cost of services as well as an increase in the numbers of individuals who feel comfortable seeking out counseling, many companies have moved toward utilizing **health maintenance organizations** (HMOs) and **employee assistance programs** (EAPs) in an effort to contain costs. HMOs are managed health care systems that offer subscribers a pool of designated providers from which they can choose. This allows HMOs to strictly oversee diagnosis and treatment, thereby cutting costs. HMOs also often provide consultation, education, and primary-prevention activities. EAPs are programs run by business and industry, or by companies hired by business and industry, that provide primary prevention and early referral for treatment.

Managed mental-health programs maintain costs in a number of ways including "[1] retrospective and prospective peer review of proposed treatment plans, [2] early detection and treatment, [3] matching treatment modality to presenting problem, [4] preauthorization for hospital admission, and [5] vigilant case management" (Foos, Ottens, & Hill, 1991, p. 332). HMOs and EAPs, along with providing integrated services of the different mental-health professions, will undoubtedly ease some of the rising costs of mental-health services (Visotsky, 1991).

The effect of these managed mental-health care programs will be great. To keep costs down, an increased emphasis on primary prevention and early detection of problems will likely occur. In the past, private-practice practitioners were the primary deliverers of services; however, with the increased usage of HMOs and EAPs, less highly trained professionals, who will be paid at lower salaries, will likely be employed to offer some of the primary-prevention services. Bachelor's- and even associate's-level human service workers will also likely be hired to do some of this work.

A Developmental Emphasis in the Human Services

Throughout this text, we have talked about the importance of understanding our own developmental maturity. We have made suggestions about how to foster our own developmental growth and have noted the importance of understanding our clients' developmental levels. The mental-health professions have increasingly highlighted the importance of understanding the developmental level of the client. This has been evidenced in many ways, including the adoption of a developmental approach to counseling in the schools (Dahir, 1991), the increased focus on wellness throughout the life span (Myers, Emmerling, & Leafgren, 1992), and the recent proliferation of developmental models of counseling (Ivey, 1989; Schwebel, Barocas, Reichman, & Schwebel, 1990). This developmental emphasis tends to have a wellness focus and views client growth or stagnation in terms of uncompleted developmental stages. In addition, it helps us determine a client's **developmental readiness** to move on to higher stages.

In the future, we are likely to continue to see new models of development as well as an increased emphasis on primary-prevention programs to assist individuals through their predictable developmental stages. Intervention strategies that emphasize help for developmental problems are likely to become more widespread, along with strategies to help clients who are ready to advance to the next developmental level.

Increased Emphasis on Consumerism and Advocacy

When I worked at a mental-health center, a client told me that she had been molested by one of the aides while she was an inpatient. This young women was diagnosed as schizophrenic, and although she was not asking me to do something about what had happened, I felt a responsibility to report this incident. I did report it to the aide's superiors and was immediately told that my client was schizophrenic and very well might have made up this story. Yet I believed her, and I persisted, despite the fact that *my* job could have been at risk. Eventually I discovered that the aide was very quietly let go from his job. To this day, I wonder if that was enough.

Increasingly, the rights of clients have been upheld in the courts. From the right not to be institutionalized against their will, to the right to services if disabled, to the right of access to services, the courts have consistently said, "Clients have rights!" Increasingly, clients today are speaking out when they do not get needed and deserved services, and this is likely to continue in the future. As human service workers, *we* also need to ask ourselves when is it time for *us* to speak up for our clients—clients who sometimes may not have the courage to speak up for themselves. This can become a particularly difficult situation; if we speak up for a client concerning conflicts that he or she may be having at the agency in which we work, such an action could potentially jeopardize our own job security.

If we are going to be advocates for our clients, Halley, Kopp, and Austin (1992) suggest three guidelines:

1. Know your agency. It is important to know whom you should contact first—who holds the power to make decisions and what the hierarchy is in the agency.

2. Be clear about the grievance. Do not make vague complaints; instead, have a clear understanding of the problem. This is often best if put in writing.

3. Be clear on what actions are being sought by the consumer. Offering a complaint without a clear sense of where it will lead can dissuade supervisors or administrators. Give them a clear sense of what the client wants.

Consumers are becoming more keenly aware of their rights. Sometimes they will advocate for themselves, and other times they might need our help. We must continually ask ourselves if we are willing to take the risk that sometimes comes along with being an advocate for our clients.

Increased Focus on Multicultural Awareness and Counseling

Chapter 7 introduced the importance of cultural awareness when working with clients. In that chapter, we examined the changing face of the United States and noted the importance of having knowledge about other cultures, the skills necessary in working with diverse populations, and the attitudes important when working with individuals of varying cultural backgrounds. As we move toward the 21st century and as the United States becomes increasingly more diverse, the human service worker will continually be challenged to meet the needs of a client population that is evermore diverse. In fact, some authors think that the increasing diversity in the United States and its impact on the mental-health professions might even represent a new forefront in the field of counseling.

Whether or not multiculturalism emerges as a truly generic approach to counseling and whether or not it emerges as a fourth force with an articulated impact on counseling equivalent to behaviorism, psychodynamics, and humanism, culture does provide a valuable metaphor for understanding ourselves and others. It is no longer possible for counselors to ignore their own culture or the culture of their clients. Until the multicultural perspective is understood as making the counselor's job easier instead of harder and increasing rather than decreasing the quality of a counselor's life, however, little change is likely to happen. (Pedersen, 1991, p. 11)

Finally, we will likely see an increased emphasis on multicultural awareness and counseling in human service programs. This is, in fact, already beginning; Mcgrath (1991–1992) found that 70% of programs now offer a course on racial/ethnic relations. This focus will greatly change the way we view ourselves and other cultures and positively affect our ability to work with clients of diverse backgrounds.

Increased Emphasis on Professionalism, Credentialing, and Professional Advocacy

A *profession* is an occupation that has gained its status by meeting certain criteria. *Professionalism*, however, is an attitude that motivates individuals to be attentive to the image and ideals of their particular profession. (VanZandt, 1990, p. 243)

The human service movement is relatively new, and the organizations that serve this field are also young. Like individuals, organizations go through developmental changes. Both NOHSE and CSHSE are two relatively young human service associations. Established in 1979, the major goals of CSHSE are to ensure "quality education through program approval, technical assistance, and publications" (Brown, 1987). A major thrust of this effort is through an approval process for human service programs; this relatively new process ensures program quality. Although a limited number of programs have so far acquired program approval, such approval will likely become increasingly more important if not essential for human service programs of the future (see Appendix C for the CSHSE National Standards for Human Service Worker Education and Training Programs).

NOHSE and CSHSE are passing out of their child stage, perhaps entering adolescence and yearning for, as Super might say, the establishment phase of their existence. However, establishment does not come easily. It calls for a clear sense of identity along with an ever-increasing understanding of the rules that govern the association. As NOHSE grapples with its professional identity and as more human service programs become nationally accredited, we will see human service associations slowly move into the establishment phase of their existence. This new phase will undoubtedly bring with it an increased sense of professionalism, which will include expansion and increased quality of professional literature; an increased number of human service programs becoming approved; movement toward registration, certification, and/or licensing of human service workers; greater attentiveness toward ethical and professional issues; and an increased number of bachelor's- and master's-level programs in human services. On a more basic level, the establishment phase almost always brings about increased salaries and more respect for those working in that field.

The psychologists, the social workers, and the counselors have all generated very powerful organizations that now do much advocacy work for their members as well as their clients. However, the human service profession is still building. When membership increases, when credentialing is established, when human service professionals are truly recognized *as* professionals, their power base will begin to build. The establishment of a profession also means power. Members pay dues. Dues hire lobbyists. Lobbyists fight for the rights of the consumer and of the member. We are not there yet, but we will be soon!

The Power of an Organization

In 1993 I saw two attempts by the Virginia legislature to "get rid of counselors." One was an attempt to do away with elementary school counselors; the second was to lessen the function and roles of the mental-health counselor. Both attempts failed. Both failures were a direct result of the power of the Virginia Counselors Association to lobby against these bills. The lobbying was through a grass roots effort on the part of the members of the association, as well as the efforts of a hired lobbyist (paid from the membership dues). An association that has members, has credibility through credentialing, and is organized can clearly change the direction of social service legislation.

Cynicism and Burnout in the Human Services

One reason that the future job outlook for the human service profession is so bright is that being a human services worker is a high-stress occupation that leads many to leave the field. Hans Selye (1956), one of the major researchers on stress, stated that stress is an adaptive response to a changing situation. Stress therefore can be seen as a healthy response in that it enables the person to be ready to take on a new situation. However, too much stress can cause psychological and physical problems including depression, anxiety, psychosomatic illnesses, heart disease, high blood pressure, the common cold, and perhaps even cancer (Friedman & Rosenman, 1959; Rosch, 1979; Rosenman, Swan, & Carmelli, 1988; Selye, 1974). Stress has also been shown to be directly related to both burnout and a cynical attitude at work (Shelton, 1993). So common is stress in professional fields that it has been described by some as a "burnout syndrome" (Maslach, 1982).

Because the human service worker is often called to intervene in particularly difficult situations (for example, individuals who may be homicidal or suicidal, individuals who have lost jobs, individuals who are dealing with the breakup of a relationship), stress is particularly high for the human service worker. Human service workers are also often placed in the middle of situations where they witness the saddest side of humanity, such as when they work with people who are homeless, hungry, or dealing with a recent loss. No wonder that many human service workers who get low pay, deal with high-stress situations, and may get minimal reinforcement for their work choose to change careers eventually.

What You Can Do about Stress and Burnout

Some authors have identified five areas related to stress and burnout, including the physical, emotional, behavioral, interpersonal, and attitudinal domains (Kahill, 1988). Each of these, either on their own or in combination, can lead to stress, burnout, and a cynical attitude on the job. Healthy human service workers are aware of their physical well-being and attend to it by eating well and taking care of their bodies through exercise, meditation, or other such activities. Such professionals also care about their emotional health through their attendance in counseling and by having supportive relationships. The activities in which healthy human service workers involve themselves are indicative of a positive lifestyle, and they take responsibility for and attend to the important relationships in their lives. Finally, healthy human service workers are aware of how their attitudes affect others and find activities such as professional workshops, personal growth groups, or the like to maintain a positive attitude.

William Glasser (1976) suggests that people need to become addicted to a positive behavior such as running or a hobby to offset some of the effects of stress. Corey, Corey, and Callanan (1993) note that it is important to have an action plan and a commitment to that plan in order to prevent stress and burnout. Finally, Carl Whitaker (1976), a well-known family therapist, suggests a number of activities to help keep the mental-health professional alive:

- Relegate every significant other to second place.
- Learn how to love.
- Listen to your impulses.
- Enjoy your significant other more than anyone else.
- Fracture role structures at will and repeatedly.
- Build long-term relations so you feel safe to express your anger.
- Enjoy being "crazy."
- Face the fact that you must grow until you die.

Ethical and Professional Issues

Continuing Education

Education never ends. Although you obtain a degree and work hard for it, to be effective throughout your career as a human service professional, it is essential that you continue your learning. Once you are in the field, you will find that there are gaps in your education—things that were not stressed that seem essential for you to know at work. Therefore, continuing education beyond your degree is essential. You can accomplish this through a variety of means. By joining your professional associations, you can participate in workshops that keep you current regarding the most recent advances in the field. You can take additional coursework, perhaps to earn an advanced degree. Sometimes agencies will have staff development workshops aimed at increasing skills in areas deemed important. Increasingly, boards of registration, certification, and/or licensing are requiring continuing education in order to maintain a professional's credentials. This ensures that the professional is continuing to learn and that he or she can offer the best services possible to his or her clients.

The Developmentally Mature Human Service Worker: Anxious about Change, Desirous of Change, Hopeful about the Future

As noted in earlier chapters, change is often not an easy process. It usually requires the giving up of an old system and the accommodation to a new way of viewing the world. Even for those who want to continue to learn and who have visions about the future, change can be a difficult process. However, effective human service workers, even if they are anxious about the future, are willing and want to take on new challenges; they look at change as crucial to their own process of living and crucial to the evolution of the profession. Human service professionals who are stressed out, burned out, cynical, and stagnated do little for themselves, probably provide poor services to their clients, and generally are not involved in positive ways with professional associations. On the other hand, human service workers who are positive, forward looking, and desirous of change are probably the people who work best with their clients and offer most to the future of the field. Which are you?

Although you may just be beginning your journey in the human services, a long and prosperous road is hopefully ahead. As a direct-service provider of tomorrow, you will offer needed services to perhaps thousands of people. The direct-service workers of tomorrow will also become the administrators and supervisors of the 21st century. Whether or not you eventually take on such a role, my hope is that you can become a change agent for the betterment of all people.

Summary

We examined some of the future trends, functions, and roles of the human service worker. We discussed some of the client populations with whom the human service worker will most likely work in the upcoming years. These included individuals who are HIV-positive; the hungry, homeless, and poor; older people; the chronically mentally ill; people with disabilities; and individuals at risk for chemical dependence.

We highlighted some of the important issues facing the human service worker as we approach the 21st century. For instance, primary prevention, which focuses on educating individuals in order to prevent future problems, was noted as a recent trend in the field. We discussed how the spread of managed mental-health services and how the expanding use of technology will affect the functions and roles of the human service worker. We highlighted how consumerism and advocacy work might affect the future of the human service worker. In addition, we noted that an understanding of developmental stages is increasingly emphasized, along with multicultural sensitivity and awareness in our work with clients.

We noted that the human service field will likely emphasize professionalism and credentialing and that a strong professional organization can affect services for clients as well as jobs for helping professionals. We discussed ways of preventing cynicism, burnout, and stagnation as a professional. Developmentally mature human service workers are individuals who look toward the future and are willing and anxious to continue their learning by joining professional associations, taking courses, and attending workshops.

Finally, as a forward-looking, continually growing individual and professional, *you* will become the change agent of the future. *You* will be the supervisor, the administrator, the legislator of tomorrow. *You* will make the difference!

Experiential Exercises

1.   Interview a Person from a Special Population

Interview an individual in one or more of the special populations listed below and ask the accompanying questions (and any other questions you think would be appropriate).

An Individual Who Has a Disability:

1. How did you become disabled?

2. What unique experiences have you had related to your disability?

3. What prejudices have you experienced?

4. What social services have you used?

5. What social services would you like to have available?

6. Is there anything you would like to have changed about your life related to your current status?

A Poor Person and/or Homeless Person:

1. How did you become homeless or poor?

2. What unique experiences have you had related to your current life situation?

3. What prejudices have you experienced?

4. What social services have you used?

5. What social services would you like to have available?

6. How do you make it financially day-to-day?

7. What financial resources are available to you?

An Individual Who Is (or Was) Chemically Dependent:

1. What led you to become chemically dependent?

2. What drugs and/or alcohol do (have) you use(d)?

3. What unique experiences have you had related to your substance abuse?

4. What prejudices have you experienced?

5. What social services have you used?

6. What social services would you like to have available?

7. How do you currently expect to handle your addiction to drugs and/or alcohol?

An Individual Who Is HIV-Positive:

1. How did you become HIV-positive?

2. What unique experiences have you had related to being HIV-positive?

3. What prejudices have you experienced?

4. What social services have you used?

5. What social services would you like to have available?

6. What changes would you like to see take place in society related to your HIV-positive status?

An Older Person

1. How do you feel about being an older person?

2. What unique experiences have you had related to your age?

3. What prejudices have you experienced?

4. What social services have you used?

5. What social services would you like to have available?

6. What attitudes related to aging would you like to see changed in society?

An Individual Who Struggles with Mental Illness:

1. When do you first remember having to deal with your mental-health problems?

2. What unique experiences have you had related to your mental illness?

3. What prejudices have you experienced?

4. What social services have you used?

5. What social services would you like to have available?

6. Has medication assisted you with your mental-health problems?

7. What changes in the mental-health care delivery system would you like to see?

2. Examining an HMO

Visit an HMO and ask the following questions concerning how mental-health treatment decisions are made:

1. Who sees clients for counseling?

2. Who decides which counselors and/or therapists can provide services for the HMO?

3. How is length of mental-health treatment decided?

4. What kind of paperwork is needed to maintain treatment for a client?

5. What kind of review of treatment is necessary for a client to continue in counseling?

6. How is the amount of payment per session decided?

7. What are the advantages and disadvantages to managed mental-health care?

3. Positive and Negative Aspects of the Developmental Emphasis

Make a list of the positive and negative aspects of the developmental focus in the human services, and answer the following questions:

1. How does this focus differ from a medical model perspective?

2. Is there a way of integrating a developmental and medical model perspective?

4.   Trends in Multiculturalism

Answer the following questions concerning muticulturalism:

1. What changes do you foresee in the future of the human service profession if, as predicted, multicultural issues continue to be stressed?

2. What are some positive and negative aspects to having same-culture helpers work with same-culture clients?

3. How do you think you will be personally affected by a more diverse group of human service workers?

5.   Trends in Credentialing

In small groups, discuss the importance of credentialing for human service workers.

1. Discuss the differences among registration, certification, and licensure.

2. Make arguments for and against the credentialing of human service workers.

3. If you think credentialing is important, do you believe it should take the form of registration, certification, or licensing?

4. How do you think credentialing will affect your work as a human service worker?

6.   Dealing with Stress and Burnout

Discuss the various ways that you deal with stress and burnout.

1. Are the ways that you deal with stress working for you?

2. Are there other ways that you might find to deal effectively with your stress?

3. What would you do if you noticed a colleague of yours was burned out and was working poorly with clients?

4. What would you do if *you* were burned out and were working poorly with clients?

7.   Focus on Continuing Education

List some continuing education activities in which you would like to get involved when you are working in the human service field, and answer the following questions:

1. Do you think continuing education should be mandated for human services workers?

2. If you think continuing education should be mandatory, how many hours per year should each human service worker undertake?

8.   Being an Advocate

Discuss the following scenarios relative to whether you believe you should take an advocacy role with a client.

1. Your client at a problem-pregnancy clinic tells you that she is being abused by her boyfriend. She would like your help in moving her belongings out of her apartment. Do you help her?

2. You work at a crisis center, and your client, who was recently released from a state hospital, tells you he was denied Social Security disability. Your experience with him tells you he is not currently capable of working. Do you advocate for him at the Social Security disability office?

3. Your client tells you that she is using illicit drugs. Your agency has a strict policy of not seeing clients who are drug users. Your client is aware of the policy, and you feel that you have made significant progress with her. Do you advocate to continue to see your client despite the fact that your supervisor strongly supports the agency policy?

4. Your agency has an unwritten policy that discourages staff from taking public stands on issues. You are an avid pro-choice (or pro-life) person and would like to take part in a local rally. What do you do?

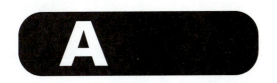

Proposed Ethical Standards of Human Service Workers (NOHSE)

Preamble

Human service workers should promote and encourage the unique values and characteristics of the human service profession. In so doing, human service workers should uphold the integrity and ethics of the profession, partake in constructive criticism of the profession, promote client well-being, and enhance their own professional growth.

The Southern Regional Education Board (1969) has identified thirteen functions and roles of the human service worker: caregiver, broker, teacher/educator, behavior changer, consultant, outreach worker, data manager, assistant to specialist, mobilizer, advocate, evaluator, administrator, and community planner. In addition, human service workers often find themselves in the role of case manager. The following standards are written in consideration of these multi-faceted roles.

The ethical guidelines presented are a set of standards of conduct which the human service worker should consider in ethical and professional decision making. Although ethical codes are not legal documents, they may be used to assist in the adjudication of issues related to ethical human service behavior. It is hoped that these guidelines will be of assistance when the human service worker is challenged by difficult ethical dilemmas.

The Human Service Worker's Responsibility to Clients

1. Human service workers have a responsibility to inform clients of the purpose, goals, and nature of the helping relationship prior to its onset.

2. The integrity and welfare of the client by the human service worker must be respected at all times; each client should be treated with humaneness and unconditional regard in a non-manipulative fashion.

3. The client has a right to confidentiality except when such confidentiality would cause harm to the client or to others, when agency guidelines state otherwise, or under other stated conditions (e.g., local, state, or federal laws). Clients should be informed of the limits of confidentiality prior to the onset of the helping relationship.

4. If it is suspected that danger or harm may occur to the client or to others, it is the responsibility of the human service worker to act in such a manner to prevent such from occurring. This may involve seeking consultation, supervision, and/or breaking the confidentiality of the relationship.

5. Human service workers should avoid any dual relationship that might negatively impact on the helping relationship with the client. Sexual relationships with clients are unethical and prohibited.

6. It is the responsibility of the human service worker to protect the integrity, safety, and security of client records. With the exception of the supervisory relationship, all client information that is shared with other professionals must have the client's prior written consent.

7. Human service workers recognize the client's right to receive or refuse services.

The Human Service Worker's Role in the Community and in Society

1. Human service workers should adhere to all local, state, and federal laws and should advocate for change if particular laws conflict with ethical guidelines and/or client rights.

2. Human service workers should be aware of multiculturalism in society and be responsive to the uniqueness of each citizen in regards to his or her cultural heritage and/or personal belief system.

3. Human service workers have the responsibility to keep informed about current social issues as they affect the client in the community.

4. Human service workers should provide a mechanism for identifying unmet client needs, calling attention to these needs, and assisting in planning and mobilizing to advocate for those needs at the local community level.

The Human Service Worker's Responsibility to the Public

1. If it is suspected that danger or harm may occur to others as a result of a client's behavior, the human service worker must act in an appropriate and professional manner to protect the safety of those individuals. When such actions conflict with other ethical guidelines (e.g., confidentiality), the human service worker has an obligation to seek out supervision to decide on the best course of action.

2. Human service workers should not misrepresent their qualifications to the public.

3. Human service workers should not make grandiose statements about the effectiveness of programs, treatments, and/or techniques.

4. Human service workers should advocate for the rights of all members of society, especially those who have been historically discriminated against.

The Human Service Worker's Relationship with Colleagues

1. The human service worker should be respectful, ethical, and professional with colleagues.

2. Human service workers should avoid duplicating an already existing helping relationship with a client. In working with a client who is involved in an additional helping relationship of a different nature, the human service worker should consult with the other mental health professional if such consultation would benefit the client.

3. If the human service worker has a conflict with a colleague, he or she should first seek out that colleague in an attempt to ameliorate the problem. If an amenable solution is not reached, the human service worker should seek mediation with a supervisor or other objective mediator.

4. Human service workers have the responsibility to report any unethical behavior of a colleague to appropriate sources. Usually, this would mean initially talking to the colleague directly, and if no resolution is forthcoming, to report the colleague to appropriate supervisory and/or administrative sources.

5. All consultations between human service professionals should be kept confidential.

The Human Service Worker's Responsibility as a Professional

1. Human service workers should know the limit and scope of their professional knowledge and seek consultation, supervision, and/or referrals when appropriate.

2. As professionals, human service workers should act with integrity, honesty, genuineness, and objectivity.

3. Human service workers should promote cooperation among related disciplines (e.g., psychology, counseling, social work) in order to foster professional growth and interests within the various fields.

4. Human service workers should promote the continuing development of their profession through any or all of the following means: membership in professional associations, support of research endeavors, pursuit of educational advancement, commitment to appropriate legislative actions, and other related professional activities.

5. Human service workers should continually seek out new and effective approaches to enhance their professional abilities.

The Human Service Worker's Responsibility to Self

1. Human service workers should strive to personify those characteristics typically associated with the helping professions (e.g., being empathic, non-judgmental, and non-dogmatic, and respecting client self-determination).

2. Human service workers have a responsibility to foster self-awareness and personal growth in order to prevent personal issues from interfering with their relationships with clients, colleagues, and the public.

3. Human service workers recognize a commitment to lifelong learning and should continually upgrade skills to serve the client population better.

The Human Service Worker's Relationship to Employer and Supervisor

1. In order to assure job satisfaction and positive client outcomes, human service workers should be presented with clear and concise job roles and functions by their employers and supervisors.

2. Human service workers have a right to be evaluated for their job performance in an objective manner on established criteria that

have been shown to be predictive of job performance. Such evaluation should be viewed as an ongoing and open process that encourages feedback and growth.

3. Human service workers have a right to have supervisors who are educated on appropriate models of supervision.

4. Human service workers and their employers have a responsibility to evaluate the effectiveness of the agency through reliable and valid assessment measures.

5. Although employers and supervisors have the right to all knowledge concerning client/human service worker interaction, they should attempt to respect the integrity of the confidential nature of the human service worker/client relationship.

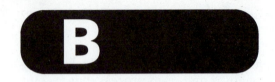

Council for Standards in Human Service Education: Summary Information Sheet

Council Membership

The Council for Standards in Human Service Education was established in 1979 to help human service educators and college administrators achieve maximum educational quality and relevance to the service delivery system in their community. Guided by the National Standards for Human Service Education, the Council formally reviews and approves educational programs whose competence warrants public and professional confidence.

To meet its goal of helping programs improve their quality, the Council has developed a wide range of services and publications for its members. New members receive a set of materials selected to provide technical assistance and information about the trends in human service education. The continuing benefits of an institution's membership include:

- the *National Standards* periodically reviewed and revised to maintain relevance to changing needs, that approved programs meet so that:

  (a) employers can be assured of a consistent "core of competence" of graduates, and

  (b) colleges can be assured that the program is meeting nationally defined essentials of quality education;

- access to *consultants* and *technical assistance*, organized nationally and within each of the Council's eight regions, to assist the program in various aspects of curriculum, maintaining community relevance, and program administration;

- *Special Reports to Members*, based on *regular surveys* of human service education programs and other information, that analyze national trends in enrollment, employment of graduates, specialized areas of study being offered in different programs, and other areas of special interest to educators;

- *The CSHSE Bulletin*, the Council newsletter, featuring current information on trends, new publications, workshops and conferences, and other issues in human service education;

- a national *Directory* of human service education programs;

- a *monograph series* exploring new developments in human service education and providing guidelines on the best administrative and program development practice currently used in the field;

- the opportunity to have your program approved by the Council for Standards in Human Service Education; this *program approval process* is itself a major source of technical assistance to your institution from some of the most experienced and successful human service educators in the country.

Program Approval

The approval process is designed to assist programs in self-study, evaluation, and continual improvement and to provide new, creative approaches to the preparation of human service practitioners at the undergraduate level. Validated standards serve as the base for guiding and reviewing programs; Council approval attests to a program's compliance with these national standards.

The first step in the approval process is for a program to apply for Council membership (if not already a member) and to complete and submit the program approval application with the one-time application fee of $250.00. The application itself can be made at any time and is a relatively simple step requring copies of material that most programs already have, such as program objectives, curriculum outline, and faculty qualifications. It is used to verify that the program is career oriented, has a significant field experience component, and is interdisciplinary. It also provides reference material for the Regional Directors in providing technical assistance during the self-study process.

Once the application is approved, the program begins the major part of the program approval process—a self-study involving faculty, students, administrators, field supervisors, and others participating in the educational program. The purpose of the self-study is two-fold: (1) it is an opportunity for a program to assess and clarify its objectives and methods and to delineate areas which need improvement, and (2) it provides the information necessary to determine program compliance with national Standards.

The applicant program has two years after the date of application to complete and submit the self-study. The Council provides informal consultation and assistance at the initial stage of application, during the self-study process, upon submission of the self-study report, or during the planning for the site visit.

Upon receipt of the self-study materials, a site visit team is selected in cooperation with the applicant program. The purpose of the site visit is to confirm the findings in the self-study document, to amplify or clarify areas that are insufficiently presented, and to explore any areas that lack documentation in the self-study summary. It is the responsibility of the program to pay the transportation and expenses of the two site visitors.

The site visit team prepares a report for the Council Board, whose function is to examine the information in the application, self-study, and site visit report and to determine whether the applicant meets the criteria for each standard. Final decision on full approval, conditional approval, or denial of approval is made by this Board of Directors. The Board meets in the spring and the fall. Full program approval is for a period of five years. Programs may apply for re-approval every five years thereafter, with a site visit required every other period.

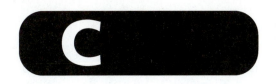

Proposed Cross-Cultural Competencies and Objectives (AMCD)

I. Counselor Awareness of Own Cultural Values and Biases

A. Beliefs and Attitudes

1. Culturally skilled counselors have moved from being culturally unaware to being aware and sensitive to their own cultural heritage and to valuing and respecting differences.

2. Culturally skilled counselors are aware of how their own cultural backgrounds and experiences and attitudes, values, and biases influence psychological processes.

3. Culturally skilled counselors are able to recognize the limits of their competencies and expertise.

4. Culturally skilled counselors are comfortable with differences that exist between themselves and clients in terms of race, ethnicity, culture, and beliefs.

B. Knowledge

1. Culturally skilled counselors have specific knowledge about their own racial and cultural heritage and how it personally and professionally affects their definitions of normality–abnormality and the process of counseling.

2. Culturally skilled counselors possess knowledge and understanding about how oppression, racism, discrimination, and stereotyping affect them personally and in their work. This allows them to acknowledge their own racist attitudes, beliefs, and feelings. Although this standard applies to all groups, for White counselors it may

mean that they understand from individual, institutional, and cultural racism (White identity development models).

3. Culturally skilled counselors possess knowledge about their social impact on others. They are knowledgeable about communication style differences, how their style may clash or foster the counseling process with minority clients, and how to anticipate the impact it may have on others.

C. Skills

1. Culturally skilled counselors seek our educational, consultative, and training experience to improve their understanding and effectiveness in working with culturally different populations. Being able to recognize the limits of their competencies, they (a) seek consultation, (b) seek further training or education, (c) refer out to more qualified individuals or resources, or (d) engage in a combination of these.

2. Culturally skilled counselors are constantly seeking to understand themselves as racial and cultural beings and are actively seeking a nonracist identity.

II. Understanding the Worldview of the Culturally Different Client

A. Beliefs and Attitudes

1. Culturally skilled counselors are aware of their negative emotional reactions toward other racial and ethnic groups that may prove detrimental to their own beliefs and attitudes and deal with those of their culturally different clients in a nonjudgmental fashion.

2. Culturally skilled counselors are aware of their stereotypes and preconceived notions that they may hold toward other racial and ethnic minority groups.

B. Knowledge

1. Culturally skilled counselors possess specific knowledge and information about the particular group that they are working with. They are aware of the life experiences, cultural heritage, and historical background of their culturally different clients. This particular competency is

strongly linked to the "minority identity development models" available in the literature.

2. Culturally skilled counselors understand how race, culture, ethnicity, and so forth may affect personality formation, vocational choices, manifestation of psychological disorders, help-seeking behavior, and appropriateness or inappropriateness of counseling approaches.

3. Culturally skilled counselors understand and have knowledge about sociopolitical influences that impinge upon the life of racial and ethnic minorities. Immigration issues, poverty, racism, stereotyping, and powerlessness all leave major scars that may influence the counseling process.

C. Skills

1. Culturally skilled counselors should familiarize themselves with relevant research and the latest findings regarding mental health and mental disorders of various ethnic and racial groups. They should actively seek out educational experiences that foster their knowledge, understanding, and cross-cultural skills.

2. Culturally skilled counselors become actively involved with minority individuals outside of the counseling setting (community events, social and political functions, celebrations, friendships, neighborhood groups, and so forth) so that their perspective of minorities is more than an academic or helping exercise.

III. Developing Appropriate Intervention Strategies and Techniques

A. Attitudes and Beliefs

1. Culturally skilled counselors respect clients' religious and/or spiritual beliefs and values, including attributions and taboos, because they affect worldview, psychosocial functioning, and expressions of distress.

2. Culturally skilled counselors respect indigenous helping practices and respect minority community intrinsic help-giving networks.

3. Culturally skilled counselors value bilingualism and do not view another language as an impediment to counseling (monolingualism may be the culprit).

B. Knowledge

1. Culturally skilled counselors have a clear and explicit knowledge and understanding of the generic characteristics of counseling and therapy (culture bound, class bound, and monolingual) and how they may clash with the cultural values of various minority groups.

2. Culturally skilled counselors are aware of institutional barriers that prevent minorities from using mental health services.

3. Culturally skilled counselors have knowledge of the potential bias in assessment instruments and use procedures and interpret findings, keeping in mind the cultural and linguistic characteristics of the clients.

4. Culturally skilled counselors have knowledge of minority family structures, hierarchies, values, and beliefs. They are knowledgeable about the community characteristics and the resources in the community as well as the family.

5. Culturally skilled counselors should be aware of relevant discriminatory practices at the social and community level that may be affecting the psychological welfare of the population being served.

C. Skills

1. Culturally skilled counselors are able to engage in a variety of verbal and nonverbal helping responses. They are able to *send* and *receive* both *verbal* and *nonverbal* messages *accurately* and *appropriately*. They are not tied down to only one method or approach to helping but recognize that helping styles and approaches may be culture bound. When they sense that their helping style is limited and potentially inappropriate, they can anticipate and ameliorate its negative impact.

2. Culturally skilled counselors are able to exercise institutional intervention skills on behalf of their clients. They can help clients determine whether a "problem" stems from racism or bias in others (the concept of health paranoia) so that clients do not inappropriately personalize problems.

3. Culturally skilled counselors are not adverse to seeking consultation with traditional healers and religious and

spiritual leaders and practitioners in the treatment of culturally different clients when appropriate.

4. Culturally skilled counselors take responsibility for interacting in the language requested by the client; this may mean appropriate referral to outside resources. A serious problem arises when the linguistic skills of a counselor do not match the language of the client. This being the case, counselors should (a) seek a translator with cultural knowledge and appropriate professional background or (b) refer to a knowledgeable and competent bilingual counselor.

5. Culturally skilled counselors have training and expertise in the use of traditional assessment and testing instruments. They not only understand the technical aspects of the instruments but are also aware of the cultural limitations. This allows them to use test instruments for the welfare of the diverse clients.

6. Culturally skilled counselors should attend to as well as work to eliminate biases, prejudices, and discriminatory practices. They should be cognizant of sociopolitical contexts in conducting evaluation and probing interventions and should develop sensitivity to issues of oppression, sexism, elitism, and racism.

7. Culturally skilled counselors take responsibility in educating their clients to the process of psychological intervention, such as goals, expectations, legal rights, and the counselor's orientation.

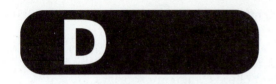

Council for Standards in Human Service Education: National Standards for Human Service Worker Education and Training Programs

General Program Characteristics

I. Primary Program Objective

STANDARD NUMBER 1: The primary program objective shall be to prepare human service practitioners to serve clients or carry out other supportive human service agency functions. Human service competencies shall be the bases for design of program goals, curriculum, and methodology.

II. Philosophical Base of Programs

STANDARD NUMBER 2: The program description shall state explicitly the philosophical and knowledge base of the program.

III. Community Needs Assessment

STANDARD NUMBER 3: The program shall conduct periodic assessments of community needs for kinds and numbers of human service workers.

IV. Program Evaluation

STANDARD NUMBER 4: The program shall use the community needs assessment, graduate follow-up studies, and evaluation of faculty and courses to determine how well the program is meeting community and student needs and to modify the program as necessary.

V. Standards and Procedures for Admitting, Retaining, and Dismissing Students

STANDARD NUMBER 5: The program shall have written standards and procedures for admitting, retaining, and dismissing students.

VI. Staffing and Resources

A. Credentials of Core Faculty/Staff

STANDARD NUMBER 6: The collective competencies of the core faculty/staff for each program shall include both a strong knowledge base and practical experience in delivery of human services to clients.

B. Essential Faculty/Staff Roles

STANDARD NUMBER 7: The program shall adequately manage the essential training program roles and provide opportunities for faculty to learn the essential staff roles and skills required for human service training programs.

C. Faculty Evaluations

STANDARD NUMBER 8: Faculty evaluations shall reflect the total role responsibilities as defined in the position description of that faculty member and shall be conducted at least every two years.

D. Program Support

STANDARD NUMBER 9: The program shall have adequate staff support and program resources to provide a complete training program.

VII. Articulation

STANDARD NUMBER 10: Each program shall make efforts to increase the transferability of credits to other academic programs and have a written policy on how a student's credits and previous learning achievements will be evaluated and accepted for admission and transfer.

Curriculum

I. Curriculum Components

A. Knowledge

1. History

STANDARD NUMBER 11: The curriculum shall provide knowledge of the historical development of human services.

2. Context and Dimensions of Human Service Work

STANDARD NUMBER 12: The curriculum shall provide knowledge of human systems—individual, group, family, organization, community, and society—and their interaction.

3. Human Service Populations

STANDARD NUMBER 13: The curriculum shall address the conditions which promote or limit optimal human functioning and identify classes of deviation from desired functioning in the major human systems.

B. Skills

1. Generic Planning and Evaluation Skills

STANDARD NUMBER 14: The curriculum shall provide skill training in systematic analysis of a service problem; in selection of appropriate strategies, services, or interventions; and in evaluation of outcomes.

2. Information Management Skills

STANDARD NUMBER 15: The curriculum shall provide skill training in information management.

3. Intervention Skills

STANDARD NUMBER 16: The curriculum shall provide training in human service intervention skills that are appropriate to the level of training.

4. Interpersonal Skills

STANDARD NUMBER 17: Learning experiences shall be provided for the student to develop his/her interpersonal skills with clients, co-workers and supervisors.

5. Administration Skills

STANDARD NUMBER 18: The curriculum shall provide skill training in the administrative aspects of the service delivery system.

C. Attitudes

1. Client Related Values and Attitudes

STANDARD NUMBER 19: The training program shall transmit the major human service values and attitudes to students in order to promote understanding of human service ethics and their application in practice.

2. Self-Development

STANDARD NUMBER 20: The training program shall provide experiences and support to enable students to develop awareness of their own values, personalities, reaction patterns, interpersonal styles, and limitations.

II. Field Experience

A. Minimum Requirements

STANDARD NUMBER 21: The program shall provide each student field experience that is integrated with the rest of the training and education.

B. Academic Credit

STANDARD NUMBER 22: The program shall award academic credit for the field experience.

C. Supervision

STANDARD NUMBER 23: It is the responsibility of the college to ensure that field placement sites provide quality training experiences and supervision.

Glossary

Italicized terms in the definitions are also defined in the glossary.

AACD *See American Association for Counseling and Development.*

ability test A test to measure an individual's cognitive capabilities. See *achievement test; aptitude test.*

ACA See *American Counseling Association.*

Academy of Certified Social Workers Established in 1965 by the *National Association for Social Work,* this organization sets standards of practice in the field for master's-level social workers.

accommodation The process of adapting new knowledge and experiences so that one's understanding of the world is altered.

accountability The evaluation that a program or an agency has accomplished or is accomplishing to show the effectiveness of the services it is offering.

ACES See *Association of Counselor Educators and Supervisors.*

achievement test A type of an *ability test* that measures what has been learned. See *diagnostic test; readiness test; survey battery test.*

ACSW See *Academy of Certified Social Workers.*

actualizing tendency The inborn, positive inner qualities and inherent traits that arise in a person when placed in a nurturing and facilitative environment. See also *humanistic counseling and education.*

acute psychotic episode Short-term loss of reality.

administrator A human service worker who supervises community service programs.

advocate A human service worker who champions and defends clients' causes and rights.

almshouses Established by the *Poor Law* of 1601, these were shelters for individuals who could not care for themselves.

American Association for Counseling and Development The renamed *American Personnel and Guidance Association* and former name of the ACA.

American Counseling Association The professional association for *counselors*.

American Personnel and Guidance Association Formed out of the *National Vocational Guidance Association* and other associations and established in the 1950s, a professional association for guidance counselors.

American Psychiatric Association The professional association for psychiatrists.

American Psychological Association The professional association for psychologists.

Americans with Disabilities Act Enacted in 1992, this act ensures that qualified individuals with disabilities cannot be discriminated against in job application procedures, hiring, firing, advancement, compensation, fringe benefits, job training, and other terms, conditions, and privileges.

anal stage Sigmund Freud's second stage of *psychosexual development*, occurring between ages 1 1/2 and 3 years, whereby a child's emotional gratification is derived from bowel movements. See also *genital stage; latency stage; oral stage; phallic stage.*

antideterministic view of human nature The view that rejects the notion that early childhood development and biological/genetic factors cause psychological problems and stresses the ability of the individual to change. This view is in opposition to the *deterministic view of human nature*.

APA See *American Psychiatric Association: American Psychological Association.*

APGA See *American Personnel and Guidance Association.*

aptitude test A type of an *ability test* that measures what one is capable of learning. See *cognitive ability test; individual intelligence test; multiple aptitude test; special aptitude test.*

assimilation The absorption of new information into an existing store of knowledge.

assistant to specialist A human service worker who works closely with the highly trained professional as an aide and helper in servicing clients.

Association of Counselor Educators and Supervisors Originally a division of the *American Personnel and Guidance Association* (now the ACA), this organization was instrumental in originally setting standards for master's-level counseling programs.

behavioral approach The use of *classical conditioning, operant conditioning,* or *modeling* to bring about behavior change.

behavior changer A human service worker who uses intervention strategies and counseling skills to facilitate client change.

block grant Federal funding to states that allows the state to decide which programs to fund.

broker A human service worker who helps clients find and use services.

Buckley Amendment See *Family Education Rights and Privacy Act.*

caregiver A human service worker who offers direct support, encouragement, and hope to clients.

case management A process that involves the ways you help a client develop goals, how you manage client contact hours, how you monitor client progress toward goals, the way you keep records, and how you evaluate client progress.

certification Usually set by states or by national organizations, a more rigorous form of credentialing as compared to registration. See also *credentialing; licensure; registration.*

charity organization society (COS) Arising in the United States in the 1800s, an organization of volunteers who tried to alleviate the conditions of poverty by entering the poorer districts of cities and helping the residents there.

classical conditioning Behavior change brought about by pairing a conditioned stimulus (such as the sound of a bell) with an unconditioned stimulus (such as the sight of food) until the conditioned stimulus alone evokes a response (such as salivation).

cognitive ability test A type of *aptitude test* that measures general intellectual ability and is usually given in group settings in schools, to assess an individual's ability to do well in school.

cognitive approach A counseling approach that stresses how the individual thinks, particularly how ideas affect our behaviors and how we feel.

collaborative effort The joint effort between helper and client that determines what goals would best meet the client's needs.

commitment to relativism The third stage of William Perry's theory of adult cognitive development, where a person maintains a relativistic outlook and commits to specific values and behaviors in his or her own life. See also *dualism; relativism.*

Community Mental Health Centers Act Passed in 1963, this act provided federal funds for the creation of comprehensive mental-health centers across the country, which greatly changed the delivery of mental-health services.

community planner A human service worker who designs, implements, and organizes new programs to service client needs.

concrete-operational stage Jean Piaget's third stage of cognitive development (ages 7–11 years) when a child starts developing logical thinking. See also *formal-operational stage; preoperational stage; sensorimotor stage.*

conditions of worth Carl Rogers's term for how conditions and opinions of significant others lead to *incongruity* in an individual because of the individual's need to be loved.

congruent The quality of being in sync with one's feelings and behaviors. See also *genuine; transparent.*

constructive model of development Robert Kegan's model of cognitive development, based on the *antideterministic view of human nature* and opposed to Freud's *deterministic view of human nature,* positing that individuals must pass through six (0–5) developmental stages (*incorporative stage, impulsive* *stage, imperial stage, interpersonal stage, institutional stage,* and *interindividual stage,* respectively) that affect the way we construct reality and understand the world. See also *subject/object theory.*

consultant   A human service worker who seeks and offers knowledge and support to other professionals and meets with clients and community groups to discuss and solve problems.

contract   A written or verbal agreement drawn by the helper and client that describes client goals.

conventional level   Lawrence Kohlberg's second level of moral development (ages 9–18 years) when a person makes a moral decision based on peer approval or disapproval (stage 3) and on established rules of what is right or wrong (stage 4). See also *postconventional level; preconventional level.*

conversion disorder   A term for the process by which emotions become transformed into physical manifestations (for example, paralysis of a limb, blindness).

COS   See *charity organization society.*

Council for Standards in Human Service Education   Founded in 1979, this organization was established to help human service educators and college administrators achieve maximum educational quality and relevance to the service-delivery system in their communities.

counseling group   Similar to a *therapy group* but with less self-disclosure and personality reconstruction expected, a meeting of individuals whose purpose is to effect behavior change and increase self-awareness.

counselor   An individual who has a master's degree in counseling, including school counselors, mental health counselors, college counselors, and rehabilitation counselors

counterconditioning   The conditioning of new adaptive behavior through the use of behavioral techniques. See also *behavioral approach.*

countertransference   The process in which the helper's own issues interfere with effectively helping his or her clients.

credentialing   Usually regulated by state or national legislation, a method of ensuring minimum competence in a field. Three types of credentialing are *certification, licensure,* and *registration.*

criterion-referenced test   A test where the examinee's score is compared to the accomplishment of specific goals the examinee must attain.

CSHSE   See *Council for Standards in Human Service Education.*

cultural mosaic   A society that has many diverse values and customs.

culture   The common values, norms of behavior, symbols, language, and life patterns that people may share.

data manager   A human service worker who develops systems to gather facts and statistics as a means of evaluating programs.

decision-making theory   The postulation that an individual's decision-making process is crucial in making career choices.

decline stage   Stage 5 of Donald Super's career development theory, occurring between age 64 and time of death, where the individual starts to separate self from the job and focuses more on retirement and avocational activities. See also *establishment stage; exploration stage; growth stage; maintenance stage.*

defense mechanism   An often unconscious mental process that allows a person to make compromises in order to avoid anxiety and to protect the ego. See *denial; projection; rationalization; regression; repression.*

deinstitutionalization   A social change occurring in the late 1970s whereby patients who were held against their will and were not in danger of hurting themselves or others were released from psychiatric hospitals.

denial   A *defense mechanism,* the refusal to admit the truth or see reality in order to protect the *ego.*

dependent variable   In *experimental research,* a quantity that is measured following manipulation of the *independent variable;* an outcome measure.

deterministic view of human nature   The view that instincts and early childhood development are so influential that there is little ability for the person to change. This view is in opposition to the *antideterministic view of human nature.*

developmental approach to career development   The concept that career development is a life-span process that involves a series of predictable stages through which people pass. Two developmental theorists are Super and Ginzberg. See also *personality approach to career development.*

developmental crisis   A predictable problem with which the family must deal.

developmental readiness   The state where the client is ready to advance to a higher *developmental stage.*

developmental stages   In the psychodynamic approach, the psychological and physical tasks an individual must accomplish in the life span.

Diagnostic and Statistical Manual III–Revised   Developed by the *American Psychiatric Association* and the *American Psychological Association,* a manual that details the different types of mental illnesses and emotional problems.

diagnostic test   A type of an *achievement test* that assesses suspected problem areas and is usually given one-to-one by a highly trained, experienced examiner.

Dictionary of Occupational Titles   Published by the federal government, a comprehensive classification system for approximately 20,000 occupations.

directive view of human nature   The view that an individual needs direction and guidance from the helper during the change process. This view is in opposition to the *nondirective view of human nature.*

discrimination   An active behavior that negatively affects individuals of ethnic, cultural, and racial groups.

DOT   See *Dictionary of Occupational Titles.*

DSM III–R   See *Diagnostic and Statistical Manual III–Revised.*

dualism   The first stage in William Perry's theory of adult cognitive development, where a person views the world in terms of black or white, or right or wrong, and has little tolerance for ambiguity. See also *commitment to relativism; relativism.*

EAP   See *employee assistance program.*

eclecticism   The selection of what appears to be the best of several methods, approaches or styles and their integration into one approach.

Education for All Handicapped Children Act   Enacted in 1975, a federal law that guarantees an education in the least restrictive environment to individuals with a disability between the ages 3 and 21 years and that mandates the states to fund the services.

ego   According to Freudian theory, the conscious portion of the *psyche* that is the mediator between the person and reality, especially in the functioning of the person's perception of and adaptation to reality. See also *id; superego.*

empathic person   An individual who has a deep understanding of another person's point of view.

empathy   The ability to show deep understanding of a client's feelings and situation.

empiricism   The practice of relying on observation and experiment.

employee assistance program   A program run by business or industry that provides primary prevention and early referral for treatment.

encounter group   A group in which expressions of feelings are encouraged, which leads to new self-awareness.

establishment stage   Stage 3 of Donald Super's career development theory, occurring between ages 24 and 44 years, where the individual stabilizes career choice and advances in the chosen field. See also *decline stage; exploration stage; growth stage; maintenance stage.*

ethnicity   Long-term patterns of behavior that have some historical significance and may include similar religious, ancestral, language, and/or cultural characteristics.

etiology   The origin(s) of a disease.

evaluator   A human service worker who assesses client programs and ensures that agencies are accountable for services provided.

existentialism   The philosophical belief centering on the individual's existence in an incomprehensible universe and on the plight of the individual to assume full responsibility for his or her acts without certain knowledge of what is moral or immoral.

exploration stage   Stage 2 of Donald Super's career development theory, occurring between ages 14 and 24 years, where the individual tentatively tests occupational fantasies through work, school, and leisure activities and later chooses an occupation or more professional training. See also *decline stage; establishment stage; growth stage; maintenance stage.*

external locus of control   A characteristic that makes a person place more importance on others' opinions, rather than his or her own, when making decisions. See also *internal locus of control*.

family counseling   Therapy that involves treating the entire family, not just an individual in the family.

Family Education Rights and Privacy Act   Also known as the *Buckley Amendment*, this 1974 federal act grants parents the right to access their children's educational records.

fixation   The condition in which maturity is hindered because of unresolved issues in earlier *developmental stages*.

formal-operational stage   Jean Piaget's fourth stage of cognitive development (ages 11–16 years) when a child can think abstractly, consider more than one aspect of problem at one time, and understand more complex meanings. See also *concrete-operational stage; preoperational stage; sensorimotor stage*.

Freedom of Information Act   Enacted in 1974, this federal law allows individuals to have access to any records maintained by a federal agency that contain personal information about the individual.

general systems theory   The postulation that any living system (individual, family, community, institution, and so on) has regulatory mechanisms that maintain *homeostasis* while it interacts with other systems.

genital stage   Sigmund Freud's fifth and final stage of *psychosexual development*, occurring at puberty and continuing through the life span, where sexual energy is focused on social activities and love relationships and where unresolved issues of earlier stages emerge. See also *anal stage; latency stage; oral stage; phallic stage*.

genuine   The quality of expressing one's true feelings. See also *congruent; transparent*.

group dynamics   The ways in which groups interact.

growth stage   Stage 1 of Donald Super's career development theory, occurring between birth and age 14 years, where the individual becomes aware of interests and abilities related to the world of work and begins to compare his or her abilities with those of peers. See also *decline stage; establishment stage; exploration stage; maintenance stage*.

guidance group   A meeting of individuals whose purpose is to educate and support group members and, unlike a *support group*, always has a designated, well-trained leader.

Head Start Program   A federally funded program, started in the 1970s, that provides an intellectually stimulating and nurturing environment to disadvantaged preschool children.

health maintenance organization   A managed health care system that offers subscribers a pool of designated providers from which they can choose.

hierarchy of needs   In Abraham Maslow's hierarchical theory, the postulation that lower-order needs must be fulfilled before higher-order needs; the order is (1) physiological needs, (2) safety needs, (3) love and belonging, (4) self-esteem, and (5) self-actualization.

HMO See *health maintenance organization.*

homeostasis The tendency for a system to maintain equilibrium.

homophobia Similar to *racism,* the irrational *prejudice* toward gay men and lesbians.

humanistic approach to counseling Developed by Carl Rogers and others, this approach to counseling is nondirective, facilitative, and present-centered; a stark contrast to the more directive and past-focus approach of psychoanalysis. See also *psychoanalysis.*

humanistic counseling and education Founded by Carl Rogers, Abraham Maslow, and others, this philosophy of counseling and education advocates that individuals are born with positive qualities that would be expressed in a nurturing environment. If such an environment was not present in early childhood, such qualities could be developed later in life in a nurturing environment. See also *actualizing tendency.*

human service worker A person who has an associate's or bachelor's degree in human services or a closely related field.

hypothesis An assumption or proposition that is derived from prior research and allows us to examine phenomena. See also *research question.*

id According to Freudian theory, the unconscious portion of the *psyche* that is the source of instinctual drives and needs. See also *ego; superego.*

identified patient In a family, the individual who is blamed for a behavior problem when in fact the family "owns" the problem.

imperial stage Stage 2 of Robert Kegan's *interpersonal model of development,* where a person can begin to control impulses and where needs, interests, and wishes become primary. See also *incorporative stage; impulsive stage; institutional stage; interindividual stage; interpersonal stage.*

impulsive stage Stage 1 of Robert Kegan's *interpersonal model of development,* where a person has limited control over his or her actions and acts spontaneously to have needs met. See also *incorporative stage; imperial stage; institutional stage; interindividual stage; interpersonal stage.*

incongruity As pertains to *conditions of worth,* the state of being inconsistent within oneself; that is, ignoring true beliefs and values and accepting significant others' beliefs and values in order to be accepted.

incorporative stage Stage 0 of Robert Kegan's *interpersonal model of development,* where a person is self-absorbed and has no sense of being separate from the outside world. See also *imperial stage; impulsive stage; institutional stage; interindividual stage; interpersonal stage.*

independent variable In *experimental research,* the variable that is being manipulated in order to examine its effect on some outcome measure. See also *dependent variable.*

individual intelligence test A type of *aptitude test* that measures general intellectual ability and is usually given one-to-one by a highly trained, experienced examiner; often given to identify individuals with learning disabilities or individuals who are gifted.

informal test   An assessment measure that varies in the way it is administered; the results may not necessarily be compared with those of a *norm group.* An example is a teacher-made test.

institutional stage   Stage 4 of Robert Kegan's *interpersonal model of development,* where a person has separated his or her values from others' and has a strong sense of personal autonomy and self-reliance. See also *incorporative stage; imperial stage; impulsive stage; interindividual stage; interpersonal stage.*

interest inventory   A type of personality test that measures an individual's likes, dislikes, and orientation to occupational choices.

interindividual stage   Stage 5 of Robert Kegan's *interpersonal model of development,* where a person maintains a separate sense of self while accepting feedback from others in order to grow and change. See also *incorporative stage; imperial stage; impulsive stage; institutional stage; interpersonal stage.*

internality   The ability of a person not to be highly affected by the views of significant people in his or her life or by societal values. See also *internal locus of control.*

internalize   To incorporate feelings and/or values within the self.

internal locus of control   A characteristic that allows a person to rely on his or her internal thoughts and beliefs when making decisions. See also *external locus of control.*

interpersonal stage   Stage 3 in Robert Kegan's *interpersonal model of development,* where a person cannot separate his or her own sense of being from family, friends, or community groups. See also *incorporative stage; imperial stage; impulsive stage; institutional stage; interindividual stage.*

intrapersonal factors   The issues within a person that affect behavior.

introjection   Unconsciously adopting significant others' beliefs and values.

introspective person   An individual who is open to his or her deeper feelings and is willing to be self-critical and receive feedback from others.

latency stage   Sigmund Freud's fourth stage of *psychosexual development,* occurring between ages 5 years through puberty, where the child replaces sexual feelings with socialization. See also *anal stage; genital stage; oral stage; phallic stage.*

LCSW   See *licensed clinical social worker.*

licensed clinical social worker   An individual who has a master's degree in social work and has met specific state requirements to obtain *licensure.*

licensed professional counselor   An individual who has a master's degree in counseling and has met specific state requirements to obtain *licensure.*

licensure   This most rigorous form of credentialing is generally set by the state and requires a minimum educational level, usually a state or national exam, and additional documentation of expertise such as evidence of post-education supervision. See also *certification; credentialing; registration.*

LPC   See *licensed professional counselor.*

loose boundary   As pertains to *general systems theory,* a framework that allows information to flow too easily into and out of the system, thus causing difficulty in the system's sense of identity. See also *rigid boundary; semipermeable boundary.*

major depression A mood disorder characterized by feelings of sadness, diminished interest in pleasure, a significant increase or decrease in appetite, diminished ability to concentrate, feelings of worthlessness, and/or suicidal thoughts.

maintenance stage Stage 4 of Donald Super's career development theory, occurring between ages 44 and 64 years, where the individual confirms career choice and hopes to avoid stagnation. See also *decline stage; establishment stage; exploration stage; growth stage.*

McKinney Act Enacted in 1987, this act provides to the poor and homeless funds for job training, literacy programs, child care, and transportation and subsidizes counseling.

mean A statistical property, the average of all test scores of the group. See also *measures of central tendency; median; mode.*

measures of central tendency Those statistical concepts that provide information about the middle range of scores. See also *mean; median; mode.*

measures of variability Those statistical concepts that provide information on how much scores vary. See also *range; standard deviation.*

median A statistical property, the middle test score—the point where 50% of examinees score above and 50% score below the group. See also *mean; measures of central tendency; mode.*

medical model The view, often held by adherents of the *deterministic view of human nature* and contrasted to the *wellness approach,* that mental illness is most likely caused by genetic/biological factors and therefore can be diagnosed and treated as an illness.

Mental Health Study Act Passed in 1955, this act was a broadly based effort to study the diagnosis and treatment of mental illness.

mobilizer A human service worker who organizes client and community support in order to provide needed services.

mode A statistical property, the most frequent test score of the group. See also *mean; measures of central tendency; median.*

modeling The acquisition of behavior patterns through the viewing of models in social situations.

moral dilemma A problem of a moral nature that has no clear-cut answer.

multiple aptitude test A type of *aptitude test* that measures a broad range of abilities and how those abilities might be associated with occupational choice.

NASW See *National Association of Social Workers.*

National Association of Social Workers Founded in 1955, the professional association for social workers.

National Defense Education Act Passed in 1958 as a direct response to the Soviet Union's launching of Sputnik, the act provided funds for the expansion of counseling programs in schools in order to identify gifted students.

National Institute of Mental Health   Created by the U.S. Congress in the late 1940s, this agency was the federal government's first real effort in confronting mental-health issues and resulted in systematic research and training in the mental-health field.

National Organization for Human Service Education   Founded in 1975, this professional association provides a link between human service organizations and practitioners, promotes the improved education of human service workers, advocates the development of human service organizations, and supports creative approaches toward meeting human service needs.

National Training Laboratory   Founded in the 1940s by Kurt Lewin and other prominent theorists, this institution examines *group dynamics* and trains individuals to understand the special interactions that occur in groups.

National Vocational Guidance Association   Founded in 1913 as a professional association for vocational guidance counselors, it is considered to be the forerunner of the ACA.

NDEA   See *National Defense Education Act.*

negative reinforcement   The removal of a stimulus that yields an increase in behavior.

NIMH   See *National Institute of Mental Health.*

NOHSE   See *National Organization for Human Service Education.*

nondirective view of human nature   The view that an individual has the ability to develop the strategies for change in the helping process. This view is in opposition to the *directive view of human nature.*

nondogmatic person   An individual who allows others to express their points of view, does not need to change others to his or her own viewpoint, and is open to criticism and change.

norm group   A peer group.

norm-referenced test   A test where the examinee's score is compared with the score of a *norm group.*

NTL   See *National Training Laboratory.*

NVGA   See *National Vocational Guidance Association.*

objective personality test   Usually given in multiple choice or true/false format, this type of personality test usually compares an individual's traits with those of a *norm group.*

Occupational Outlook Handbook   Published by the federal government, a sourcebook on approximately 300 occupations that includes future outlook, nature of the work, type of training needed, and wage/employment conditions.

OOH   See *Occupational Outlook Handbook.*

operant conditioning   The shaping of behavior, which is brought about through the use of *positive reinforcement* and/or *negative reinforcement.*

operationalize   To take an abstract construct (for example, empathy) and develop a means to define, measure, and quantify it.

oral stage Sigmund Freud's first stage of *psychosexual development,* occurring between birth and age 1 1/2 years, whereby a child's emotional gratification is derived from intake of food, by sucking, and later by biting. See also *anal stage; genital stage; latency stage; phallic stage.*

outcome evaluation The assessment of a program after it is completed. See also *process evaluation.*

outreach worker A human service worker who might go into communities to work with clients.

paradigm shift The concept that knowledge builds upon itself, that new discoveries are based on past knowledge, and that when current knowledge no longer explains the way things work, a new view of understanding the world is in order.

participant observation Research where information is gathered by the researcher who joins and interacts with a group.

personal growth group A special kind of *support group* that offers support to group members while encouraging expression of feeling and exploration of individual growth.

personality approach to career development The concept that career choice is greatly affected by personality development. Two personality theorists are Ann Roe and John Holland. See also *developmental approach to career development.*

person-centered approach Developed by Carl Rogers and part of the *humanistic approach to counseling,* this is a way to facilitate change through the counseling relationship, whereby *empathy, unconditional positive regard,* and *genuineness* are necessary and sufficient personality characteristics to effect growth.

phallic stage Sigmund Freud's third stage of *psychosexual development,* occurring between ages 3 and 5 years, when the child becomes aware of his or her and the opposite sex's genitals and receives pleasure from self-stimulation. See also *anal stage; genital stage; latency stage; oral stage.*

phenomenology The philosophical study of the development of human consciousness and self-awareness.

Poor Law Established by the English government in 1601, this was one of the first attempts at legislating aid for the poor. In many ways, the American system of social welfare was modeled after this law.

positive reinforcement The presentation of a stimulus that yields an increase in behavior.

postconventional level Lawrence Kohlberg's third level of moral development (age 14 years and older) when a person makes a moral decision based on universally recognized truths, principles, and laws (stage 5) and on personal acceptance or rejection of those matters (stage 6). See also *conventional level, preconventional level.*

power differentials The control, authority, or influence over others.

power dynamics   The force of individuals, institutions, and/or society that places, on some individuals, undue demands that cause stressful behaviors that many people call abnormal.

practicality   The usefulness of a test, considering such factors as cost, length, ease of administration, and ease of interpretation.

preconventional level   Lawrence Kohlberg's first level of moral development (ages 2–9 years) when a person makes a moral decision based on punishment (stage 1) and reward (stage 2). See also *conventional level; postconventional level.*

prejudice   As pertains to *stereotyping* and *racism*, negative opinions and attitudes held about members of ethnic and/or cultural groups.

preoperational stage   Jean Piaget's second stage of cognitive development (ages 2–7 years) when a child develops language ability and can maintain mental images. A child in this stage responds intuitively as opposed to acting in a manner that might seem to be logically correct. See also *concrete-operational stage; formal-operational stage; sensorimotor stage.*

privileged communication   As determined by the state, the legal right of a professional (lawyer, priest, physician, or licensed therapist) to not reveal information about a client.

process evaluation   The assessment of an ongoing program to rate its effectiveness so as to make changes as needed. See also *outcome evaluation.*

professional disclosure statement   A written statement, given to the client, describing such issues as the limits of confidentiality, the length of the interview, the helper's credentials, the limits of the relationship, the helper's theoretical orientation, legal concerns, fees for service, and agency rules that might affect the client.

projection   A *dense mechanism,* the viewing of one's own unacceptable qualities (ideas, emotions, attitudes) as belonging to others in order to protect the *ego.*

projective test   A type of personality test where the individual gives an unstructured response to a stimulus. These responses are then interpreted by an experienced clinician for personality characteristics. Examples are the Rorschach inkblot test and sentence-completion tests.

psyche   The conscious and unconscious emotions, thoughts, and sensations of an individual.

psychiatrist   A physician who generally has completed a residency in psychiatry—that is, has completed extensive training in some kind of mental-health setting.

psychoanalysis   Developed by Sigmund Freud, a method of analyzing psychological problems, based on early childhood experiences and instinctual aggressive and sexual drives, where the client talks freely about himself or herself—especially about childhood experiences. See also *psychosexual stages of development; structures of personality.*

psychobiology   The study of the mind/body interactions that influence the development and functioning of the personality.

psychodynamic approach   The belief that drives (instinctual like sex and aggression, social, attachment/separation), which are at least somewhat unconscious, motivate behavior.

psychologist   Generally, a person who has a doctoral degree in psychology, has completed an internship at a mental-health facility, and has passed specific state requirements to obtain licensure as a psychologist.

psychosexual stages of development   As posited by Sigmund Freud, the five stages of individual development: *oral stage, anal stage, phallic stage, latency stage,* and *genital stage.* See also *psychoanalysis.*

psychosocial model of development   Erik Erikson's model of human development, based on the *antideterministic view of human nature* and opposed to Freud's *deterministic view of human nature,* positing that both psychological and social forces are major motivators in individual development throughout the life span.

psychotherapist   Although generally not licensed by states, on a practical level, a person who has an advanced degree in psychology, social work, or counseling and who works in a mental-health setting or in private practice, providing individual, marital, or group counseling.

quasi-experimental research   Undertaken when *true experimental research* is impractical or impossible, research where one examines intact groups instead of randomly assigning subjects to groups.

race   Traditionally, a division of people who share common genetic and biological characteristics.

racism   The irrational dislike or hate held about and/or directed at people of a particular *race.*

range   A statistical property, the spread of test scores from highest to lowest for the group. See also *measures of variability; standard deviation.*

rationalization   A *defense mechanism,* attributing one's actions and thought to apparent, but not real, creditable motives in order to protect the *ego.*

readiness test   A type of an *achievement test* that measures an individual's readiness to advance to the next educational level.

reality therapy   Developed by William Glasser, a proponent of the *antideterministic view of human nature,* a treatment that helps the individual cope with the stress of living through the use of behavior-change strategies.

registration   The most basic form of ensuring minimum competence for a profession by requiring individuals to register their credentials, usually with the state. See also *certification; credentialing; licensure.*

Rehabilitation Act   Enacted in 1973, this law ensured access to vocational rehabilitation for adults, based on three conditions: a severe physical or mental disability, a disability that interferes with obtaining or maintaining a job, and employment that is feasible.

regression   A *defense mechanism* of reverting to an earlier stage of development with less demanding ways of responding to anxiety.

reinforcement contingencies   Those stimuli in the environment that shape (reinforce) one's behavior.

relativism   The second stage in William Perry's theory of adult cognitive development, where a person begins to think abstractly, allows for differing opinions, and understands there are many ways to view the world. See also *dualism; commitment to relativism.*

reliability   The consistency of test scores; a measure of the accuracy of a test.

repression   A *defense mechanism*, the result of thrusting painful memories—usually early childhood experiences—into the unconscious.

research design   After developing a *hypothesis* or *research question* and doing a *review of the literature*, the approach one takes to study and evaluate a particular question. See also *quasi-experimental research; sociological research; true experimental research.*

research question   Based on prior research and theory, a question that is developed to examine a particular problem. See also *hypothesis.*

review of the literature   A thorough examination of major research done in a particular area, found in books, articles, and computerized abstracts.

rigid boundary   As pertains to *general systems theory*, a framework that does not allow information to flow easily into and out of the system, thus causing difficulty in a change process. See also *loose boundary; semipermeable boundary.*

role-playing   Acting out the thoughts and beliefs of another person.

scapegoat   An individual within a system who is unconsciously given the blame for problems in the system.

schemata   The organized, mental ways of perceiving and responding to complex situations or stimulants.

schizophrenia   A psychotic disorder characterized by misrepresentation of and retreat from reality, delusions, hallucinations, and withdrawn, bizarre, or regressive behavior; popularly and erroneously called split personality.

self-actualized person   Abraham Maslow's term for a person who is in touch with himself or herself, can hear feedback from others, is nondogmatic, has a strong *internal locus of control*, and is empathic and introspective.

self-disclosure   The act in which the helper reveals to the client personal information about himself or herself in order to show more effective ways of coping.

self-efficacy theory   The postulation that an individual's belief system greatly affects the types of choices he or she makes.

semipermeable boundary   As pertains to *general systems theory*, a framework that allows information to enter the system and be processed and incorporated. See also *loose boundary; rigid boundary.*

sensorimotor stage   Jean Piaget's first stage of cognitive development (ages birth–2 years) when the child responds to only physical and sensory experiences. See also *concrete-operational stage; formal-operational stage; preoperational stage.*

settlement movement   Arising in the United States in the 1800s, the attempt by social activists, while living with the poor, to change communities through community action and political activities.

situational crisis An unexpected problem, with which the family must deal, that is condition-specific.

situational theory The postulation that often the career choices we make are out of our control and are related more to conditions in society.

social casework Having its roots in *charity organization societies,* the process by which the needs of a client are examined and a treatment plan is designed to facilitate client growth.

social class The grouping of people according to such things as wealth, ancestry, rank, and status.

social learning The learning gained from watching the behavior of others and then acting out those behaviors.

social worker Generally, a person who has a master's degree in social work.

sociological research The systematic gathering of information to determine patterns of behavior. See also *participant observation; survey research.*

special aptitude test A type of *aptitude test* that measures a specific ability (for example, hand/eye coordination) and is often used for job placement and acceptance into specialty schools.

spontaneous recovery During treatment for behavior change, the recurrence of former behaviors after the use of a specific intervention that seems successful.

standard deviation A statistical property, the amount, on average, that test scores vary from the *mean.* See also *measures of variability; range.*

standardized test An assessment instrument that is administered in the same way every time it is given; the test results may be compared with those of a *norm group.* An example is the Scholastic Aptitude Test (SAT).

stereotyping One of the leading causes of *racism,* the ascribing of characteristics, usually negative, onto a group of people.

structures of personality The *id, ego,* and *superego.* See also *psychoanalysis.*

subception Carl Rogers's term for the professional's ability to perceive feelings and deeper meanings beyond what the individual experiences.

subculture A group of people whose behaviors and values may differ from the larger *culture.*

subject/object theory The basis for Robert Kegan's *constructive model of development,* the conjecture that individuals pass through specific developmental stages in constructing a system that makes meaning of the world.

superego According to Freudian theory, the partly conscious portion of the *psyche* that *internalizes* parental and societal rules and serves as the rewarder or punisher through a system of moral attitudes, conscience, and a sense of guilt. See also *ego; id.*

support group A meeting of individuals whose purpose is to educate and affirm group members; an example is Alcoholics Anonymous.

survey battery test A type of an *achievement test* that measures general knowledge and is usually given in large-group settings in schools.

survey research   Research where specific information is gathered from a target population, using a questionnaire.

tabula rasa   From the Latin meaning "smoothed or erased tablet," the mind in its blank, or empty, state before receiving outside impressions.

teacher/educator   A human service worker who tutors, mentors, and models new behavior for clients.

therapy group   Similar to a *counseling group* but with more self-disclosure and personality reconstruction expected, a meeting of individuals whose purpose is to effect behavior change and increase self-awareness.

token economy   A technique to bring bout positive behavior changes. The client is given a token for each success, and at the end of a specified time, the tokens are turned in for a higher-level reinforcer (for example, money).

trait-and-factor approach to vocational guidance   As developed by Frank Parsons, a systematic approach to vocational guidance that involves knowing oneself, knowing job characteristics, and making a match between the two through "true reasoning."

transference   The redirection of both negative and positive feelings and desires, especially those unconsciously retained from childhood, toward a helper.

transparent   The quality of embodying genuineness and congruence. See also *genuine; congruent*.

triad model   A training model that provides a safe environment for the counselor so that he or she can learn to better understand culturally different clients. The team members are the client; the counselor; the anticounselor, who highlights the differences in values and expectations between the counselor and client; and a procounselor, who highlights the similarities.

true experimental research   Research where one manipulates the variables by random assignment of subjects to particular groups, to measure the effect of the outcome. See *dependent variable; independent variable*.

unconditional positive regard   Carl Rogers's term for the characteristic of the helper to unconditionally accept the helpee, with "no strings attached."

unconscious factors   A concept that much of our behavior is caused by factors beyond our everyday awareness.

unfinished business   Unresolved problems and experiences brought from an earlier life stage that affect interpersonal relationships.

validity   The ability of a test to measure what it is supposed to measure.

values clarification   An approach to help a person understand and accept his or her own perspectives and worldview while encouraging openness to view the world in other ways.

wellness approach   The view, supported by adherents of the antideterministic view of human nature and contrasted to the *medical model*, that espouses the ability of the individual to change.

References

ACA (American Counseling Association). (1988). *Ethical standards for the American Counseling Association* (rev. ed.). Alexandria, VA: Author.

Addams, J. (1910). *Twenty years at Hull House*. New York: Macmillan.

ADL (Anti-Defamation League). (1992). *Anti-defamation league survey on anti-semitism and prejudice in America*. New York: Author.

Adler, A. (1963). *Understanding human nature* (4th ed.). Greenwich, CT: Fawcett.

Adler, A. (1964). *Social interest: A challenge to mankind*. New York: Capricorn.

Alinsky, S. (1970). *The professional radical: Conversations with Saul Alinsky*. New York: Harper & Row.

Alinsky, S. (1971). *Rules for radicals*. New York: Random House.

Allen, J. P., & Turner, E. J. (1988). *We the people: An atlas of America's ethnic diversity*. New York: Macmillan.

American Psychiatric Association. (1987). *Diagnostic and statistical manual of mental disorders* (3rd ed., rev.). Washington, DC: Author.

Americans with Disabilities Act. (1992, July). Americans with Disabilities Act. *The Resource*, p. 1. Norfolk, VA: Old Dominion University Office of Personnel Services.

Ansell, C. (1984). Ethical practices workbook. In *Preparatory course for the national and state licensing examinations in psychology* (Vol. IV). Los Angeles: Association for Advanced Training in the Behavioral Sciences.

APA (American Psychological Association). (1954). *Technical recommendations for psychological tests and diagnostic techniques*. Washington, DC: Author.

APA (American Psychological Association). (1989). *Ethical principles of psychologists* (rev. ed.). Washington, DC: Author.

Appignanesi, R. (1979). *Freud for beginners*. New York: Pantheon Books.

Assouline, M., & Meir, E. I. (1987). Meta-analysis of the relationship between congruence and well-being measures. *Journal of Vocational Behavior, 31,* 319–332.

Atkinson, D. R. (1985). A meta-review of research on cross-cultural counseling and psychotherapy. *Journal of Multicultural Counseling and Development, 13,* 138–153.

Atkinson, D. R., Poston, W. C., Furlong, M. J., & Mercado, P. (1989). Ethnic group preferences for counselor characteristics. *Journal of Counseling Psychology, 36*(1), 68–72.

Axelson, L. J., & Dail, P. W. (1988). The changing character of homelessness in the United States. *Family Relations, 37,* 463–469.

Bach, M. (1959). *Major religions of the world: Their origins, basic beliefs, and development.* New York: Abingdon Press.

Baker, S. B., & Shaw, M. C. (1987). *Improving counseling through primary prevention.* Columbus, OH: Merrill.

Bandura, A. (1977). *Social learning theory.* Englewood Cliffs, NJ: Prentice-Hall.

Bandura, A., Ross, D., & Ross, S. A. (1963). Imitation of film-mediated aggressive models. *Journal of Abnormal and Social Psychology, 67,* 3–11.

Baruth, L. G., & Huber, C. H. (1984). *An introduction to marital theory and therapy.* Pacific Grove, CA: Brooks/Cole.

Baruth, L. G., & Manning, L. M. (1991). *Multicultural counseling and psychotherapy: A lifespan perspective.* New York: Macmillan.

Basse, D. T., & Greenstreet, K. L. (1991). On counseling men. *Journal of the Colorado Association for Counseling and Development, 19,* 3–6.

Beck, A. T. (1976). *Cognitive therapy and emotional disorders.* New York: International Universities Press.

Bell, W. (1987). *Contemporary social welfare.* New York: Macmillan.

Benack, S. (1988). Relativistic thought: A cognitive basis for empathy in counseling. *Counselor Education and Supervision, 27*(3), 216–232.

Benjamin, A. (1981). *The helping interview* (3rd ed.). New York: Houghton Mifflin.

Bennett, B. D., Bryant, B., VandenBos, G. R., & Greenwood, A. (1990). *Professional liability and risk management.* Washington, DC: American Psychological Association.

Bertalanffy, L. von. (1934). *Modern theories of development: An introduction to theoretical biology.* London: Oxford University Press.

Bertalanffy, L. von. (1968). *General systems theory.* New York: Braziller.

Best, J. W., & Kahn, J. V. (1986). *Research in education.* Englewood Cliffs, NJ: Prentice-Hall.

Biegeleisen, J. I. (1976). *Job résumés: How to write them, how to present them, preparing for interviews.* New York: Grosset & Dunlap.

Binswanger, L. (1962). *Existential analysis and psychotherapy.* New York: Dutton.

Binswanger, L. (1963). *Being-in-the-world. Selected papers.* New York: Basic Books.

Black, C. (1979). Children of alcoholics. *Alcohol Health and Research World,* Fall, 23–27.

Blasi, G. L. (1990). Social policy and social science research on homelessness. *Journal of Social Issues, 46*(4), 207–219.

Bolles, R. N. (1993). *What color is your parachute?: A practical manual for job-hunters and career changers.* Berkeley, CA: Ten Speed Press.

Bowman, J. T., & Allen, B. R. (1988). Moral development and counselor trainee empathy. *Counseling and Values, 32*(2), 144–146.

Bowman, J. T., & Reeves, T. G. (1987). Moral development and empathy in counseling. *Counselor Education and Supervision, 26*(4), 293–299.

Bray, J. H., Shepherd, J. N., & Hays, J. R. (1985). Legal and ethical issues in informed consent to psychotherapy. *American Journal of Family Therapy, 13*(2), 50–60.

Brislin, R. W. (1981). *Cross-cultural encounters: Face-to-face interaction.* New York: Pergamon Press.

Brown, C. (1987). Council for standards in human service education: Update on regionalization. *Human Service Education, 8*(1), 32–34.

Brown, D. (1984). Trait and factor theory. In D. Brown & L. Brooks (Eds.), *Career choice and development, applying contemporary theories to practice* (Chap. 2). San Francisco: Jossey-Bass.

Brown, N. (1992). *Teaching group therapy: Process and practice.* New York: Praeger.

Burck, H. D., & Petersen, G. W. (1975). Needed: More evaluation, not research. *Personnel and Guidance Journal, 53*, 563–569.

Burgess, R. G. (1984). *In the field: An introduction to field research.* Boston: Allen & Unwin.

Buscaglia, L. (1972). *Love.* Thorofare, NJ: Slack.

Capuzzi, D., & Gross, D. R. (1992). *Introduction to group counseling.* Denver: Love Publishing.

Carkhuff, R. R. (1969). *Helping and human relations* (Vol. 2). New York: Holt, Rinehart & Winston.

Carkhuff, R. R. (1983). *The art of helping* (5th ed.). Amherst, MA: Human Resource Development Press.

Cayleff, S. E. (1986). Ethical issues in counseling, gender, race, and culturally distinct groups. *Journal of Counseling and Development, 64*(5), 345–347.

Chandras, K. V. (1991, April). *Changing role of father in the United States.* Paper presented at the annual convention of the American Association for Counseling and Development, Reno Nevada.

Claiborn, C. D. (1991). The Buros tradition and the counseling profession. *Journal of Counseling and Development, 69*, 456–457.

Clubok, M. (1984). Four-year human services programs: How they differ from social work. *Journal of the National Organization of Human Service Educators, 6*, 1–6.

Clubok, M. (1987). Human services: An "aspiring" profession in search of a professional identity. In R. Kornick (Ed.), *Curriculum development in human aervices education.* Council for Standards in Human Service Education, Monograph Series, Issue 5.

Code of Virginia (1950). *Communications between physicians and patients,* 8.01–399, p. 439.

Cogan, D. B. (1989). A theoretical perspective on the supervision of field work students. In C. Tower (Ed.), *Field work in human service education* (pp. 40–52). Knoxville, TN: Council for Standards in Human Service Education.

Cogan, D. B., & O'Connell, G. R. (1982). Models of supervision: A five-year review of the literature. *Journal of the National Organization of Human Service Educators, 4*, 12–17.

Cogan, D. B., & Wood, A. C. (1987). A survey of the introductory course in mental health and human services. *Human Service Education, 8*(2), 1–8.

Cohen, E. D. (1990). Confidentiality, counseling, and clients who have AIDS: Ethical foundations of a model rule. *Journal of Counseling and Development, 68*(3), 282–286.

Cohen, G. D. (1984). Counseling interventions for the late twentieth century elderly. *Counseling Psychologist, 12*(2), 97–99.

Cole, S. (1975). *The sociological method.* Chicago: Rand McNally.

Collison, B. B., & Garfield, N. J. (Eds.). (1990). *Careers in counseling and human development.* Alexandria, VA: American Association for Counseling and Development.

Committee on Government Operations. (1991). *A citizen's guide on using the Freedom of Information Act and the Privacy Act of 1974 to request government records* (4th report). House Report 102–146. Washington, DC: Government Printing Office.

Corey, G. (1992). *Theory and practice of counseling and psychotherapy.* (5th ed.). Pacific Grove, CA: Brooks/Cole.

Corey, G., & Corey, M. (1987). *Groups, process & practice* (3rd ed.). Pacific Grove, CA: Brooks Cole.

Corey, G., Corey, M., & Callanan, P. (1993). *Issues and ethics in the helping professions.* Pacific Grove, CA: Brooks/Cole.

Croteau, J. M., & Morgan, S. (1989). Combating homophobia in AIDS education. *Journal of Counseling and Development, 68*(1), 86–91.

D'Andrea, M., & Daniels, J. (1991). Exploring the different levels of multicultural counseling training in counselor education. *Journal of Counseling and Development, 70*(1), 78–85.

D'Andrea, M., & Daniels, J. (1992, September). *The structure of racism: A developmental framework.* Paper presented at the Association for Counselor Education and Supervision National Conference, San Antonio, TX.

Dahir, C. (1991). *State Department of Education Comprehensive Developmental School Counseling Survey. Report of the ASCA Developmental School Counseling Task Force.* Alexandria, VA: American School Counseling Association.

Danish, S. J., D'Augelli, A., Brock, G., Conter, K., & Meyer, R. (1978). A symposium on skill dissemination for paraprofessionals: Models of training, supervision, and utilization. *Professional Psychology, 9*(1), 16–37.

Davis, F. J. (1978). *Minority-dominant relations: A sociological analysis.* Arlington Heights, IL: AHM Publishing.

Deutsch, C. J. (1984). Self-reported sources of stress among psychotherapists. *Professional Psychology: Research & Practice, 15*(6), 833–845.

DeVoe, D. (1990). Feminist and nonsexist counseling: Implications for the male counselor. *Journal of Counseling and Development, 69*(1), 33–38.

Dinkmeyer, D. C., Dinkmeyer, D. C., Jr., & Sperry, L. (1987). *Adlerian counseling and psychotherapy* (2nd ed.). Columbus, OH: Merrill.

Donaho, M. W., & Meyer, J. L. (1976) *How to get the job you want: A guide to résumés, interviews, and job-hunting strategy.* Englewood Cliffs, NJ: Prentice-Hall.

Donaldson v. O'Connor, 422 U.S. 563 (U.S. Supreme Ct., 1975).

Doyle, R. E. (1992). *Essential skills and strategies in the helping process.* Pacific Grove, CA: Brooks/Cole.

Dworkin, S. H., & Gutierrez, F. (1989). Counselors be aware: Clients come in every size, shape, color, and sexual orientation. *Journal of Counseling and Development*, *68*(1), 6–8.

Edelrich, J., & Brodsy, A. (1980). *Burn-out stages of disillusionment in the helping professions*. New York: Human Sciences Press.

Educational Testing Services. (1993). *SIGI*. Princeton, NJ: Author.

Ellis, A. (1988). *How to stubbornly refuse to make yourself miserable about anything—yes anything!* Secaucus, NJ: Lyle Stuart.

Ellis, A., & Harper, R. A. (1961). *A guide to rational living*. Hollywood, CA: Wilshire Book.

Encyclopedia of Associations. (1993). Detroit: Gail Research.

Encyclopedia of Black America. (1981). New York: McGraw-Hill.

Engelkes, J. R., & Vandergoot, D. (1982). *Introduction to counseling*. Boston: Houghton Mifflin.

Erikson, E. H. (1963). *Childhood and society* (2nd ed.). New York: Norton.

Erikson, E. H. (1968). *Identity: Youth and crisis*. New York: Norton.

Erikson, E. H. (1982). *The life cycle completed*. New York: Norton.

Evans, D. R., Hearn, M. T., Uhlemann, M. R., & Ivey, A. E. (1993). *Essential interviewing* (4th ed.). Pacific Grove, CA: Brooks/Cole.

Federal Register. (1977). Regulation implementing Education for All Handicapped Children Act of 1975 (PL94–142), *42*(163), 42474–42518.

Flavell, J. H. (1963). *The developmental psychology of Jean Piaget*. New York: Van Nostrand.

Foos, J. A., Ottens, A. J., & Hill, L. K. (1991). Managed mental health: A primer for counselors. *Journal of Counseling and Development*, *69*(4), 332–336.

Foundation Grants Alert. (1992). Supplement to Federal Grants and Contracts Weekly, *5*(11). Alexandria, VA: Capitol Publications.

Fowler, J. W. (1991). *Stages in faith and religious development: Implications for church, education, and society*. New York: Crossroad.

Frank, J. D. (1979). The present status of outcome studies. *Journal of Consulting and Clinical Psychology*, *47*, 310–316.

Frankl, V. E. (1984). *Man's search for meaning: An introduction to logotherapy*. New York: Simon & Schuster.

French, M. (1993, April). *How to get the job you want: Using a portfolio*. Symposium conducted at the annual Spring conference of the Southern Organization for Human Services Education, Port Richey, FL.

Freud, S. (1947). *The ego and the id*. London: Hogarth Press.

Friedman, M., & Rosenman, R. (1959). Association of specific overt behavior patterns with blood cholesterol level, blood clotting time, incidence of arcus senilis and clinical artery disease. *Journal of the American Medical Association*, *169*(12), 1286–1296.

Fullerton, S. (1990). A historical perspective of the baccalaureate-level human service professional. *Human Service Education*, *10*(1), 53–62.

Gable, R. A., & Hendrickson, J. M. (Eds.). (1990). *Assessing students with special needs: A sourcebook for analyzing and correcting errors in academics*. New York: Longman.

Gallup, G. (1989). *The Gallup Poll: Public opinion 1989*. Wilmington, DE: Scholarly Resources.

Gallup, G. (1991). *The Gallup poll: Public opinion 1991*. Wilmington, DE: Scholarly Resources.

Gallup, G., & Castelli, J. (1989). *The people's religion*. New York: Macmillan.

Ganikos, M. L. (Ed.). (1979). *Counseling the aged: A training syllabus for educators*. Washington, DC: American Personnel and Guidance Association.

Garcia, M. H., Wright, J. W., & Corey, G. (1991). A multicultural perspective in an undergraduate human services program. *Journal of Counseling and Development, 70*(1), 86–90.

Gilligan, C. (1982). *In a different voice: Psychological theory and women's development*. Cambridge, MA: Harvard University Press.

Ginzberg, E. (1972). Toward a theory of occupational choice: A restatement. *Vocational Guidance Quarterly, 20*(3), 169–176.

Gladding, S. T. (1991). *Group work: A counseling specialty*. New York: Macmillan.

Gladding, S. T. (1992). *Counseling: A comprehensive profession*. New York: Macmillan.

Glasser, W. (1961). *Mental health or mental illness?* New York: Harper & Row.

Glasser, W. (1965). *Reality therapy: A new approach to psychiatry*. New York: Harper & Row.

Glasser, W. (1976). *Positive addiction*. New York: Harper & Row.

Glasser, W. (1985). *Control theory: A new explanation of how we control our lives*. New York: Harper & Row.

Gompertz, K. (1960). The relation of empathy to effective communication. *Journalism Quarterly, 37*, 535–546.

Gottfredson, G. D., Holland, J. L., & Ogawa, D. K. (1982). *Dictionary of Holland occupational codes*. Palo Alto, CA: Consulting Psychologists Press.

Guy, J. D., & Liaboe, G. P. (1986). Personal therapy for the experienced psychotherapist: A discussion of its usefulness and utilization. *Clinical Psychologist, 39*(1), 20–23.

Haley, A. (1992). *The autobiography of Malcolm X*. New York: Ballantine.

Halley, A. A., Kopp, J., & Austin, M. J. (1992). *Delivering human services: A learning approach to practice* (3rd ed.). New York: Longman.

Hammer, A. L., & Hile, M. G. (1985). Factors in clinicians' resistance to automation in mental health. *Computers in the Human Services, 1*(3), 1–25.

Hammond, L. A., & Fong, M. L. (1988, August). *Mediators of stress and role satisfaction in multiple role persons*. Paper presented at the annual meeting of the American Psychological Association, Atlanta, Georgia.

Handelsman, M. M., Kemper, M. B., Kesson-Craig, P., McLain, J., & Johnsrud, C. (1986). Use, content, and readability of written informed consent forms for treatment. *Professional Psychology: Research & Practice, 17*(6), 514–518.

Hannon, J. W., Ritchie, M. R., & Rye, D. A. (1992, September). *Class: The missing dimension in multicultural counseling and counselor education*. Presentation made at the Association for Counselor Education and Supervision national conference, San Antonio, TX.

Hansen, J. C., Stevic, R. R., Warner, R. W. (1978). *Counseling: Theory and process*. Boston: Allyn & Bacon.

Harrington, T., & O'Shea, A. (1988). *CDM interpretative folder*. Circle Pines, MN: American Guidance Service.

Harris-Bowlsby, J., Spivack, J. D., & Lisansky, R. S. (1986). *Take hold of your future* (Leader's Manual) (2nd ed.). Towson, MD: American College Testing Program, Career Planning Services, Towson State University.

Havighurst, R. J. (1972). *Developmental tasks and education* (3rd ed.) New York: McKay.

Heinrich, R. K., Corbine, J. L., & Thomas, K. R. (1990). Counseling Native Americans. *Journal of Counseling and Development, 69*(1), 128–133.

Herr, E. L., & Cramer, S. H. (1988). *Career guidance and counseling through the life span: Systematic approaches* (3rd ed.). Boston: Scott, Foresman.

Holland, J. L. (1985). *Manual for the self-directed search*. Odessa, FL: Psychological Assessment Resources.

Hollis, J. W., & Wantz, R. A. (1993). *Counselor preparation: Programs and personnel* (8th ed.). Muncie, IN: Accelerated Development.

Hothersall, D. H. (1984). *The history of psychology*. Philadelphia: Temple University Press.

Isaacson, L. E. (1986). *Career information in counseling and career development* (4th ed.). Newton, MA: Allyn & Bacon.

Isaacson, L. E., & Brown, D. (1993). *Career information, career counseling, and career development* (5th ed.). Newton, MA: Allyn & Bacon.

Ivey, A. (1980). *Counseling and psychotherapy: Skills, theories and practice*. Englewood Cliffs, NJ: Prentice-Hall.

Ivey, A. E. (1989). Mental health counseling: A developmental process and profession. *Journal of Mental Health Counseling, 11*(10), 26–35.

Ivey, A. (1991). *Developmental strategies for helpers: Individual, family, and network interventions*. Pacific Grove, CA: Brooks/Cole.

Jagger, L., Neukrug, E., & McAuliffe, G. (1992). Congruence between personality traits and chosen occupation as a predictor of job satisfaction for people with disabilities. *Rehabilitation Counseling Bulletin, 36*(1), 53–60.

Jayakar, P. (1986). *Krishnamurti: A biography*. New York: Harper & Row.

Johansson, C. (1982). *Manual for career assessment inventory*. Minneapolis: National Computer Systems.

Johnson, A. B. (1990). *Out of bedlam: The truth about deinstitutionalization*. New York: Basic Books.

Kahill, S. (1988). Symptoms of professional burnout: A review of the empirical evidence. *Canadian Psychology, 29*(3), 284–297.

Kain, C. D. (Ed.) (1989). *No longer immune: A counselor's guide to AIDS*. Alexandria, VA: American Association for Counseling and Development.

Kaplan, M., & Cuciti, P. L. (Eds.). (1986). *The Great Society and its legacy: Twenty years of U.S. social policy*. Durham, NC: Duke University Press.

Kazantzakis, N. (1952). *Zorba the Greek*. New York: Simon & Schuster.

Kegan, R. (1982). *The evolving self*. Cambridge, MA: Harvard University Press.

King, P. M. (1978). William Perry's theory of intellectual and ethical development. In L. Knefelkamp, C. Widick, & C. L. Parker (Eds.), *Applying new developmental findings* (pp. 34–51). San Francisco: Jossey-Bass.

Kinsey, A. C. (1948). *Sexual behavior in the human male*. Philadelphia: Saunders.

Kohlberg, L. (1969). *Stages in the development of moral thought and action*. New York: Holt, Rinehart & Winston.

Kohut, H. (1984). *How does analysis cure?* Chicago: University of Chicago Press.

Krogman, W. M. (1945). The concept of race. In R. Linston (Ed.), *The science of man in world crisis*. New York: Columbia University Press.

Krumboltz, J. D., Mitchell, A. M., & Jones, G. B. (1976). A social learning theory of career selection. *Counseling Psychologist, 6*(1), 71–81.

Kuhn, T. S. (1962). *The structure of scientific revolutions*. Chicago: University of Chicago Press.

Laing, R. D. (1967). *The politics of experience*. New York: Ballantine Books.

Lamar, J. (1992). The problem with you people. *Esquire, 117,* 90–91, 94.

Lambert, M. J., Ogles, B. M., & Masters, K. S. (1992). Choosing outcome assessment devices: An organizational and conceptual scheme. *Journal of Counseling and Development, 70,* 527–534.

Lao-tzu. (1919). *Lao-tzu's Tao and Wu Wei*. New York: Brentano.

Lee, J. L., & Pulvino, C. J. (1988). Computer competency: A means for learning to be a better counselor. *Counselor Education and Supervision, 28*(2), 110–115.

Lee, V. E., Brooks-Gunn, J., Schnur, E., & Liaw, F. (1990). Are Head Start effects sustained? A longitudinal follow-up comparison of disadvantaged children attending Head Start, no preschool, and other preschool programs. *Child Development, 61,* 495–507.

Leiby, J. (1978). *A history of social welfare and social work in the United States*. New York: Columbia University Press.

Libby, B., & Walz, G. (1988). *9 for the 90's: Counseling trends for tomorrow*. Ann Arbor: School of Education, University of Michigan. (ERIC Documentation Reproduction Service No. ED 291 012)

Linzer, N. (1990). Ethics and human service practice. *Human Service Education, 10*(1), 15–22.

Lipps, T. (1935). Empathy, inner-imitation of sense feelings. In *Radar: A modern book of esthetics*. New York: Holt.

Locke, D. (1992). Counseling beyond U.S. borders. *American Counselor, 1*(2), 13–17.

Loewenberg, F., & Dolgoff, R. (1988). *Ethical decisions for social work practice* (3rd ed.). Itasca, IL: Peacock.

Lombana, J. H. (1989). Counseling persons with disabilities: Summary and projections. *Journal of Counseling and Development, 68*(2), 177–179.

Ludwigsen, K., & Enright, M. (1988). The health care revolution: Implications for psychology and private practice. *Psychotherapy, 25,* 424–428.

Lum, D. (1986). *Social work practice and people of color: A process-stage approach*. Pacific Grove, CA: Brooks/Cole.

Mabe, A. R., & Rollin, S. A. (1986). The role of a code of ethical standards in counseling. *Journal of Counseling and Development, 64*(5), 294–297.

Magolda, M. B., & Porterfield, W. D. (1988). *Assessing intellectual development: The link between theory and practice*. Alexandria, VA: American College Personnel Association.

Mandel, B. R., & Schram, B. (1985). *Human Services: Introduction and interventions*. New York: Macmillan.

Maslach, C. (1982). *Burnout—The cost of caring*. Englewood Cliffs, NJ: Prentice-Hall.

Maslow, A. H. (1954). *Motivation and personality*. New York: Harper & Row.

Maslow, A. (1968). *Toward a psychology of being* (2nd ed.). Princeton, NJ: Van Nostrand.

Maslow, A. (1970). *Motivation and personality* (rev. ed.) New York: Harper & Row.

May, R., Angel, E., & Ellenberger, H. F. (Eds.). (1958). *Existence: A new dimension in psychiatry and psychology*. New York: Basic Books.

McAuliffe, G. (1992). Assessing and changing career decision making self-efficacy expectations. *Journal of Career Development, 19*, 25–36.

McCarthy, M. (Ed.). (1991). *Chesapeake community services directory*. Chesapeake, VA: Chesapeake Community Services Board.

McClam, T., & Woodside, M. R. (1989). A conversation with Dr. Harold McPheeters. *Human Service Education, 9*(1), 1–9.

McGrath, P. R. (1991–1992). *Human service education: Stage of the discipline—a survey of faculty members of the National Organization for Human Service Education*. Unpublished doctoral dissertation, National Louis University, Evanston, IL.

Mead, M. (1961). *Coming of age in Samoa: A psychological study of primitive youth for Western civilization*. New York: Morrow.

Mehrens, W. A. (1992). Leadership to researchers and practitioners. *Journal of Counseling and Development, 70*(3), 439–440.

Midgette, T. E., & Meggert, S. S. (1991). Multicultural counseling instruction: A challenge for faculties in the 21st century. *Journal of Counseling and Development, 70*(1), 136–141.

Milgram, S. (1965). Some conditions of obedience and disobedience to authority. *Human Relations, 18*, 56–76.

Milgram, S. (1974). *Obedience to authority*. New York: Harper & Row.

Miller, J. B. (1976). *Toward a new psychology of women*. Boston: Beacon Press.

Miller, C. D., Morrill, W. H., & Uhlemann, M. R. (1970). Microcounseling: An experimental study of pre-practicum training in communicating test results. *Counselor Education and Supervision, 9*(3), 178–182.

Miller v. California, 413 U.S. 15 (U.S. Supreme Ct., 1973).

Minuchin, S. (1974). *Families and family therapy*. Cambridge, MA: Harvard University Press.

Montgomery, M. (1988). Shrink mental health costs. *Personnel Journal, 67*, 89–91.

Mussen, P. H., Conger, J. J., & Kagan, J. (1969). *Child development and personality*. New York: Harper & Row.

Myers, J. E. (1983). Gerontological counseling training: The state of the art. *Personnel and Guidance Journal 61*(7), 398–401.

Myers, J. E., Emmerling, D., & Leafgren, F. (Eds.). (1992). Wellness throughout the life span [Special issue]. *Journal of Counseling and Development, 71*(2).

Myers, J. E., Loesch, L. D., & Sweeney., T. J. (1991). Trends in gerontological counselor preparation. *Counselor Education and Supervision, 30*(3), 194–204.

Myers, J. E., & Salmon, H. E. (1984). Counseling programs for older persons: Status, shortcomings, and potentialities. *Counseling Psychologist 12*(2), 39–53.

Napier, A., & Whitaker, C. (1978). *The family crucible*. New York: Harper & Row.

NASW (National Association of Social Workers). (1990). *Code of ethics of the National Association of Social Workers.* Washington, DC: Author.

Neukrug, E. (1980). *The effects of supervisory style and type of praise upon counselor trainees' level of empathy and perception of supervisor.* Unpublished doctoral dissertation, University of Cincinnati. Cincinnati, OH.

Neukrug, E. (1987). The brief training of paraprofessional counselors in empathic responding. *New Hampshire Journal for Counseling and Development, 15*(1), 15–19.

Neukrug, E. (1991). Computer-assisted live supervision in counselor skills training. *Counselor Education and Supervision, 31*(2), 132–138.

Neukrug, E. S., Barr, C. G., Hoffman, L. R., & Kaplan, L. S. (1993). Developmental counseling and guidance: A model for use in your schools. *The School Counselor, 5,* 356–362.

Neukrug, E., & Bonner, A. (1993). *The development of ethical guidelines for human service workers.* Manuscript submitted for publication.

Neukrug, E., Healy, M., & Herlihy, B. (1992). Ethical practices of licensed professional counselors: An updated survey of state licensing boards. *Counselor Education and Supervision, 32*(2) 130–141.

Neukrug, E., & McAuliffe, G. (1993). Cognitive development and human service education. *Human Service Education,* in press.

Neukrug, E., & Williams, G. (1993). Counseling counselors: A survey of values. *Counseling and Values 38* (October), 51–62.

NOHSE (National Organization for Human Service Education). (1990). *Human Service Education, 10*(1), 72.

Norcross, J. C., Strausser, D. J., & Faltus, F. J. (1988). The therapist's therapist. *American Journal of Psychotherapy, 42*(1), 53–66.

Nurius, P. S. (1990). Computer literacy in automated assessment: Challenges and future directions. *Computers in the Human Services, 6*(4), 283–297.

Nurius, P. S., & Hudson, W. (1989a). Computers and social diagnosis: The client's perspective. *Computers in the Human Services, 5*(1–2), 21–35.

Nurius, P. S., & Hudson, W. W. (1989b). Workers, clients, and computers. *Computers in Human Services, 4*(1–2), 71–83.

Nye, R. D. (1986). *Three psychologies: Perspectives from Freud, Skinner, and Rogers.* Pacific Grove, CA: Brooks/Cole.

Ohlsen, M. M. (1983). Evaluation of the counselor's services. In M. M. Ohlsen (Ed.), *Introduction to counseling* (pp. 357–372). Itasca, IL: Peacock.

Parsons, F. (1909). *Choosing a vocation.* Boston: Houghton Mifflin.

Peck, M. S. (1985). *People of the lie.* New York: Simon & Schuster.

Pedersen, P. B. (1981). Triad counseling. In R. Corsini (Ed.), *Innovative psychotherapies.* New York: Wiley.

Pedersen, P. B. (1983). Cross-cultural training of mental health providers. In R. Brislin & D. Landis (Eds.), *Handbook of intercultural training.* Elmsford, NY: Pergamon Press.

Pedersen, P. B. (1985). Intercultural criteria for mental-health training. In P. Pedersen (Ed.), *Handbook of cross-cultural counseling and therapy.* Westport, CT: Greenwood Press.

Pedersen, P. B. (1991). Multiculturalism as a generic approach to counseling. *Journal of Counseling and Development 70*(1), 6–12.

Pedersen, P. B., Draguns, J. G., Lonner, J., & Trimble, J. E. (1989). *Counseling across cultures* (3rd. ed.). Honolulu: University of Hawaii Press.

Perry, M. A., & Furukawa, M. J. (1986). Modeling methods, In F. H. Kanfer & A. P. Goldstein (Eds.), *Helping people change: A textbook of methods* (3rd ed.) (pp. 66–110). New York: Pergamon Press.

Petrie, D. (1987). Life cycle simulation: Human growth and development course design and method. *Human Service Education, 8*(1), 21–25.

Petrie, R. D. (1984). Competence and curriculum. *Journal of the National Organization of Human Service Educators, 6*, 8–13.

Petrie, R. D. (1989). Entry-level skills of human service work. *Human Service Education, 9*, 37–41.

Piaget, J. (1954). *The construction of reality in the child.* New York: Basic Books.

Porter, R. E., & Samovar, L. A. (1985). Approaching intercultural communication. In L. A. Samovar & R. E. Porter (Eds.), *Intercultural communication: A reader* (pp. 15–30). Belmont, CA: Wadsworth.

Pottick, K. J. (1988). Jane Addams revisited: Practice theory and social economics. *Social Work with Groups, 11*, 11–26.

Prochaska, J. O., & Norcross, J. C. (1983). Contemporary psychotherapists: A national survey of characteristics, practices, orientations, and attitudes. *Psychotherapy: Theory, Research and Practice, 20*(2), 161–173.

Prospero, A. (1987, December). Selecting a case manager for psychiatric care. *Business and Health*, 32–33.

Psychological Corporation. (1977). *The differential aptitude test and career planning program.* New York: Author.

Rabinowitz, F. E. (1991). The male-to-male embrace: Breaking the touch taboo in a men's therapy group. *Journal of Counseling and Development, 69*(6), 574–576.

Randolph, D. L., & Lassiter, P. S. (1985). A directory of graduate and undergraduate internships in human services agencies. *Journal of the National Organization of Human Service Educators, 7*, 7–11.

Raths, L. E., Harmin, M., & Simon, S. B. (1966). *Values and teaching.* Columbus, OH: Merrill.

Reeves, T. G., Bowman, J. T., & Cooley, S. L. (1989). Relationship between the client's moral development level and empathy of the counseling student. *Counselor Education and Supervision, 28*(4), 299–305.

Reynolds, J. F., Mair, D. C., & Fischer, P. C. (1992). *Writing and reading mental health records: Issues and analysis.* Newbury Park, CA: Sage.

Rice, F. P. (1992). *Human development: A life-span approach.* New York: Macmillan.

Richan, C. (1988). *Human services: Beyond altruism: Social welfare policy in American society.* Binghamton, NY: Haworth Press.

Riverside Publishing Company (1992). *Guidance information systems.* Chicago: Author.

Robertiello, R. C., & Schoenewolf, G. (1987). *Common therapeutic blunders: Countertransference and counterresistance in psychotherapy.* Northvale, NJ: Jason Aronson.

Roe, A. (1956). *The psychology of occupations.* New York: Wiley.

Rogers, C. R. (1942). *Counseling and psychotherapy.* Boston: Houghton Mifflin.

Rogers, C. R. (1951). *Client-centered therapy.* Boston: Houghton Mifflin.

Rogers, C. (1957). The necessary and sufficient conditions of therapeutic personality change. *Journal of Consulting Psychology, 21*(2), 95–103.

Rogers, C. R. (1959). A theory of therapy, personality and interpersonal relationships as developed in the client-centered framework. In S. Koch (Ed.), *Psychology: A study of science*: Vol. 3. *Formulations of the person and the social context* (pp. 184–256). New York: McGraw-Hill.

Rogers, C. R. (1961). Ellen West—and Loneliness. In H. Kirschenbaum & V. L. Henderson (Eds.), *The Carl Rogers Reader* (pp. 157–167). Boston: Houghton Mifflin.

Rogers, C. R. (1970). *Carl Rogers on encounter groups*. New York: Harper & Row.

Rogers, C. (1980). *A way of being*. Boston: Houghton Mifflin.

Rogers, C. R. (1986). Reflection of feelings. *Person-Centered Review, 1*(4), 375–377.

Romano, G. (1992). Description of D. Locke's "Counseling beyond U.S. borders." *American Counselor, 1*(2), 13–17.

Rosch, P. J. (1979). Stress and cancer: A disease of adaptation? In J. Toche, H. Selye, & S. Day (Eds.), *Cancer, stress, and death* (pp. 187–212). New York: Plenum.

Rose, P. I. (1964). *They and we: Racial and ethnic relations in the United States*. New York: Random House.

Rosenman, R., Swan, G., & Carmelli, D. (1988). Some recent findings relative to the relationship of type a behavior pattern to coronary heart disease. In S. Maes, C. Speilberger, P. Defares, & I. Sarason (Eds.), *Topics in health psychology* (pp. 21–29) New York: Wiley.

Rossi, P. H. (1990). The old homeless and the new homelessness in historical perspective. *American Psychologist, 45*(8), 954–959.

Sadow, D., Ryder, M., Stein, J., & Geller, M. (1987). Supervision of mental health students in the context of an educational milieu. *Human Service Education, 8,*(2), 29–36.

Sang, B. E. (1989). New directions in lesbian research, theory, and education. *Journal of Counseling and Development, 68*(1), 92–96.

Satir, V. (1967). *Conjoint family therapy*. Palo Alto, CA: Science & Behavior Books.

Schaef, A. W. (1981). *Women's reality: An emerging female system in the white male society*. Minneapolis: Winston Press.

Schmolling, P., Youkeles, M., & Burger, W. R. (1993). *Human services in contemporary America* (3rd ed.). Pacific Grove, CA: Brooks/Cole.

Schwebel, A. I., Barocas, H., Reichman, N., & Schwebel, M. (1990). *Personal adjustment and growth: A life-span approach*. Dubuque, IA: Brown.

Sears, S. (1982). A definition of career guidance terms: A national vocational guidance association perspective. *Vocational Guidance Quarterly, 31*(2), 137–143.

Selye, H. (1956). *The stress of life*. New York: McGraw-Hill.

Selye, H. (1974). *Stress without distress*. New York: Lippincott.

Shaffer, J. B. P., & Galinsky, M. D. (1974). *Models of group therapy and sensitivity training*. Englewood Cliffs, NJ: Prentice-Hall.

Shartle, C. L. (1959). *Occupational information—Its development and application* (3rd ed.). Englewood Cliffs, NJ: Prentice-Hall.

Sheehy, G. (1976). *Passages: Predictable crises of adult life*. New York: Bantam Books.

Shelton, J. (1993). *A construct validity study of the MMPI-II cynicism scale*. Unpublished doctoral dissertation, Old Dominion University, Norfolk, VA.

Short, R. L. (1965). *The Gospel according to Peanuts*. Richmond, VA: John Knox Press.

Shostrum, E. (1974). *Manual for the Personal Orientation Inventory: An inventory for the measurement of self-actualization*. San Diego: Educational and Industrial Testing Service.

Simon, P. (1969). *The boxer*. New York: Paul Simon Music.

Simon, S. B., Howe, L. W., & Kirschenbaum, H. W. (1991). *Values clarification: A handbook of practical strategies for teachers and students* (rev. ed.). Hudley, MA: Values Press.

Skillings, J. H., & Dobbins, J. E. (1991). Racism as a disease: Etiology and treatment implications. *Journal of Counseling and Development, 70*(1), 206–215.

Skinner, B. F. (1953). *Science and human behavior*. New York, MacMillan.

Skinner, B. F. (1960). Pigeons in a pelican. *American Psychologist, 15*, 28–37.

Skinner, B. F. (1971). *Beyond freedom and dignity*. New York: Knopf.

Skynner, A. C. (1976). *Systems of marital and family psychotherapy*. New York: Brunner/Mazel.

Smith, D. (1982). Trends in counseling and psychotherapy. *American Psychologist, 37*(7), 802–809.

Smith, T. W., & Pope, M. K. (1990). Cynical hostility as a health risk: Current status and future directions. *Journal of Social Behavior and Personality, 5*(1), 77–88.

Sommer, B., & Sommer, R. (1991). *A practical guide to behavioral research: Tools and techniques*. New York: Oxford University Press.

Special Committee on Aging, U.S. Senate. (1983). *Developments in aging. 1983*. Washington, DC: Government Printing Office.

Speight, S. L., Myers, J., Cox, C. I., & Highlen, P. S. (1991). A redefinition of multicultural counseling. *Journal of Counseling and Development, 70*(1), 29–36.

Spiegler, M. D. (1983). *Contemporary behavior therapy*. Palo Alto, CA: Mayfield.

Spokane, A. R. (1985). A review of research on person-environment congruence in Holland's theory of careers. *Journal of Vocational Behavior, 26*, 306–343.

Sprinthall, R. C., & Sprinthall, N. A. (1990). *Educational psychology: A developmental approach* (5th ed.). New York: McGraw-Hill.

SREB (Southern Regional Educational Board). (1969). *Roles and functions for different levels of mental health workers*. Atlanta: Author.

Steinem, G. (1992). *Revolution from within: A book on self-esteem*. Boston: Little, Brown.

Stokes, D., Rowe, D., Romero, D., Gonzales, M., Adams, M., & Lyons, S. (1987). Establishing a university multicultural peer counseling program: A brief description. *Human Service Education, 8*, 26–29.

Strong, E. K., Hansen, D. P., & Campbell, D. P. (1985). *The Strong Interest Inventory*. Stanford, CA: Consulting Psychologists Press.

Sue, D. W. (1992). The challenge of multiculturalism: The road less traveled. *American Counselor, 1*(1), 6–15.

Sue, D. W., Arredondo, P., & McDavis, R. J. (1992). Multicultural counseling competencies and standards: A call to the profession. *Journal of Multicultural Counseling and Development, 20,* 64–88.

Sue, D. W., Bernier, J. E., Durran, A., Feinberg, L., Pedersen, P., Smith, E. J., & Vasquez-Nuttall, E. (1982). Professional forum: Position paper: Cross-cultural counseling competencies. *Counseling Psychologist, 10,*(2), 45–52.

Sue, D. W., & Sue, D. (1990). *Counseling the culturally different: Theory and practice.* New York: Wiley.

Super, D. E. (1957). *The psychology of careers.* New York: Harper & Row.

Super, D. (1976). *Career education and the meaning of work.* Monographs on Career Education. Washington, DC: Office of Career Education, U.S. Office of Education.

Super, D. (1984) Career and life development. In D. Brown, L. Brooks, & Associates (Eds.), *Career choice and development.* San Francisco: Jossey-Bass.

Super, D. E. & Hall, D. T. (1978). Career development: Exploration and planning. *Annual Review of Psychology, 29,* 333–372.

Sweitzer, H. F., & McKinney, W. L. (1991). A survey of human service graduates: Implications for curriculum planning. *Human Service Education, 11*(1), 3–16.

Swenson, L. C. (1993). *Psychology and law for the helping professions.* Pacific Grove, CA: Brooks/Cole.

Szaz, T. (1961). *The myth of mental illness.* New York: Hoeber.

Szaz, T. (Speaker). (1990). *A conversation with an officially dominated schizophrenic patient* (Cassette Recording No. PC289-W9AD). Phoenix: Milton H. Erickson Foundation.

Taeuber, D. M. (1991). *Statistical handbook on women in America.* Phoenix: Oryx Press.

Tarasoff v. *Regents of University of California,* 529 P.2d 553 (Calif. 1974), vacated, reheard en banc, and affirmed 551 P.2d 334 (1976).

Thompson, J. J. (1973). *Beyond words: Nonverbal communication in the classroom.* New York: Citation Press.

Thorndike, R. M., Cunningham, G. K., Thorndike, R. L., & Hagen, E. P. (1991). *Measurement and evaluation in psychology and education.* New York: Macmillan.

Tiedeman, D. V. (1983). Flexible filing, computers, and growing. *Counseling Psychologist, 11*(4), 33–47.

Tiedeman, D. V., & O'Hara, R. P. (1963). *Career development: Choice and adjustment.* New York: College Entrance Examination Board.

Trotzer, J. P. (1989). *The counselor and the group* (2nd ed.). Muncie, IN: Accelerated Development.

Tuckman, B. W. & Jensen, M. A. C. (1977). Stages of small-group development revisited. *Group and Organizational Studies, 2,* 419–427.

U.S. Department of Commerce, Bureau of the Census. (1990). *Statistical abstracts of the United States* (110th ed.). Washington, DC: Government Printing Office.

U.S. Department of Commerce, Bureau of the Census. (1991). *Statistical abstracts of the United States* (111th ed.). Washington, DC: Government Printing Office.

U.S. Department of Commerce, Bureau of the Census. (1992a). *Census bureau releases 1990 decennial counts for persons enumerated in emergency shelters and observed on streets* (CB91–117). Washington, DC: Government Printing Office.

U.S. Department of Commerce, Bureau of the Census. (1992b). *Current population reports: Poverty in the United States* (Series P–60, No. 181). Washington, DC: Government Printing Office.

U.S. Department of Health and Human Services. (1991). *Summary of findings from the 1991 national household survey on drug abuse*. Rockville, MD: National Institute of Drug Abuse.

U.S. Department of Justice. (1992). *Americans with Disabilities Act requirements fact sheet*. Washington, DC: Civil Rights Division, Coordination and Review Section.

U.S. Department of Labor. (1991). *Dictionary of occupational titles* (5th ed.). Washington, DC: Government Printing Office.

U.S. Department of Labor, Bureau of Labor Statistics. (1992–1993). *Occupational outlook handbook published*. Washington, DC: Government Printing Office.

Usher, C. H. (1989). Recognizing cultural bias in counseling theory and practice: The case of Rogers. *Journal of Counseling and Development, 17*(2), 62–71.

Vander Kolk, C. J. (1990). *Introduction to group counseling and psychotherapy*. Prospect Heights, IL: Waveland Press.

VanZandt, C. E. (1990). Professionalism: A matter of personal initiative. *Journal of Counseling and Development, 68*(3), 243–245.

Viney, L. L., Allwood, K., Stillson, L., & Walmsley, R. (1992). Caring for the carers: A note on counseling for the wider impact of AIDS. *Journal of Counseling and Development, 70*(3), 442–444.

Visotsky, H. M. (1991). Courage, creativity, and cost-effectiveness: The challenge for a psychiatric program administration. *New Directions for Mental Health Services, Spring*(49), 51–59.

Vroman, C. S., & Bloom, J. W. (1991). A summary of counselor credentialing legislation. In F. Bradley (Ed.), *Credentialing in counseling* (pp. 86–102). Alexandria, VA: Association for Counselor Education and Supervision.

Wallerstein, J. S., & Blakeslee, S. (1989). *Second chances: Men, women, and children a decade after divorce*. New York: Ticknor & Fields.

Walsh, W. B., & Betz, N. E. (1985). *Tests and assessment*. Englewood Cliffs, NJ: Prentice-Hall.

Ward, D. E. (1982). A model for the more effective use of theory in group work. *Journal for Specialists in Group Work, 7*, 224–230.

Warnath, C. F. (1975). Vocational theories: Direction to nowhere. *Personnel and Guidance Journal, 53*, 422–428.

Waxman, L. D., & Reyes, L. M. (1988). *A status report on hunger and homelessness in America's cities: A 27 city survey*. Washington, DC: United States Conferences of Mayors. (ERIC Document Reproduction Service No. ED315465.)

Webster. (1975). *The living Webster Encyclopedic Dictionary of the English language*. Chicago: English Language Institute of America.

Wertheimer, M. (1978). *A brief history of psychology*. New York: Holt, Rinehart & Winston.

Westwood, M. J., & Ishiyama, F. I. (1990). The communication process as a critical intervention for client change in cross-cultural counseling. *Journal of Multicultural Counseling and Development, 18*, 163–171.

Whitaker, C. (1976). The hindrance of theory in clinical work. In P. J. Guerin (Ed.), *Family Therapy* (pp. 154–164). New York: Gardner Press.

Whitfield, W., McGrath, P., & Coleman, V. (1992, October). *Increasing multicultural sensitivity and awareness*. Symposium presented at the annual conference of the National Organization for Human Service Education, Alexandria, Virginia.

Wicks, R. J. (1977). *Counseling strategies and intervention techniques for the human services*. New York: Lippincott.

Widick, C. (1975). The Perry scheme: A foundation for developmental practice. *Counseling Psychologist, 6*(4), 35–38.

Williams, R. J., & Stafford, W. B. (1991). Silent casualties: partners, families, and spouses of persons with AIDS. *Journal of Counseling and Development, 69*(5), 423–427.

Wise, R., Charner, I., & Randour, M. A. (1978). A conceptual framework for career awareness in career decision-making. In J. Whiteley & A. Resnikoff (Eds.), *Career counseling* (pp. 216–231). Pacific Grove, CA: Brooks/Cole.

Woititz, J. G. (1983). *Adult children of alcoholics*. Hollywood, FL: Health Communications.

Wolpe, J. (1969). *The practice of behavior therapy*. New York: Pergamon Press.

Woodside, M., & McClam, T. (1990). *An introduction to human services*. Pacific Grove, CA: Brooks/Cole.

World Almanac. (1992). New York: Scripps Howard Company.

Yalom, I. D. (1985). *The theory and practice of group psychotherapy* (3rd ed.). New York: Basic Books.

Zimbardo, P. G. (1988). *Psychology and life* (12th ed.). Boston: Scott, Foresman.

Zwelling, S. S. (1990). *Quest for a cure: The public hospital in Williamsburg, Virginia, 1773–1885*. Williamsburg, VA: Colonial Williamsburg Foundation.

Index

TO THE OWNER OF THIS BOOK:

We hope that you have found *Theory, Practice, and Trends in Human Services: An Overview of an Emerging Profession* by Edward Neukrug useful. So that this book can be improved in a future edition, would you take the time to complete this sheet and return it? Thank you.

Instructor's name: _____

Department: _____

School and address: _____

1. The name of the course in which I used this book is: _____

_____

2. My general reaction to this book is: _____

_____

_____

3. What I like most about this book is: _____

_____

_____

4. What I like least about this book is: _____

_____

_____

5. Were all of the chapters of the book assigned for you to read?   Yes   No

   If not, which ones weren't? _____

6. Do you plan to keep this book after you finish course?   Yes   No

   Why or why not? _____

_____

7. On a separate sheet of paper, please write specific suggestions for improving this book and anything else you'd care to share about your experience in using the book.

Optional:

Your name: _____ Date: _____

May Brooks/Cole quote you either in promotion for *Theory, Practice and Trends in Human Services: An Overview of an Emerging Profession* or in future publishing ventures?

Yes: _____ No: _____

Sincerely,

Ed Neukrug

Brooks/Cole is dedicated to publishing quality publications for education in the human services fields. If you are interested in learning more about our publications, please fill in your name and address and request our latest catalogue.

Name: _____

Street Address: _____

City, State, and Zip: _____

FOLD HERE

NO POSTAGE
NECESSARY
IF MAILED
IN THE
UNITED STATES

FOLD HERE